W9-AMC-741

Superstorm

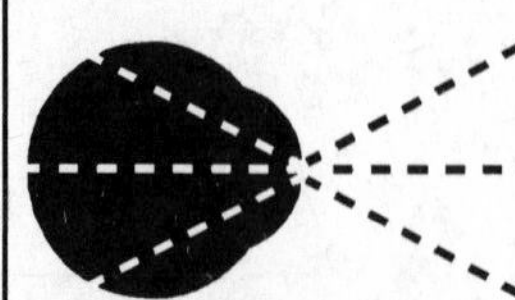

This Large Print Book carries the Seal of Approval of N.A.V.H.

SUPERSTORM

NINE DAYS INSIDE HURRICANE SANDY

KATHRYN MILES

THORNDIKE PRESS
A part of Gale, Cengage Learning

GALE
CENGAGE Learning®

Farmington Hills, Mich • San Francisco • New York • Waterville, Maine
Meriden, Conn • Mason, Ohio • Chicago

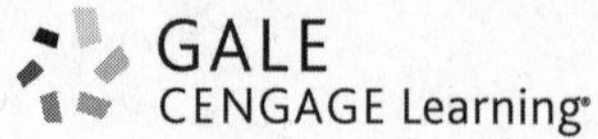

Thorndike Press, a part of Gale, Cengage Learning.

Thorndike Press® Large Print Nonfiction.
The text of this Large Print edition is unabridged.
Other aspects of the book may vary from the original edition.
Set in 16 pt. Plantin.

LIBRARY OF CONGRESS CATALOGING-IN-PUBLICATION DATA

Miles, Kathryn, 1974–
Superstorm : nine days inside Hurricane Sandy / by Kathryn Miles. — Large print edition.
pages (large print) ; cm. — (Thorndike Press large print nonfiction)
Includes bibliographical references.
ISBN 978-1-4104-7686-9 (hardcover) — ISBN 1-4104-7686-3 (hardcover) 1. Hurricane Sandy, 2012. 2. Hurricanes—United States—History—21st century. 3. Weather broadcasting—United States. 4. Large type books. I. Title.
QC945.M46 2014b
551.55'2—dc23 2014040952

Published in 2015 by arrangement with Dutton, a member of Penguin Group (USA) LLC, a Penguin Random House Company

Printed in the United States of America
1 2 3 4 5 6 7 19 18 17 16 15

For Hayden,
who helped write the first word

In the eye of a hurricane, you learn things other than of a scientific nature. You feel the puniness of man and his works. If a true definition of humility is ever written, it might well be written in the eye of the hurricane.

— Edward R. Murrow

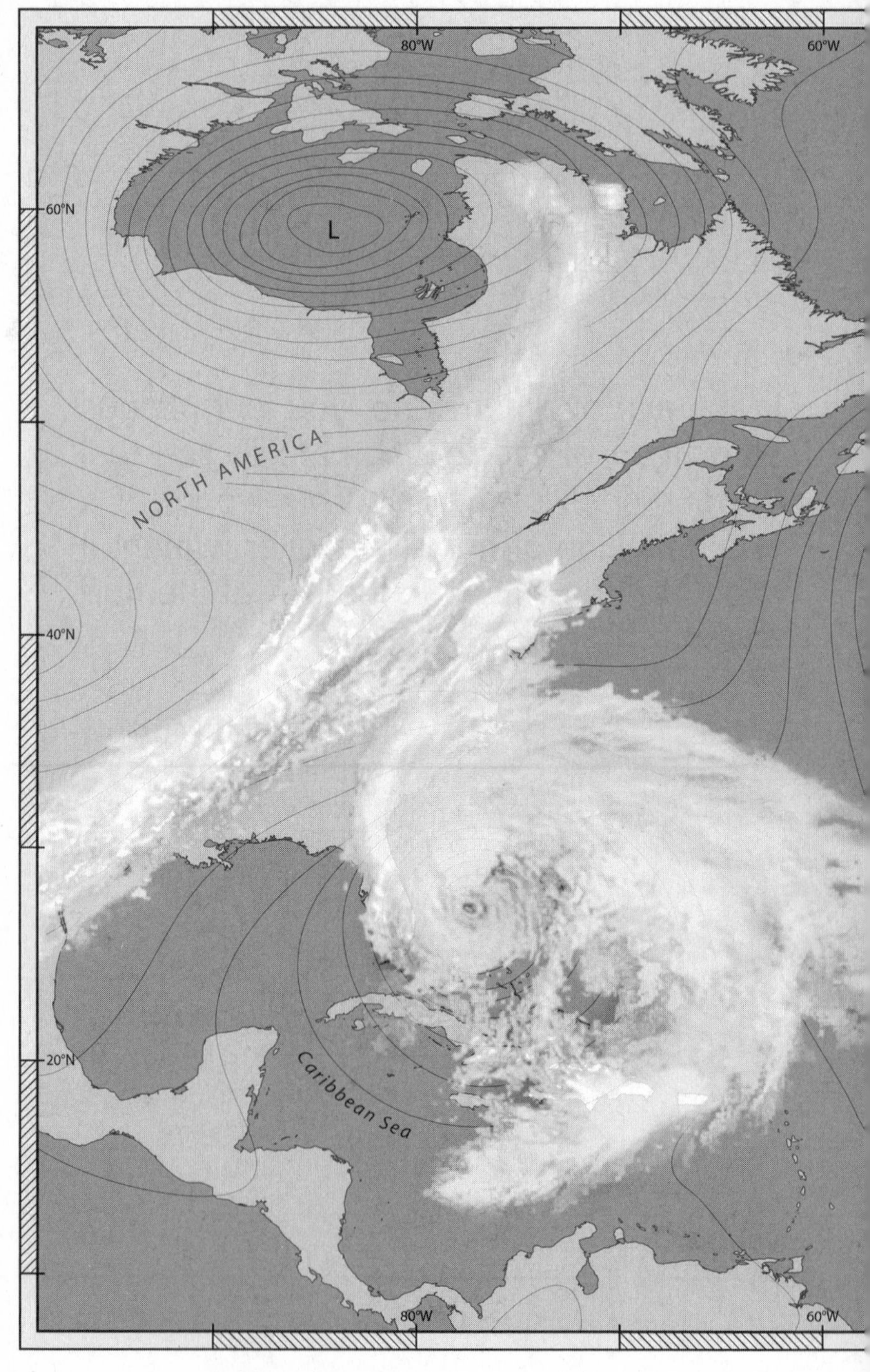
80°W
60°W
60°N
L
NORTH AMERICA
40°N
20°N
Caribbean Sea
80°W
60°W

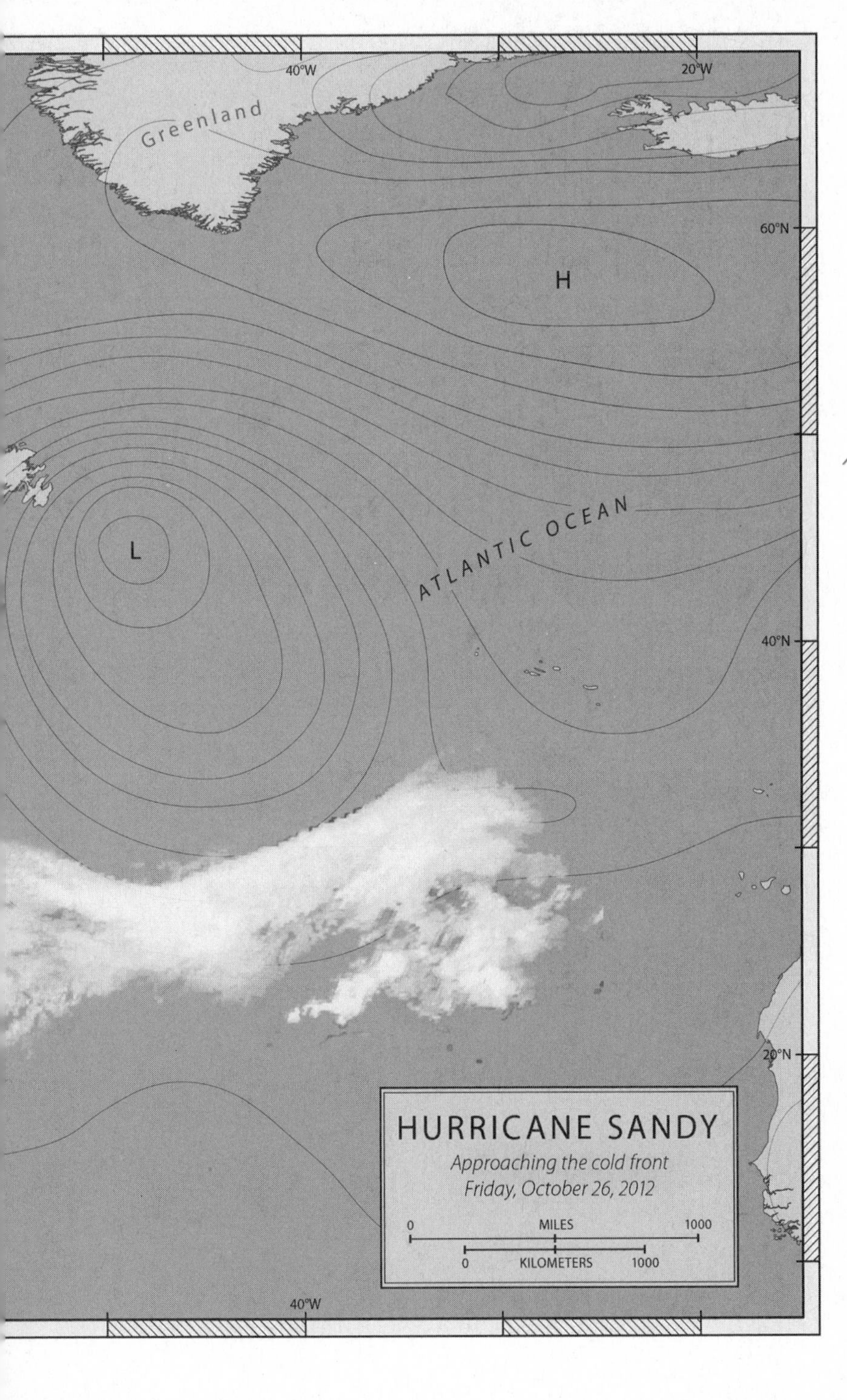

40°W
20°W
Greenland
60°N
H
L
ATLANTIC OCEAN
40°N
20°N
HURRICANE SANDY
Approaching the cold front
Friday, October 26, 2012
0
MILES
1000
0
KILOMETERS
1000
40°W

CONTENTS

Landfall

The sky was lit by a full moon that night, but no one could see it. Everything — the enormous harvest moon, the stars, the horizon — had been consumed by cloud. The storm was so immense it caught the attention of scientists on the International Space Station, who stopped what they were doing and peered out their windows. From there, the cloud cover seemed almost limitless: 1.8 million square feet of tightly coiled bands so huge they filled the windows of the station, so thick they showed only the briefest insinuation of an eye. It was the largest storm the planet had ever seen — a storm big enough to consume the entire Eastern Seaboard and beyond.

It had already wreaked devastation in the Caribbean, taking lives and destroying families. Now the storm was marching up the Atlantic, turning the ocean into unimaginable chaos. Waves the size of a two-story house collided against one another, exploding in foam and fury and blocking everything else from view as millions of pounds of water rose and crashed and fell, only to rise again. Those same waves fueled the machine that created them, sending more and more moisture into the storm's core, where energy exploded with the force of a nuclear bomb. Gale-force winds rose and then spread out for 870 nautical miles, threatening everything in their path. The system was growing.

Nightfall came by imperceptible degrees. The wind and rain did not. They were soon punctuated by an omnipresent moaning: a kind of dark, low hum that made it seem as if the entire world was haunted. Within minutes, that moan became a constant, pervasive shriek as gusts of 90 miles per hour were recorded everywhere from Washington, D.C., to New York City. Barometers plummeted to unseen lows, heralding the force of the storm. So, too, did the apocalyptic precipitation that began to follow: almost thirteen inches of rain in Bellevue, Maryland; nearly six in Cleveland, Ohio. Twenty inches of snow fell in places like Kentucky and Newfound Gap, a low pass in the Great Smoky Mountains that divides North Carolina and Tennessee. In West Virginia, more than three feet of snow fell near the town of Richwood, collapsing roofs and collecting into barricade-like drifts six feet tall.

At the National Zoo in Washington, D.C., keepers scrambled to corral their charges inside, wrangling elephants and clouded leopards, the facility's iconic pandas, and even a spindly, two-week-old dama gazelle. As they did, the storm turned inland, fixing a bead on the mid-Atlantic coast. Heralded by hurricane-force winds, the storm announced its arrival long before it made landfall, knocking down power lines and exploding transformers. A woman in Toronto was killed when a large illuminated sign pulled from its supports, then plummeted thirty feet to the ground. An eight-year-old Pennsylvania boy died when a tree fell in his Franklin Township yard. Not long after, an enormous oak fell through a home in North Salem, New York, crushing two best friends, ages eleven and thirteen, but leaving the rest of the home's occupants unharmed.

And still the storm continued its relentless beat to shore, charging across three hundred miles of open ocean, picking up strength with every step. Meteorologists and scientists, officials and emergency managers stood baffled: What *was* this thing? By the time many of them decided, it was too late to issue warnings, too late to persuade millions of people their lives were in danger.

Gusts rose to 83 knots, building the waves higher, blowing off their tops and sending cataracts of salt water through the air for miles. Across Manhattan, those residents who resisted the call to evacuate struggled to walk down rain-swept streets, where litter tornadoed around telephone poles and newspaper kiosks. Awnings sheared off of storefronts and took flight. Flags stood straight and solid; trees rippled as if suddenly liquefied. Nearly a thousand miles away, spray from twenty-foot surf on Lake Michigan crashed onto Chicago museumgoers and commuters. At the international airport in Gary, Indiana, 50-mile-per-hour winds grounded planes. Hundreds of stranded passengers sat packed in terminals from Baltimore to Oklahoma City — and beyond.

By 6:00 P.M. that evening, three million people were without power, most of them in Manhattan and the surrounding boroughs. The lights went out on Broadway. Wall Street ground to a standstill and would remain closed for two days — the first time weather had shut down stock markets for consecutive days since the Great Blizzard of

1888. Out on Ellis Island, the Statue of Liberty — whose newly renovated crown had reopened to visitors just one day before — lost her torchlight and went dark.

At New York University's Langone Medical Center, hospital officials were certain their patients would be safe, despite the deteriorating conditions outside. But the facility's backup power system soon failed, shrouding the eighteen-story complex in blackness and requiring the evacuation of three hundred patients into a caravan of ambulances that extended blocks down rain-torn streets. The first to emerge from the darkened hospital were twenty infants from the neonatal intensive care unit, each one cocooned in blankets and heating pads and carried down nine flights of stairs by nurses, administrators, and maintenance workers. They worked by flashlight and feel, delivering first the babies and then the most critical patients, some of whom weighed well over two hundred pounds. They moved silently, synchronized, and often arm in arm, working together in teams of five or ten and stopping frequently to check breathing tubes and vitals. The only audible sound, some would report later, was that of the growing wind and surf. Waves so big they hardly seemed real rolled through streets. It was like being in a movie, said the staff, only much, much scarier.

That same surge swamped beaches and shoreline from Florida to Nova Scotia. It sank boats in Bar Harbor, Maine, and swept as far inland as Albany, New York — nearly 150 miles from the coast.

And then the storm itself arrived.

It hit land like . . . what? Like a freight train or an atomic explosion or an alien invasion? People tried to find a comparison, but everything fell short. It was a hurricane that wasn't a hurricane. A superstorm. And as it hit like whatever it was, the storm sheared away sections of Atlantic City's iconic boardwalk before inundating the streets with a wall of wave eight feet high. Within minutes, more than 75 percent of the city was underwater. Sixty miles away, in Seaside Heights, the storm ripped the Jet Star Roller Coaster — a massive structure with seventeen hundred feet of steel track and fifty-foot drops — from its pier and relocated it in the ocean shallows. It swept entire houses from their foundations and pulled cars into the surf. In Fall River, Massachusetts, the storm peeled away roofs and flooded Battleship Cove. In New London, Connecticut, it pulled the town's iconic bathhouse from its pilings and left in its place a household stove, along with cords of splintered timber. The weather station atop New Hampshire's Mount Washington registered gusts of 139 miles per hour.

Back in Manhattan, seawater poured down stairs and vents into subway stations, filling tunnels from track to ceiling. At the NYU medical center, the most critical patients had been safely evacuated, but thousands of animals used for medical testing had not. More than ten thousand mice and rats, many of which had been genetically altered for cancer and mental illness research, drowned in their basement cages. Seven thousand trees fell in New York City parks. More than sixty-five thousand boats were destroyed in New York alone. The city, one meteorologist said, was living its own worst-case scenario.

The force of the wind and sea exploded electrical transformers and caused massive fires that destroyed both fin de siècle mansions in Old Greenwich, Connecticut, and more than one hundred working-class homes in Queens. Other damage created a kind of cruel *carnivàle:* As the storm marched across the region, it neatly piled sailboats at the end of a dry pier and left floating taxicabs in their slips. It relocated a fishing vessel onto railroad tracks and pushed pickup trucks into backyard pools. Dining rooms filled with sand. Floodwaters plucked the New York Aquarium's resident three-foot American eel from its tank and deposited it, unharmed, in a staff shower stall.

But those were the easy stories. Most were far more grim.

More than ten feet of salt water flooded the low-lying areas of Staten Island. There, neighbors banded together and decided to make a last-minute run for it. They set out down their street, but were soon stopped by a wave of dark water bearing down on them. They turned and raced the opposite way, only to stop dead in their tracks. An angry wall of water was coming from that direction, too. It snaked, leapt, spun, and crashed, picking up bits and pieces of people's lives: toilets and kitchen sinks, pianos and sewing machines, lawn mowers and bicycles, porches and chimneys. Jack-o'-lanterns bobbed their way through the storm-churned water by the hundreds, a parade of ghoulish faces amid the chaos.

There was no escape.

The waves continued to grow, cannoning through windows and doors and deluging homes. Within minutes, that water was lapping at attic floors.

In the Oakwood neighborhood, two men sought shelter on the second story of a home after their car stalled on the street below. Within minutes, floodwater was above their chests. They jimmied open the attic window and looked into the surge of water, now at eye level. A car floated by, then a Dumpster. And then — what was that? The roof of an entire house. Still attached to the house. The whole damn thing was floating on the angry tide. They agreed to take a chance. On three, they leapt out the window and onto the floating roof. There, they dug their nails into the shingles, trying not to get dizzy as the building spun its way through the crashing water.

Not everyone was so lucky.

The same rising sea caught several elderly people unawares and trapped them in their homes. The residents screamed for help, but neighbors couldn't reach them: The waters were just too high, too fast. The bodies of the trapped would be found floating in living rooms and bedrooms days later. So, too, would the body of an off-duty police officer who relocated his family, including his fifteen-month-old son, to their attic before retreating back downstairs to secure the rest of the house. The family waited for hours, but he never returned. Another father and son were found in their basement, their bodies locked in a tight embrace, the dead father's arms still shielding his son's head.

In Tottenville, Staten Island, a family of three who had been robbed during Hurricane Irene also chose to remain in their home, despite the evacuation orders. As they finished dinner, the waters began flooding their house, lifting the dining room from its foundation and eventually shearing it away. They ran to their second-story master bedroom, but within minutes the water began pouring in through the windows and doors there as well. They retreated to the bathroom, where the mother and her thirteen-year-old daughter clung to the sink faucet as storm water lapped at their chins. And then the entire wall of their house gave way, pouring them out into the churning surge. Waves tore them from each other. The mother called — no, shrieked — her daughter's name, but the plea evaporated in the roar of water. She kept calling, clinging to the sink, flinching each time another house slid into the waves. Hours later, she was deposited on a pile of debris. She was severely hypothermic but otherwise unharmed. It would be days before the bodies of the father and daughter were found.

As news of the rising water began to

intensify, another mother bundled her two boys, ages two and four, and tucked them into their car seats, then set out for a family member's house in Brooklyn. She thought she was doing the right thing — keeping her boys safe. But their SUV was soon overtaken by swell. The car stalled. Water began to pour in. She struggled with her seat belt, slipped into the back and wrestled both boys out of their car seats, took a deep breath, and crashed into the surge. The waves were unrelenting. They crashed upon her, pulling the mother and boys down. She clung more tightly. The waves kept coming. And then the biggest one of all struck. It tore the boys from her arms before sweeping her away, too. She clung, first to a tree, and then to the hope that someone would help. But no one would answer their door — no one would take that risk, no matter how much she begged and cried. Exhausted, she collapsed on a stranger's porch and waited until daybreak, then walked the flooded streets until she found a police officer. Days later, the bodies of the boys were found less than twenty feet from each other, tangled in reeds and debris in a marsh at the end of a dead-end street.

On average, about six hurricanes develop

each year. Fewer than two of them strike the United States. Major storms — storms with winds greater than 110 miles per hour — occur even less frequently: one every eighteen months, give or take. The chance that one of those storms will strike New York City is 3.2 percent. None of these statistics mattered at all with Superstorm Sandy. There was no precedent, no authoritative model or soothing data to help make sense of what was happening. The world had simply never witnessed a storm like this one.

Barometric pressures that day, October 29, 2012, were the lowest ever recorded north of the Carolinas. Surge levels were their highest. And the damage wrought by this storm was immense. Sandy damaged or destroyed a million homes. More than half of those were in the United States, located in a damage area roughly the size of all of Europe. Nearly nine million households were without power from South Carolina to Maine. Rain from the storm reached as far west as the Dakotas and as far south as Texas. Thousands of acres of shoreline were severely eroded. By the time Sandy dissipated somewhere over western Pennsylvania, at least 147 people had lost their lives in places as far-ranging as Jamaica and

Canada.

This storm — this superstorm — wasn't supposed to be that deadly. And it certainly wasn't supposed to make landfall in the most populated region of North America. Nor was it supposed to morph into a monstrous hybrid the likes of which our oceans had never born. And that's what was so terrifying about this storm. Hurricane Sandy broke all the rules.

Its story began just more than a week before it made landfall.

Sunday

3:00 A.M.
National Weather Service Forecast Office
Mt. Holly, New Jersey
45°F
Barometer: 29.93 inches (rising)
Winds: 4 mph (WNW)
Skies: Clear

The absence of any windows and a constant, humming fluorescence give the forecasting floor of the Mt. Holly National Weather Service bureau a timeless quality not unlike that of an Atlantic City casino, where day and night are marked by the same pulsing light. Thirty computer monitors and four sixty-inch flat-screen TVs flank the walls, filling the room with cool blue light. There's a vibration there, too. The combined workings of dozens of strong hard drives and the equally strong fans required to keep them from overheating give off a kind of alien-spaceship buzz. The entire effect can feel like one of inhuman sensory deprivation — or at least sensory reassignment, dialing you in to the constant flash of radar and innumerable, incomparable graphs. A special way of looking at our planet's nature.

Watching this data shift and stream were two young forecasters, dressed in the requisite National Weather Service uniform: faded jeans, a T-shirt, and a fleece pullover. She wore pink socks and a ponytail. He had wire-rimmed glasses and running sneakers. They sat, as they did most midnight shifts, with their backs to each other. She was working the short-term forecasting desk, crunching line after line of data to generate the forecasts that would keep the Philadelphia International Airport and the ports of New Jersey running for the next twenty-four hours. He was working the long-term desk: generating a far more general forecast that would keep the mid-Atlantic thinking about the next five days. Their shift had been quiet. Uneventful. Outside the cavernous brick building, another perfect autumn day would soon be dawning — warm, sunny, with barely a ripple of wind. Perfect autumn days tend to bore forecasters. Especially at 3:00 A.M. It can be a struggle not to get a little sleepy on a shift like that.

He rubbed his eyes, pushed back his chair.

There wouldn't be much happening for the next half hour — not until the European Centre for Medium-Range Weather Forecasts Integrated Forecast System (or ECMWF) sent out its forecast. Based in Reading, England, this European forecasting system boasts one of the largest supercomputers in the world (#41, to be precise: behind NASA, several Chinese supercomputer centers, and the University of Edinburgh, but ahead of the US Army Research Laboratory and the French Alternative Energies and Atomic Energy Commission). Twice a day, the ECMWF supercomputer generates one of the planet's most dependable weather forecasts. That information comes by way of a series of spatial maps, and forecasters on both sides of the Atlantic know to wait for them. On a quiet graveyard shift, it's the highlight of the night — particularly during hurricane season. The forecaster toggled over to the ECMWF display, then got up and went to the vending machine to get himself a snack.

At precisely 3:30 A.M., the maps began to stream in. He sat at attention. She wheeled her chair over to the computer so they could watch together. The forecasters glanced. Then glanced again. And then they laughed. It just seemed so absurd. A system had begun building deep in the southern Caribbean. That was a little unusual, given how late it was in the hurricane season. But what really seemed ludicrous was what ECMWF said the system would do next: grow. And not just grow, but become enormous. So enormous, in fact, that it would become unstoppable, even after it left the warm waters of the Caribbean. So enormous that it would keep marching up into the colder waters of the Atlantic, eventually turning not out to sea, like practically every other storm in recorded history, but inland instead. According to the ECMWF, this storm was going to do the almost unthinkable: It was going to slam directly into the mid-Atlantic seaboard. Preposterous. No storm had done anything like this since 1903, when a hurricane named the Vagabond assaulted New York and New Jersey, killing dozens and endangering the life of President Theodore Roosevelt, who had the misfortune to be aboard his yacht in Long Island Sound. That hurricane was the first to make landfall in New Jersey in recorded history, and everyone agreed it was a freak occurrence. The chances of such a thing happening again were minuscule. This forecast must be a giant mistake. A wonky anomaly — a reminder about just how fallible even the best prediction can be. The two forecasters at Mt. Holly felt certain of this.

"Well, at least we know what's *not* going to happen next week," he said.

"I know," she agreed. "That's totally off the wall. Absurd."

They laughed a little more, and then they put it out of mind. *The model will resolve itself tomorrow,* they said. *I mean, how could it possibly be accurate?*

5:00 A.M.
Boothbay, Maine
Barometer: 29.74 (rising)
Winds: 6 mph (WNW)
Skies: Clear
Seas: Calm

In the summertime, the coastal town of Boothbay bustles with tourists and nautical groupies making their way down the commercial district's narrow streets and into gift shops with names like Two Salty Dogs, Joy to the Wind, and Sweet Bay. Down near the wharves, taffy and ice cream shops vie for a tourist's attention alongside attractive girls hawking whale and puffin tours. But the real attraction here is not so much the town itself as it is the harbor, a narrow and deeply set port well protected by rocky crags and spruce-swept islands. When the days are long, the harbor positively hums with controlled chaos, as yachts and day cruisers zip between lobster boats and the iconic schooners that have made the region famous.

By Columbus Day, though, much of this seaside town slips into hibernation. The fried-clam stands are stowed away in inland barns; stores hang cheerful signs promising they'll reopen in the spring; schooners sleep quietly at the dock, swaddled in white plastic. Even the Boothbay Harbor Shipyard stood all but vacant that early Sunday morning in late October. The predawn air was thick with chill, and remnants of the previous day's fog still pushed against the harbor's floating docks, making everything feel low and close and damp.

Just after 5:00 A.M., alarm clocks and cell phones began ringing on board the *Bounty.* A few lights began to shine out of the portholes and the windows of the great cabin. Several minutes later, groggy bodies spilled out onto the deck, dressed in Carhartts and sweatshirts, with hoods and stocking caps pulled low to cover dreadlocks and piercings. They wore headlamps and gloves. They fired up the ship's two aging engines; they fiddled with lines for the ship's enormous square sails; they hauled off the last of the trash and anything else they couldn't take with them.

Standing near the rear of the ship, their captain looked on. His hair was thinning, but he wore it in a wisp of a ponytail anyway. He also wore thick glasses, attached to a heavy cord so he wouldn't lose them, and beat-up Teva sandals with wool socks, even though his wife told him they looked silly. He didn't care about that, he said. And he liked having warm feet. It never occurred to him to try closed shoes. His jeans were dirty, his canvas jacket a little worn. But he didn't care about that, either. He was quiet. Almost shy. And his two hearing aids could make it seem like he was ignoring you. Sometimes, he actually was. But he knew his ship better than anything, and his crew knew that, too. They loved him. Worshipped him, almost.

His name was Robin Walbridge. He'd been master of the *Bounty* for almost twenty years. She was, he was fond of saying, his greatest love. His wife, Claudia, didn't mind being runner-up. Robin, she says, always had plenty of love to spread around. There was a charisma to him — an energy. It drew you in. Made you want to stay. Crew members thought of him as the dad they'd always hoped to have. They depended upon his calm good nature. It takes that and something more to work on a tall ship. Certainly it's not the paycheck — about $100 a week for a deckhand. But tall-ship sailors aren't the kind of people who worry about money. They're environmental studies majors taking a semester off from school and tattooed wanderers who never really fit in (at least, not until they found their ship). They spend their winters running day trips out of the Florida Keys or couch surfing in Puerto Rico or skiing Jackson Hole on their last twenty bucks. They eat ramen and hot sauce and drink cheap beer out of tall cans. Those things are all good. But nothing makes them nearly as happy as being under way.

Their captain knew that. He banked on it. *Shore spoils a crew,* he always said. The prospect of heading back to sea made him almost giddy that morning. The crew was stumbling a little — it'd been six weeks since they'd sailed their ship. Robin teased them when they tangled a line. He spoke to them in rhyme when they had a hard time shaking off too little sleep and one too many beers at the House of Pizza: "Wakey, wakey, little snakies," he said. "Wakey, wakey, eggs and bacy." They laughed. Even with the fatigue and the little hangovers, they were excited. They were itching to be back on the water. It was where they belonged. It was home.

At that time in the morning, just about everyone on the working waterfront blended in. The blond woman who tumbled onto the *Bounty*'s deck wearing an oversize green stocking cap and humming the Rolling Stones did not. She had the body and the kind of charisma that stopped traffic, whether she was in a Miami club or on an L.A. beach. In a Maine sailing town, a jut of her pinup-girl hip was enough to silence an entire boatyard.

Her name was Claudene Christian. She'd come to the *Bounty* because she was lost. Because she was looking for something tangible — structure and truth. And yes, okay, she wanted a little adventure, too. That morning in Boothbay, she was more certain than ever that she had found all of those things. And she was nothing if not utterly enamored with her shipmates.

That stocking cap she wore — the one embroidered with the word *Bounty* in big gold letters — had been given to her by her watch supervisor, Doug Faunt. He'd bought hats for all of them after their first night sleeping in the New England chill. That's just the kind of thing he did. At sixty-six,

Faunt was the oldest member of the crew, and a successful career in computers had allowed him to join the ship as a volunteer rather than as a paid employee. It also made him a wiz at wiring and electrical systems and entitled him to play the role of curmudgeon when needed. But that was really just skin deep. Faunt adored both his ship and his fellow crew members: He'd often put electrical parts for the former on his own credit card; he'd take the latter out for donuts, give them his frequent-flyer miles, or buy big wheels of expensive cheese for them all to share.

For the first time all year, there was time for that. The season was over. No more dockside tours, no more pirate-themed festivals or answering tourists' questions. The ship had just one more stop to make before it returned to its onetime home in St. Petersburg, Florida. Claudia would be waiting. So, too, was a possible benefactor. The captain's best friend, Ralph McCutcheon, a longtime fixture on the ship, was planning a massive party for them. After that, a couple of them would stay on the ship at its winter home in Texas. The rest would disperse to those day sailers and couches and chairlifts. Until then, they had nothing to worry about.

The crew's numbers had dwindled to seventeen: Several of the younger sailors were heading back to school; others were returning to jobs or beginning winter work. Faunt asked Walbridge if that made them shorthanded (the ship's manual said it did), but the captain assured him he'd sailed with fewer. To replace the departing crew, Jess Hewitt, a twenty-five-year-old graduate of the Maine Maritime Academy with the soul of a rock star, had joined the ship just two weeks before it began its month-long dry dock at the Boothbay Harbor Shipyard. Already she was known for her fabulous flair: big sunglasses, slim jeans, braided captain's caps, and bikini tops on workdays. Chris Barksdale, a fifty-six-year-old handyman with a background in horticulture, arrived a few weeks later to replace the ship's engineer. The crew loved his decorum and southern drawl: the soft consonants of a Vah-ginian gentleman, the way he put "Miss" before women's names.

Barksdale had arrived while the *Bounty* was in dry dock. He wasn't sure what to make of the ship — it seemed worn to him. But the rest of the crew agreed it was in the best shape ever. Most of them had worked together on the ship during the previous season. They were tight. Walbridge told them they were the best crew he'd ever had, and they believed him. Throughout that whole summer, they had moved up the Eastern Seaboard, stopping in places like Savannah and New York and Boston and Philadelphia. They scraped and painted historic buildings in exchange for free dock space. They hung hand-painted advertisements, gave endless tours, and entertained streams of tourists, answering the same questions every day with a smile. During their downtime, they played Twister and grilled hamburgers on deck; they had movie nights and slumber parties down below. They took cities by storm and drank rum. Most of the time, they moved as a single unit, playing around wherever they went, whether it was jumping in bouncy houses or staging impromptu jam sessions on deserted streets late at night.

The sheer energy of it all both surprised and delighted Claudene Christian, who called the scene "Booty on the *Bounty.*" It was exactly her cup of tea. She was a former beauty queen. A cheerleader. A sorority girl. The kind of woman men adore and women love to hate. Except, of course, for the fact that it was nearly impossible to hate Claudene. She was outgoing and unassuming and funny. She never had a bad word to say about anyone, and always made you feel like you were her best friend — even if she had just met you.

The *Bounty,* Claudene was certain, would be the greatest adventure of her life. She talked on and on about how capable her fellow crew members were — that they could literally build, fix, or engineer anything. She said that they were super cool and super intelligent, which, she admitted, kind of surprised her. Her family and friends were skeptical. It had been a rough several years for Christian. She had been diagnosed with bipolar disorder. She was drinking too much. She suffered a nasty lawsuit with Mattel and an even worse relationship with a boyfriend named Sasha.

Christian had always been obsessed with sailing and the Knights Templar. Her family claimed direct descent from Fletcher Christian, the famous mutineer on the original *Bounty.* Her father encouraged her to try life on a tall ship. With his help, she signed on as cook of the *Niña,* a re-creation of Christopher Columbus's famed ship. But Claudene did not fit into the regimented culture of the *Niña:* Policies on board prohibit tattoos and piercings, and "extreme hair" — including dreadlocks and colors other than those naturally endowed at birth

— was not permitted. The ship's captain adhered to age-old nautical hierarchy, forbidding people to sit at his table unless expressly invited or to speak to him unless he spoke to them first. When Claudene appeared to work her way into his little world, jealousies erupted. By the time the ship reached Florida, Claudene was miserable and soon called her new boyfriend, Brad Leggett, to help her escape.

It wasn't long after that she found the *Bounty* on the Internet. Claudene felt certain she would be bringing history full circle if she could manage to join that organization: *Imagine! A descendant of Fletcher Christian willingly stepping aboard the ship!* And she'd be smarter this time — of that she felt certain. The *Niña* had enlightened her about the realities of life at sea — enough for her to know that that kind of life wouldn't be sustainable for someone like her. Instead, she said she had bigger aspirations: to find a way to market the ship and, eventually, to become its owner. But to do that, she'd first have to get aboard. She wrote to the organization, playing up her marketing experience. They agreed to accept her as a volunteer.

Her father drove Claudene from Oklahoma to North Carolina that May, where they rendezvoused with the *Bounty* in Wilmington. He was a little apprehensive when they arrived. The ship needed a major overhaul, he told Brad, and would certainly never pass an inspection.

Rex Christian wasn't the only one who was concerned. Coast Guard Sector Commander Anthony Popiel was on the ship that day, too. Popiel's job is a heavy one: He's captain of a major port, and has the authority to close it when serious weather — like a hurricane — bears down on the region. It's a serious decision, and one that can cost hundreds of millions of dollars in lost trade, fuel, and sailor wages. But Popiel is also in charge of monitoring the safety of the waters beyond that port, and his team at sector must oversee all search-and-rescue or recovery operations that happen therein. Risk is his life, and he's seen a lot of it — enough to know it should be avoided at every opportunity.

Popiel and his son spent that May day aboard the *Bounty.* John Svendsen, the ship's first mate, gave them a tour, showing them all the nooks and crannies of the ship. Svendsen is a soft-spoken guy who, with his long blond hair and trim beard, looks a little like he stepped out of a nineteenth-century novel. Like his captain, he tends to stand in the shadows when faced with a crowd. But he and Popiel hit it off at once and spent the day sharing stories about their experiences at sea. Popiel was impressed by Svendsen's experience and expertise: The first mate really seemed to know his stuff. So did the other five or six crew members Popiel met on board. Still, the ship had limitations. Unlike sailing school vessels, the *Bounty* had only a dockside coast guard inspection, which meant it wasn't certified to take passengers to sea. Popiel could tell it had been built as a movie prop instead of as a seagoing ship. There wasn't a lot of organization concerning where things ought to go, and space was tight — especially in the crew quarters.

That alone, he says, wasn't really cause for serious concern. But Popiel says he was also "fresh off Irene," the hurricane that hammered North Carolina the previous year. It had been a big storm and had taken a lot out of the coast guard — not to mention the people and the vessels in his coastal state. The day Popiel visited the *Bounty,* he checked the marine forecast (he *always* checks the marine forecast), and he didn't like what he saw: An early-season tropical storm was heading their way. He tried, gently, to persuade the crew of the *Bounty* to stay. “Hey,” he remembers saying, “don’t you want to hang out here for a while?” Popiel added he was even sure he could find dockage for them as long as they needed. But John Svendsen declined, saying the storm would be good for the ship. Popiel remembers that the first mate told him the ship “likes wind,” that she “moves well” in a big storm. That, the sector commander says, was what got him worried. “The takeaway from a storm, when you’ve had that experience, should be to heed warnings and seek safe shelter,” says Popiel.

Svendsen told Popiel he felt confident his ship could beat Mother Nature. And if his newest deckhand knew about the storm or worried about it, she didn’t say so. Instead, Claudene pulled out her guitar and sang songs. She flirted. She was enthralled. Her spark had returned.

The *Bounty* crew took a little time warming up to their new shipmate. But once they did, they fell head over heels. They called her their spy, because she could find out anything about anyone. She’d talk up visitors and crews from other vessels and invariably find out where the best party was that night. During the yard period, she wiggled into tight spaces with a Shop-Vac, and led the crew in gymnastics sessions. At the

House of Pizza, she'd buy everyone's rounds. When her credit card was declined, Barksdale happily lent her fifty bucks. She promised she'd repay him — and promised, and promised. He said he didn't care either way. How could you? She was just so happy.

That particular October morning, Claudene was one of the first on deck. She sang a couple of Juice Newton songs and tried to look busy. She winked at fellow crew members as they walked by. She texted her mom to say she was doing great.

Walbridge was happy, too. He was on his way home to Claudia. He hadn't seen her in weeks. He made a show of tucking away the jewelry he had purchased for her the day before at Patty Stone's gift shop, just half a block up from the shipyard. He told everyone the ship looked great. They'd worked really hard in the yard. He was proud of them.

The sun wouldn't rise for over an hour. But by 5:45 A.M., they were making their way out of the deserted harbor, past Mouse Island and the Burnt Island Lighthouse, motoring on the strong outgoing tide — there wasn't enough wind to sail. Everything was calm. Flat calm, Walbridge said. He seemed a little disappointed. So did the crew. The trip to New London, Connecticut, would be boring. Mundane. At least there was work to do. Temporary lights still hung below deck, and Doug Faunt was still working on much of the wiring. The crew quarters were in shambles. But no one looked worried. After all, they trusted one another — and their captain. He had the traditional maritime knowledge and personal experience to deal with whatever the sea threw at them. And they were a family.

11:00 A.M.
Miami, Florida
Barometer: 30.00 inches (falling)
Winds: 7 mph (NNE)
Skies: Mostly cloudy
Seas: 2–4 feet

By all meteorological accounts, the 2012 hurricane season was not going to be throwing much at anyone. Chris Landsea, the Science and Operations Officer at the National Hurricane Center, was inclined to agree.

Outside his office window at the NHC headquarters, cars streamed by on the Florida Turnpike, casting blinding reflections of light off their bumpers and windows. Even convertibles were rolled up tight — it was too hot for anything other than maxed-out air-conditioning. Twenty miles to the east, South Beach's perennial parade of bikers and Rollerbladers had already stripped down to the barest of tropical essentials: thongs and short shorts, bare chests, visors, and lots of oversize sunglasses. Families crowded onto towels and into the lapping waves. West of the city, out among the cream-and-pink-colored buildings of Florida International University, the heat was a different story altogether. It pressed down, made everything come to a standstill. By noon, the temperature had reached 90 degrees Fahrenheit, and the dew point was almost as high. Even the super-industrial air conditioners at the National Hurricane Center were having a hard time keeping apace.

The NHC is a relatively new organization by US governmental standards — and one that often operates with more questions than answers. The Hurricane Center is the storm trooper of the National Oceanic and Atmospheric Administration (NOAA), an organization not much older than its youngest meteorologists. NOAA was formed by President Nixon in October 1970, with the goal of streamlining the country's major scientific branches: the Coast and Geodetic Survey, the Weather Bureau, and the Bureau of Commercial Fisheries, each of which had profound impact on environmental policy, and each of which was seen as crucial in our understanding of how we move through the world. The idea of uniting these disparate branches was based in the realization not only that the oceans and atmosphere are inextricably linked, but that we are utterly dependent upon both. Nixon summed it up this way in his 1970 proposal to create a new organization: "We face immediate and compelling needs for better protection of life and property from natural hazards, and for a better understanding of the total environment — an understanding which will enable us more effectively to monitor and predict its actions, and ultimately, perhaps to exercise some degree of control over them."

Control appealed to just about everyone that year. It was already a calendar marked by uncontrollable disasters: That spring, a freak avalanche killed 39 tourists in the French Alps; a month later, another killed 74 boys at a French sanitarium. An F5 tornado struck Lubbock, Texas, killing 28. Landslides killed 200 in Colombia and a staggering 47,000 people in Peru. More than 500,000 people died after a late-season cyclone struck East Pakistan. An unusually wet monsoon season in Vietnam left 200,000 people homeless and did what no treaty had been able to accomplish: It forced a temporary end to the Vietnam War. Cholera was sweeping across Eastern Europe. Revolutionary groups with names like the Weather Underground were surfacing to protest governmental policy.

Still, those in power did their damnedest to eke out a sense of autonomy. England announced plans to build a revolutionary flood barrier on the Thames. Not to be outdone, the United States decided to build the scientific organization to end all organizations — one that would acknowledge, at long last, that our fate is tied to both the weather and the sea. At the center of it all would be the National Weather Service. Nixon placed the new organization, known as NOAA, within the Department of Commerce: a decision, as it is apocryphally recorded, that was based more on spite than a sense of organization. As the story goes, the Republican president was so incensed by the antiwar sentiment expressed by his secretary of the interior that he made a point of denying that office the opportunity to house NOAA. Instead, the agency was bestowed upon the Department of Commerce. Whether or not that story is true has been lost to history, but it has enough traction that President Obama trucked it out in a 2012 State of the Union address, when announcing that he intended to restore NOAA to its rightful place in the Department of the Interior.

Meanwhile, the Hurricane Center continues to define itself in reaction to storms that got the better of us all. It's a process of fits and starts, says Chris Landsea: Each storm shows them another place where they need to improve. After FEMA, the Federal Emergency Management Agency, underwent harsh criticism for its slow response to Hurricane Katrina in 2005, the federal government decided to locate a FEMA office at the NHC so that relief efforts could be coordinated more quickly and efficiently: Instead of having to call the NHC to find out about a storm, FEMA managers would have their own on-site representative with the most advanced teleconferencing equipment available. In 1992, when Hurricane Andrew sent satellite dishes careering off the NHC roof, disabling meteorologists' ability to communicate, they decided they needed new digs. And so they traded their original building — a commercial site in the southern part of Miami — for a plot of land offered to them by Florida International University. The new headquarters they built there is nothing short of a bunker, and it stands out like a weird braces-wearing kid among the genteel architecture of the rest of the campus, what with its collection of satellites and communication towers perched atop the concrete structure.

But the NHC building isn't intended to look pretty, says Landsea. It was built to withstand major hurricanes. That's why its foundation is four feet higher than any other building on the campus — computers don't tend to work well when they're wet. That's why imposing metal shutters can be dropped over the building's few doors and windows at a moment's notice. And why, inside those doors and windows, there's a kind of inner sanctum, a building inside a building as it were, built out of still more concrete and rebar. There, two enormous generators can keep the whole operation running for days. When a major storm is approaching, they'll actually switch off from the public grid so that no operations are interrupted by service blips. Fiber optics laid well below its foundation allow forecasters to tap into different information lines, even when hurricane winds are upon them. A secondary roof made of poured concrete and reinforced with steel bars keeps forecasters safe. They also have independent sewer and water systems, and the two generators make sure at least a few creature comforts are met during a cataclysmic storm — like the vending machines in the lounge. In fact, this inner sanctum is so regulated, so removed from anything approaching the natural elements, that the meteorologists working there regularly have to consult sources like the Weather Channel to know what's happening right outside their door. There are no seasons, no dips in temperature or darkening storms at the NHC — just fluorescent light and 72-degree canned air. They may as well be miles underground.

And that, says Landsea, is precisely how you want to feel when a hurricane is barreling down on you. He's seen the building put through its paces — enough to know that all the concrete in the world isn't enough when a major storm comes knocking. In 2005, Hurricane Wilma thrashed Florida, killing twenty-two people and leaving millions without power. The National Hurricane Center would have gone dark, too, had they not disconnected from the grid and switched over to generator power. Not certain that would be enough, they also dispatched a team of forecasters to Washington, D.C. — just in case the hurricane proved too much for their new headquarters.

It remained standing. Their generators continued to power their computers and radios, but both were drowned out by the ferocity of the winds, which blew through the satellite guy wires so hard that the whole building was screaming. "It was like being on a battleship," says Landsea. "A battleship during a really, really ugly storm. It's not a pleasant feeling." And it's made all the more intense by an architect's whimsy: At NHC headquarters, large metal doors with portholes mark egresses, and ship's lanterns illuminate hallways outside the restrooms. A ship, says Landsea, is the last place you want to be in a hurricane. The second-to-last, he says, is on the lawn outside the National Hurricane Center. Their satellite dishes can really only withstand winds under 100 miles per hour. Any higher, says Landsea, and "those things are going to go sailing like giant Frisbees."

The question for Landsea is not so much whether that will happen as it is when. "Florida sticks out like a sore thumb. We know we're going to get hit again."

That's one reason the NHC is deadly serious about storm protection. It's equally serious about security, but there are surprising moments of whimsy there as well. The guard's station is militaristic in its configuration, but also includes a wholesale club–size tub of cat food. They leave a few scoops out each morning for a cat who skulks around in the bushes just outside the front door. The staff has named the cat Pit because, explains the guard, the long-haired tabby is clearly tougher than all of the other feral cats in the area. Beyond the guard's station, and at moments when you least expect it, ABBA's "Dancing Queen" will come blaring out of the marine forecasting room. Over and over again. In their spare time, forecasters send around hilarious cartoons that only a meteorologist would get. They daydream about sharknados.

Marine forecasters, say the hurricane specialists, are like that. They move at a pace not unlike what you'd see at a bank or an insurance office. On particularly routine days, one of the large TV monitors will be tuned to ESPN or CNN. The hurricane forecasting side of the building is more feast-or-famine. The forecasting desk there stands largely empty for six months of the year, as the forecasters travel throughout the hurricane region educating families about storms or while they conduct training workshops on everything from new satellite technology to emergency management. Both, they say, are efforts to mitigate the stress felt during an actual storm. Stress they want the rest of us to understand — especially if you work in the realm of disaster response. "If you really want to freak out a first responder guy," says Landsea, "put them in the forecast seat with some real-time hurricane data and tell them to predict the track of a storm."

Frankly, he says, that freaks out the hurricane specialists sometimes, too.

On that particular Sunday, Chris Landsea wasn't freaked out yet, but he was really interested. And hot. That the heat was enough to try Landsea's patience says quite a lot about the National Hurricane Center's most cheerful employee, who is — not coincidentally — also the agency's most charismatic star. At academic and press conferences alike, Landsea prefers bright Hawaiian shirts to suit jackets or NOAA's traditional uniform of a navy-blue golf shirt (though he does pair even his brightest prints with creased slacks and European dress shoes). He's famous for taking basketball breaks at lunch and is an unabashed Jimmy Buffett groupie (hence the Hawaiian shirts). He refers to politicians and high-level administrators as "critters." He plays water polo in his spare time. He's also hurricane *obsessed:* his three kids are all named after major storms; his idea of a great vacation is a cyclone conference in Key West, where he'll walk from session to session like the celebrity he is, often talking to admiring grad students while simultaneously holding a cell phone with a reporter or a science writer conducting an interview on the other end. If someone is sitting at a computer station and sees Landsea, they get up and offer him the seat.

That afternoon, Landsea was thinking less about conferences and more about water polo and time with his kids. The hurricane season seemed all but over, and no one at the National Hurricane Center minded at all. It had been a weird year — tied for the third most active in history, but without a major storm. Months had passed without a single system threatening land — not even hurricane-prone Florida. And then there was all this lingering, record-breaking heat.

Sitting at his computer station, Landsea was trying hard not to sweat through his thinnest Hawaiian shirt as he watched the satellite data streaming in. Something had caught his interest. Ten days earlier, an easterly wave had formed off the coast of the Western Sahara and was now being buffeted by the trade winds. On a fair day, those winds funnel toward the equator, then coalesce into a steady conveyor belt, pushing air (and everything in it) across the Atlantic. They are relentless in their singular pursuit, moving westward — always westward — making them the most consistently powerful force on the planet. But every once in a while, there is a hiccup — a kind of ripple — in their movement. In meteorological parlance, it is a "migratory disturbance," which is to say that some of the winds zig, while the rest of the trades zag. That's when real weather begins to form.

The hiccup's gap creates an easterly wave — a pocket in which unstable air can form. And that unstable air can create anything from a brief rain shower to a catastrophic hurricane. On average, about sixty easterly waves form each year. Most of them (90 percent, in fact), dissipate with a few thunderclaps somewhere over the Atlantic Ocean. A small handful of them grow into a system of clouds with organized movement (what meteorologists call a "tropical disturbance"). An even smaller handful of these disturbances continue to grow, eventually coalescing into a swirling circle of thunderstorms capable of feeding themselves (a "tropical depression"). Every once in a while, that depression continues to intensify, eventually becoming a tropical storm or, in the rarest of cases, a full-fledged hurricane. But going from a wave to a hurricane is about as likely as making it from Little League to the majors. If you've been in the tropical weather business for a while, that means you tend not to get too excited when you see a wave forming out there.

The process by which a wave develops into a tropical storm or hurricane is called "tropical cyclone genesis," and it requires a very particular set of complex meteorological circumstances. Most of our weather occurs between sea level and about forty thousand feet up — a region of the atmosphere known as the troposphere. For a tropical wave to become a hurricane, it must build itself up into a giant, menacing tower of swirling thunderstorms that brush the tropopause, or uppermost ceiling of the troposphere. For that to happen, the hurricane — perhaps paradoxically — needs calm, fair weather wherever one of its many thunderstorms is developing, and that requires a kind of synchronicity not often found in our atmosphere. The troposphere is really just a giant layer cake of different wind fields (which is why airplanes often change altitude during a flight — they're always on the lookout for the most favorable wind conditions). Some of these tropospheric winds can be severe: It's not at all uncommon for even private pilots of single-engine planes to encounter 100-mile-per-hour winds as low as ten thousand feet. Those sorts of winds are more than enough to disrupt cloud formation or to prevent a system from developing. In fact, winds as high as 25 miles per hour will easily shear off a developing thunderstorm as it begins to form. Sometimes, even 10 or 15 miles per hour of wind is enough to stunt a developing storm, particularly if the air is cool and dry. Hurricanes thrive on warm, moist air; once that air cools or begins to dry, the storm wilts.

Initially, Landsea's wave had been encountering plenty of wind and low-pressure air as it bounced across the Atlantic. And Hurricane Rafael, which was churning east of the Bahamas, was throwing in its own complications, too. Both sets of factors had been preventing the wave from growing into much of anything. And for all Landsea knew, this new wave would fizzle out completely. Still, he couldn't help but look at the data streaming in. Two days earlier, that wave had split into two systems — one was now meandering around the Azores, while the other was on a more deliberate path toward the Caribbean. As it moved westward, the wave encountered the second in the series of specific circumstances required for a tropical system to grow: deep, warm ocean waters — at least 80 degrees Fahrenheit and of a "sufficient depth," though just how deep no one knows. That warm water is the lifeblood of a storm — it's what allows it to build, to move, and, ultimately, to unleash its fury.

As a developing system passes over warm water, it sucks up the moist air around it, creating a vacuum that is quickly filled by more warm, moist air: food for the growing storm. This air pushes upward and is cooled by the surrounding atmosphere. As it does, two things happen: First, the water vapor it contains condenses — releasing latent heat to fuel the storm and causing massive rain showers; second, low pressure forms at the surface, creating a vacuum that the surrounding air rushes in to fill. The Coriolis effect forces that air to swirl — counterclockwise in the northern hemisphere; clockwise in the southern — so as it rises, it begins to circulate around a developing eye, looping its way up to the tropopause. As long as the air is warmer than its surroundings, it will continue to rise. If it meets a high-pressure system sitting atop the growing storm, its winds will continue to intensify. (Pressure differentials create wind. The greater the pressure difference between two areas, the stiffer the wind.) A high-pressure system can also help prevent wind shear from lopping off the growing clouds and pushing them away, where they will quickly dissipate. Instead, these clouds continue to expand, heaping upon one another and defined by the winds within, which mold the clouds into organized, swirling bands. Once they have a full circular rotation, the system is considered "closed." And that's when it really begins to grow.

The system Landsea was watching hadn't become a tropical depression yet. But there was always the chance it could. That chance was increasing by the moment, thanks to a developing high-pressure system in the Caribbean. What had been a 10 percent likelihood was now up to 60 percent. Those are the sorts of odds that get Landsea excited.

Forecasters are gamblers. They live in the realm of probability. Sixty percent is like a strong deal at a blackjack table. Every so often, Landsea would get up from his seat at the marine forecasting station and wander over to see his colleague Lixion Avila, who was nursing a cup of coffee at the main hurricane forecasting desk. The senior hurricane specialist loves ritual and says he never peeks at weather data overnight. Instead, Avila says he likes the drama and surprise of letting the past twelve hours unfold in brilliant color. There's a romance to it, he says, and that appeals to him a great deal.

"Hey, Lixion."

Avila was so absorbed by the satellite images that it took him a while to process that Landsea was standing beside him.

"Christopher," said Avila, rolling out the *R*s with an exaggerated Cuban accent.

Avila was in his first hour of what was supposed to be an eight-hour shift, though he says they always have a way of going longer. He doesn't mind. And he was enjoying his morning routine. There was data to gather and numbers to crunch and, eventually, a forecast to write that would be read by millions. That's where Avila has earned his stardom. Weather advisories can seem almost robotic in their construction. But Avila bucks that trend, and he loves to quote musical lyrics or make wry comments. When announcing the development of 2002's fourth tropical storm, he wrote: "The bell just rang in the Atlantic. Hello

Dolly!" Weather junkies everywhere went crazy. In 2007, he wrote, "If some of the dynamical models have their way . . . Juliette could meet her less-than-Shakespearean demise sooner than indicated." Those same junkies swooned. In early December 2005, when Hurricane Epsilon, a relentless storm that had been building and then weakening for days, finally showed signs of dying out, Avila quipped in his forecast, "I've heard that before about epsilon . . . haven't you?"

Most of the time, Avila's levity comes from self-deprecating jokes about the frustrating unknowability of storms. "I hope there will be no more surprises," he wrote when Hurricane Kyle teased the Carolinas in 2002. "Famous last words," he rued after calling for Hurricane Bertha to diminish. "Neither I nor the models are good enough to precisely know if Ernesto will have an intensity of 64 knots at landfall," he admitted.

That kind of honesty is one reason why Avila is the only NHC forecaster to have his own Wikipedia page. At sixty-one, he is also the senior-most forecaster at the National Hurricane Center. He jokes that that honor entitles him, like Landsea, to one of the few offices with a view of the Florida Turnpike. From his desk in the NHC bunker, if you tilt your head and lean a little, you can see palm trees and cloud formation in addition to the flow of traffic out there in the natural Florida light. Frankly, says Avila, he'd set up shop in the basement if he had to (even though the building doesn't have a basement). As far as Avila is concerned, working at the NHC is a dream come true for someone who grew up watching the storm-churned sea off Cuba's northeastern coast. Storms are his greatest obsession.

His second is dance. And if he was thinking about anything that afternoon, it was his upcoming trip to the International Ballet Festival in Cuba. His colleagues had agreed to cover him. An easy trade, he says, since he's the only one who never wants to take time off for Dolphins or University of Miami football games.

As the morning progressed, however, Avila was beginning to have second thoughts about heading off on a vacation. The heat wave was continuing to push across the region, and that was making the atmosphere south of Florida unstable. Out over Grenada, one of the disturbances began to throw thunderheads high into the air. The enormous clouds broke upon themselves, unleashing a shower of heavy warm rain on the Spice Island Resort that flattened palms and sent vacationers scurrying away from the pool. At the Hewanorra International Airport on the southern tip of St. Lucia, that rain was joined by lightning and thunder — enough to delay a few flights, but hardly unusual in this sultry climate, where humid air regularly makes for afternoon showers. What was unusual was the fact that this system was clearly growing. And it was on the move. Once past the Windward Islands, it continued its messy slog — an amorphous system with sloppy edges and no real sense of direction.

Avila squinted at the radar. He was playing a guessing game now, hoping these clouds might drop some clues about just how menacing it, whatever it was, intended to become. But the images gave away nothing. He needed to know what was going on closer to the surface — what the winds were doing. And that presented a challenge. Meteorologists have very few tools that can provide that kind of information. For years, the forecasters at the National Hurricane Center relied upon a tool called the quick scatterometer (or Quick-Scat, for short), which used microwave sensors to gauge wind speeds near the ocean surface. Attached to an orbiting satellite, it could give meteorologists a sense of winds across the globe, but it broke in 2009. Ask forecasters at the NHC how or why and they'll shrug. *It just broke,* they'll say. *That's all we know.*

Their boss, James Franklin, says it's more like the Quick-Scat died of old age. He's heard rumors that there is another one lying around somewhere that might get fixed to the exterior of the International Space Station at some point, but he's not holding his breath. For a while, he and his staff relied upon a Canadian scatterometer, but it failed recently, too. And so now the forecasters content themselves with a European version, called the A-scat, which they all agree is far inferior to the previous two. The A-scat takes pictures much like an old 35-millimeter camera does, which is to say that it takes fractions of a second for its shutter to open and close. Given how fast the satellite moves (about 15,000 miles per hour), that means forecasters end up with ribbons of data separated by large swaths of empty space — some as wide as three hundred miles.

It's frustrating, says Franklin. But not nearly so much as the data that does come in. The images forecasters get aren't very precise: They'll show you the presence of wind, but don't expect the images to distinguish between 60 and 100 miles per hour.

And forget about reading gusts over 100 miles per hour — that's just too sophisticated for the European scatterometer's technology. There's also the problem of time: The scat's images take an eternity to load. But the most infuriating aspect of the A-scat is that, for each point the scatterometer reads, it offers three or four potential wind directions, called ambiguities. Franklin says you have to be a real masochist to enjoy figuring out which direction represents what is actually happening. But if you get good at it, you can learn a lot about whether or not a system has become organized enough to become a tropical depression. And if you know whether or not that system has become a tropical storm, you can get a decent sense of intensity sometimes, too. The technology exists for a more sophisticated scatterometer to be launched, and the forecasters get a hopeful look in their eyes when they talk about the possibility of having access to a tool like that. Franklin says he's asked — repeatedly — but the budget just never seems to be there. Without it, the only way they can really know if a tropical depression is forming is to send an aircrew into the storm. And that comes with obvious negative side effects, too, so NHC officials tend to wait until they're pretty sure about a storm before dispatching crews.

That meant that, for the time being at least, Lixion Avila really had only one tool available to him. And if he wanted to know anything at all about this new system, he also knew he'd have to wait. Avila's a pretty patient guy. He sat at the desk, tapping his fingers. Landsea returned.

"I think there's something out there," said Avila.

Landsea looked over his shoulder. The data was still loading. Landsea sighed.

Avila lobbed a few jokes about how even old guys are faster than their technology.

Landsea laughed. Still no data. He wandered back to the marine forecasting desk. Avila thought about ballet.

And then, one strand at a time, the scatterometer began to reveal the winds of the Caribbean. Avila was really paying attention now. In between gaps of missing information, the forecaster could see the thunderstorms heaping on top of one another, releasing more moisture as they coalesced and began wrapping their winds around one another.

A cyclone was building. Or so it seemed. He called Landsea back over. They both leaned close to the screen. Neither of them said anything for a while. Then Avila pointed to the center of the storm. There, bands of clouds appeared to be orbiting around one another. Circulating. The system was organizing itself into a tropical depression. Landsea sighed. Clearly, the season wasn't over yet. And it was time to get somebody inside this storm. Avila picked up the phone. In an instant, he was patched through to Lieutenant Colonel Jon Talbot, Chief Meteorologist for the 53rd Weather Reconnaissance Squadron.

"Hey," asked Avila, "do you guys see what we see?"

"Yep," said Talbot. "I think we do."

Monday

7:45 A.M.
Keesler Air Force Base
Biloxi, Mississippi
68°F
Barometer: 30.14 inches (steady)
Winds: 9 mph (E)
Skies: Clear

Jon Talbot hadn't been able to sit still since receiving the call from Avila the night before. In the hours since, he'd been hopping from one satellite image to another. This was the kind of thing he lives for. Talbot isn't just obsessed with weather; he is utterly consumed and created by it. He loves to start sentences with "As a weather guy," or "Weather people like me," the way some people might claim their astrological sign or hometown or ethnicity. Like Avila and Landsea, Talbot has attracted some serious fans in his years as a meteorologist. It doesn't hurt that he sports a marathon runner's build, a movie-star face, and close-cropped silver hair. If there were to be a film about the Hurricane Hunters, a director would cast Jon Talbot as Jon Talbot. And that would delight a lot of female moviegoers. Already, his constant smile and patient encouragement of any and all weather questions make him a favorite for newspaper interviews, school programs, and TV shows like the Weather Channel's wildly popular *Hurricane Hunters.* And when Talbot stands there in a well-fitting green flight suit, explaining wind speed and cyclonic systems, people really listen. They want to know what he knows. And they really, really want to know what it's like to fly through a hurricane.

Talbot didn't set out to do this for a living. He'd been working for years as a meteorologist in the navy when a general approached him and asked if he'd like to take a different kind of desk job. One of the new hurricane-hunter meteorologists kept getting airsick. The general thought Talbot could probably take the extreme turbulence and still read a radar screen. More important, he thought Talbot might really like it.

He was right.

Talbot acknowledges that enjoying this work makes him something of an odd duck, even in the world of meteorologists. If a storm becomes a verified tropical depression, the 53rd Squadron will remain with it, flying constant flights until the system dissipates or is no longer a threat. It's the only way the National Hurricane Center can know what's really going on out there. And so they keep going, even if a system grows to herculean dimensions. As far as the 53rd is concerned, there is no hurricane too risky to fly in.

"Once that system develops," says Talbot, "we're going to stay with it until the end. End of story."

Theirs is a seventy-year-old pursuit, which began somewhat infamously in a bar, where army air corps pilots dared Joe Duckworth, already a noted pilot — and kind of a hotshot — to fly into a hurricane. Duckworth wasn't the kind of guy to say no to such a challenge (what air corps pilot in a bar really is?), so he strapped himself into a single-engine trainer and flew through the storm twice. On the second flight, he took with him a white-knuckled weather officer, who discovered, once he was past the abject terror, that there was quite a lot to be learned about a storm from being inside it.

The US government agreed and formed the 53rd Weather Reconnaissance a year later. The Great Atlantic Hurricane of 1944 was the first that included regular plane reconnaissance, and forecasters involved agreed it was a great boon to their work. When World War II ended, the navy donated decommissioned bombers, giving the 53rd the kind of hard-core aircraft needed to penetrate storms. This was before the real start of the space race, before test pilots like John Glenn and Alan Shepard of Mercury 7 or the air force's Chuck Yeager won the hearts of America with their courage. In a decade divided between baby-booming exuberance and increasing fears about the cold war, the Hurricane Hunters gave the country a new kind of hero. Most were decorated fighter pilots reassigned to an even more dangerous task. They flew daring missions. They delivered letters to Santa at the North Pole. They lived rock-and-roll lifestyles, drinking hard and living on the edge. They were legends.

But their flights weren't without consequences. Turbulence was severe enough to injure crew members. Sometimes, they'd lose consciousness. In 1965, *Snowcloud Five,* part of the air force's Airborne Early Warning Squadron, disappeared in Hurricane Janet. Nine crew members and two reporters were lost. Then, in 1974, a Hurricane

Hunter C-130 crashed in the South China Sea while attempting a reconnaissance flight of Typhoon Bess. The crew was unable to send any kind of distress call, leading investigators to conclude that their plane suffered from a problem so immediate and catastrophic that the crew simply did not have time to react. All six crew members were listed as "killed in action."

The federal government deactivated the 53rd in 1991, but soon learned we really need them to understand storms. So they were placed back on duty two years later, but in a diminished capacity as part of the air force reserves. Ever since, they've fought budget cuts and assignments that have absolutely nothing to do with weather reconnaissance.

It's a tough line to walk, especially since the meteorologists at the National Hurricane Center are emphatic that they can't be very good at forecasting without the 53rd. Even the world's best scatterometer can't tell you what's happening on the ocean surface — at least, not when a growing tropical system is blocking that view. Data buoys are few and far between: Sometimes hundreds or even thousands of miles separate them. The only way to know what's going on in a system — the only way to assess wind speeds and barometric pressure and just how powerful a storm has become — is to put yourself in that storm. Not many people are willing to do that: Lixion Avila says he frankly thinks the Hurricane Hunters are a little crazy. "There's no way I'm going in there," he says. "I'd rather wait until the storm comes to me."

But Hurricane Hunters aren't just anybody. They know what their planes can do. They know what they can do. They love the adrenaline rush. They get antsy when they're not up there — they worry they might be missing something.

That is how Jon Talbot was feeling when he got Avila's late-night call. The flight meteorologist was glued to the computer screen in his small office at Keesler Air Force Base, tapping his foot as he scanned the satellite images. Like the folks at the National Hurricane Center, he'd been watching the building disturbance throughout the weekend. The Hurricane Hunters had already flown fifty-three missions that year — making it one of the busiest seasons in years. But October had been marked by an unexpected lull in storms: plenty of weather, says Talbot, "but not a single storm out there that was going to bother anybody." That meant flight teams had been confined to training missions and public outreach. Two of the planes — and their crews — were out on air-show tours, hopping from one small airport to another. The others were undergoing maintenance checks. It was hard to stay busy. The crews were getting restless.

The call from the NHC changed all that. And by Monday morning, the system was showing even more signs of organization. Winds had grown to around 25 miles per hour, making the system an official tropical depression. That warranted the assignment of a number — 18 — and increasing attention from the meteorological world. Talbot had a hunch they'd be following Tropical Depression 18 for quite some time.

"I was seeing things that made me believe that this could be a really big storm. This storm could mean business," says Talbot. Chief on his mind was Hurricane Mitch, which began precisely the same way — and fourteen years earlier to the very day. A massive Category 5 hurricane, Mitch remains one of the deadliest on record. The storm began to frustrate forecasters as soon as it formed in late October 1998: It trudged rather than surged, and zigged when everyone thought it would zag. The resulting devastation was almost unimaginable. Honduras and Nicaragua were all but leveled. More than eleven thousand people were pronounced dead in the days after the storm. By the end of the year, another eleven thousand were still missing, including the thirty-one crew members of the *Fantome,* a 282-foot, four-masted schooner that played hide-and-seek with the storm — and lost in the worst way.

Whether or not it is warranted, the Hurricane Hunters feel a certain responsibility for numbers like these. What they find — or don't find — in a system has an immediate impact when it comes to issuing warnings or evacuation orders. If they miss a hurricane's strongest winds, it'll be categorized as a lesser storm. Residents may stay when they should go. Public action can be delayed or aborted altogether. People will die. That's a lot of pressure to carry with you into an already adrenaline-drenched situation. Talbot does everything he can to make sure they get it right.

Each Hurricane Hunters mission is staffed by a team of five: a pilot and copilot, who must hold the plane as steady as possible against storm-force winds; a navigator, who helps them pick the least dangerous route (though in truth they're all dangerous); the weather officer; and a lodemaster, who deploys the state-of-the-art recording equipment used to test conditions. The base employs twenty crews, and that meant there were twenty meteorologists champing at the bit to get out into this new storm. The lucky straw was drawn by Rich Harter, a San Diego native with oversize glasses, wide eyes, and thirty years of experience in the air force.

At fifty-nine, Harter was the most senior meteorologist at Keesler. A year shy of his mandatory retirement, he had already logged six thousand flying hours. He had passed through hurricane eyes more than 250 times. However, it wasn't enough. "If I could keep going, I would," he readily admits. Nothing about him suggests that retirement would suit him. Still, he says (with reluctance), an aging body can't handle the turbulent abuse of these flights nearly as well as a younger one can. "There comes a time when you've got to hang it up."

Knowing that time was approaching made Harter all the more glad his number was called for the first reconnaissance mission into Tropical Depression 18. There wasn't a cloud in the sky that morning, and the unusually temperate weather meant that Harter could keep the windows open in his car as he drove to Subway to collect his customary turkey sub before making his way to Keesler for their 9:00 A.M. departure. It'd be a long day in the air, he knew, and he didn't like flying hungry. Once at the base, he set to work creating a flight package, which would guide the plane and its crew into the storm. He called the National Hurricane Center and conferred about satellite data. The system was getting big and messy — there would be a lot of ground to cover on this flight, and not much time to do it. So the crew was working extra hard to get the plane prepped for takeoff.

A Hercules C-130 isn't just a workhorse; it's a juiced-up warhorse — and an expensive one. Driving one off the lot will set you back $48.5 million, and that's without any add-ons. It's a price plenty of countries and their militaries are willing to pay. The C-130 has room enough for a helicopter or a couple of Humvees, or a Humvee and an armored personnel carrier, along with the army needed to drive and maintain it. The plane can take off from and land on a variety of unprepared surfaces, which is part of why militaries love it (groomed runways are often in short supply in places militaries need to go). Its thrust comes from four Rolls-Royce turboprop engines, and it pushes through the air at speeds well over 300 miles per hour. That is modest compared to jet engine aircraft; nevertheless, that reliable speed, along with one of the toughest riveted aluminum alloy fuselages ever made, is why the Hurricane Hunters trust it.

But trusting in it also means trusting that it is running perfectly.

As the crew prepared to take off, Colonel Jeff Van Dootingh, the base's operations group commander, was certain he heard an abnormal noise in the engine. Anything that could be construed as irregular is considered a major threat to the Hurricane Hunters and their planes: Their missions come with so much inherent risk that even something as simple as a sticky door hinge can shut down a mission.

Van Dootingh's observations were more than enough to abort this flight, and his orders sent the maintenance crews scrambling to prep another plane. Harter's crew was getting rattled. Pilot John Wagner, already apprehensive about the length of this mission and the conditions awaiting them, looked agitated. "We've got to start from scratch now," he told a *Hurricane Hunters* cameraman. Time was getting away from them.

It was 9:30 A.M. before Harter and the crew were taxiing down the runway in their replacement plane. A few minutes later, they leveled off at twenty-four thousand feet. Tropical Depression 18 was now just three hundred miles north of Colombia. "That's a long way away from Biloxi, Mississippi," says Harter. The Hurricane Hunters would be pushing it to get back with any fuel left. In the meantime, they'd have a four-hour flight to endure — just to reach the edge of the storm.

Being inside a 53rd Reconnaissance C-130 is a little bit like being inside Adam West's Batcave: It is packed with gadgets of every possible sort, and most of them are labeled. Unlike the Batcave, though, everything in a weather reconnaissance plane is also strapped down — and for good reason. An Igloo cooler — the kind, when filled with Gatorade, that football players like to pour over winning coaches — appears suspended in the air, tethered to the plane's interior with industrial-grade straps. Data-collection kits are bungeed and double bungeed. Even the microwave is all but bolted down, though it gets enough use that its door is rarely secured. The Hurricane Hunters have become adept at gourmet dining in even the most inhospitable conditions and rarely fly a mission without at least one hot meal. In one of the most popular episodes of the Weather Channel's *Hurricane Hunters,* the crew is seen eating bowls of hot gumbo someone made from scratch and then warmed up in that microwave. Viewers throughout the South went crazy for that scene, further solidifying the almost mythic status of the 53rd.

Today, though, the crew settled for potato chips. They passed the bags around like they were watching an afternoon baseball game instead of flying one of the most sophisticated scientific devices of the modern world across a storm-tossed sea. As the pilots and navigator considered routes, Harter squared aviation charts with satellite images of the growing storm. His station on the plane is small, but it has the screens and electronics he needs, not to mention an almost anachronistically grand seat, which looks like the unholy offspring of a CEO's leather throne and an electric chair, what with its elaborate straps and shackles.

Harter wasn't strapped in yet — he likes to be able to look around for as long as he can, usually moving between his computer and the nearby window with a callisthenic energy and precision that would please any fitness instructor. And he barely noticed the casual banter around him. The meteorologists at the National Hurricane Center needed Harter to tell them precisely what was happening inside the system, and that meant Harter had a lot of puzzle pieces he had to put together — and no discernible way to do it.

Once a hurricane or tropical storm has been identified, the Hurricane Hunters' regular reconnaissance paths follow "alpha" patterns: They fly the lines of a boxed X, with the center of the X at the center of the storm. It's a standard transect the 53rd practices hundreds of times each year, and one in which there are rarely any surprises. This mission, on the other hand, would have no such regularity. Instead, the crew was on a sleuthing expedition, hoping they could find the center of the storm. That tiny center of low pressure was somewhere in an already massive, sloppy weather cell. To confirm that they really had a cyclonic system on their hands, the NHC would also need proof of what Harter calls "the four winds" — gusts coming from the northeast, northwest, southwest, and southeast directions, which would indicate a fully developed and circulating system.

But how do you find the invisible? Radar is of no use in systems like this — it lacks the definition needed and mostly just depicts dramatic thunderstorms that show up as dangerous bands and splotches on an instrument panel in more developed storms. Satellite images weren't much use, either, since they just showed a pile of white soup. That's part of the reason Harter relies as much on his window as on the state-of-the-art equipment at his station: Sometimes, he says, you can learn more from watching ocean waves than from crunching numbers. For that kind of observation to work, though, the plane has to be perilously close to the ocean's surface, which is part of why his pilots had been on edge. They balked when Harter asked them to drop down below the clouds.

"There's a lot that can go wrong at that altitude," pilot John Wagner warned Harter. "And I'm only going to have five hundred feet to correct a problem." Wagner added that he was feeling really uncomfortable about being that low — especially in a system as unknown as Tropical Depression 18.

Harter conceded that he could probably get what he needed from 750 feet. That helped allay Wagner's concerns — a little. But before the plane could dip down to that altitude, they needed clearance from Jamaica's air traffic controllers, and Wagner's repeated attempts to hail anyone covering the airspace went unanswered. The crew was forced to maintain their position at twenty-four thousand feet. Minutes passed. Wagner tried hailing Jamaica again. "Kingston, this is Teal 7-1. Position."

No answer. He tried a third time. "Kingston, Teal 7-1."

More dead air. The crew was running out of time.

Back in his executive chair, Harter was straining against the side window, trying to make out the ominous horizon still several hundred miles ahead of them. At this rate, there wouldn't be enough time to get there and back.

Wagner scanned the radar, looking for anyone else who might be able to help. A commercial jet was within hailing range to their east. He picked up the radio and called.

"Any aircraft on 128.35, this is Teal 7-1, requesting relay."

Somewhere, out in the distance, the commercial jet pilot responded.

"This is American 9-2-5 checking in."

The commercial pilot agreed to patch them through. A few seconds later, a distinctly Caribbean voice acknowledged the C-130.

"Teal 7-1, we have you."

"We do appreciate the relay," said Wagner.

"Not a problem," shot back the American Airlines pilot.

Cleared by the Jamaican air traffic controller, Wagner pitched the C-130 into a sharp descent through leaden clouds. Down below, enormous Venezuelan oil platforms rose above the storm chop. The light had grown flat. Visibility was worsening by the minute. The pilot strained to make out obstacles and what looked like another plane on his radar screen. It was inconceivable to him that anyone would be out in these conditions; still, that dot kept moving toward them. Frustrated, Wagner pulled the plane up to one thousand feet and waited for the small aircraft to pass. As he did, Harter studied the rain shafts streaking down into the growing surf. The C-130 had been in the air for five hours. Finally, they were getting close.

Harter and the crew have access to all sorts of high-tech equipment, including the Stepped Frequency Microwave Radiometer (SFMR, known colloquially among some Hurricane Hunters as the "Smurf"), which sits on the wing of a Hercules C-130 and measures surface wind speed, even when that plane is thousands of feet above the surface. Jon Talbot was instrumental in creating it. They also use sophisticated barometers and thermometers, along with dozens of little devices called dropsondes, which read temperature, pressure, and humidity at various elevations. Placed in a tube that looks a whole lot like a cardboard paper-towel roll, these little gadgets are dropped by the plane's lodemaster at specific intervals, and immediately relay the conditions as they cascade down. They cost about $700 apiece and can be deployed only once. In a typical hurricane season, the Hurricane Hunters will deploy more than a thousand of them. That's nearly a million dollars a year in cardboard tubes, but Chris Landsea says the cost is more than worth it. They've improved hurricane forecasting immensely, decreasing prediction error by at least 25 percent during the first forty-eight hours of a storm. Forecasting error grows exponentially from day to day, and a mistake made in the first hours of data collection can result in a five-day forecast that is hundreds — if not thousands — of miles off course.

Harter knew this, but it didn't concern him. He says his available technology, along with thirty years of experience, instill great confidence.

"If there's a closed system out there," says Harter, "I'll find it."

As the plane entered the outer edges of the depression, though, the flight meteorologist began to wonder if his assuredness was misplaced. A large band of clouds had begun to form what clearly looked like a semicircle around the base of the system. Below, ocean temperatures were warm — plenty of heat to generate a hurricane. Nevertheless, the SFMR kept insisting that winds were light — no matter where the crew put the plane. As they passed over a second quadrant, the ocean surface looked almost glassy. The crew was getting frustrated.

"You could water ski down there," quipped Wagner.

"Off the back of a C-130?" retorted another crew member. "That'd be cool."

"Sweet," agreed a third.

Harter didn't say a word. At that point, anything he did seemed like a guess. And the clock was ticking: They'd have less than two hours to verify all four winds before the plane would hit bingo fuel and force their retreat.

Harter, now beginning to show fatigue,

craned to look outside the small window at his station. What he saw didn't look overly impressive: no bands of clouds, and certainly no eye. He began to doubt whether they'd find anything on this trip. The radar was just a mottle of yellow and green.

Harter asked Wagner to descend to a couple hundred feet above sea level. The pilot balked again. Downdrafts, the number one cause of plane crashes, were common at that level. Lightning was erupting around them. The crew talked it over. They'd proceed, but cautiously. And slowly. As the plane began to drop, the scene outside Harter's window changed instantly. Clear skies gave way to thick clouds and scattered thunderstorms. The nose of the C-130 began to buck as winds built around them. Each time the plane pitched and rolled, Harter caught a glimpse of the telltale white crescents of waves breaking below the wing of the plane. At this level, they were too low to employ the dropsondes, so the only thing Harter had at his disposal to determine surface wind direction was the SFMR.

It took an hour for Harter to find any winds strong enough to register as storm-force. Once he found them, though, he could tell they were organized. "That's when we knew we had something," says

Harter. He would need to find winds moving in the remaining three cardinal directions, however, before he'd have a verifiable tropical storm. The crew had less than forty-five minutes of fuel and flying time to do that: barely enough to explore another section of the storm.

Satellite images were suggesting that the most likely place to go next was farther north and east than Harter wanted to go. But the meteorologist was resolute: He was certain they were nearly on top of the winds they needed to find. He told Wagner they should stay put, despite what the images suggested.

That was all Van Dootingh needed to hear. Rich Harter, he says, is not just one of the most experienced meteorologists in the business: He's also one of the most intuitive.

"In some cases," Van Dootingh says, "the people are a lot more important than the science. A hunch can be worth a thousand sweeps of a radar."

This was one of those days. With less than thirty minutes of flying time remaining, Wagner edged the plane toward the section of the system Harter had identified. The meteorologist was sweating now, his face red and creased as he leaned hard between the window and his workstation. The satellite showed tapering clouds here, but Harter was more interested in what the sea was doing: the way waves were breaking in angry white streaks, making the surface look like shattered glass. That's exactly what Harter wanted to see. Big breakers mean big wind.

Wagner announced bingo fuel: In another few minutes, they'd have to turn back. Harter kept pushing. And then, with what felt like just seconds remaining, he found the last of the four winds. It measured just 39 miles per hour — the lowest possible wind speed for a tropical storm, but it was enough for the flight meteorologist. He sent his data streaming to Miami, then took off his glasses and rubbed his weary eyes.

Wagner banked north, beginning their long return flight. As he did, Harter received word from Lixion Avila at the National Hurricane Center. He quickly relayed it to the rest of the crew.

"They've named the storm," he said. "They've named it Sandy."

"Sandy?" asked Wagner, his voice incredulous. He paused, then tried out the name again. "Tropical Storm Sandy," he said, rolling the name around on his tongue. He shook his head and angled the plane back toward Mississippi. Meanwhile, announcements of the system's elevated stature as a named storm prompted a flurry of Internet jokes: The storm was nothing more than the female lead from a throwback soda-fountain musical, a two-bit squirrel from a cartoon about a square-pants-wearing sponge. The cyberworld reveled in its levity: How could such a sweet-sounding name possibly wreak much damage?

No one remained incredulous for long.

Naming storms is not a particularly new convention. The Mayans dubbed the storms Kukulkan, a manifestation of their supreme deity: a force capable of both creation and unimaginable destruction, good and evil, wind and rain. Other Caribbean cultures created their own variations — yuracan, haurachana, foracan, uracano — derivations, perhaps, from the Taino word *huracán* and often representing an evil spirit. Once European exploration reached the Caribbean, those cultures devised their own organizational system, giving specific storms the names of Christian saints — a convenient West Indian convention that allowed people to track storms based on the day they arrived, since just about every day on the Catholic calendar included a patron saint. At the dawn of the twentieth century,

Clement Wragge, director of the Queensland state meteorological department in Australia, began assigning cyclones the names of his least favorite politicians. Fifty years later, the US National Weather Service adopted the convention and introduced its own classification system. Some of the names selected in 1950 seemed random at best, others hopelessly inappropriate: titles like Dog, Easy, and Love. Had that season been a busier one, we might have had Hurricanes Oboe, Sugar, and Zebra, too.

But coming up with random words from the alphabet soon proved inefficient, and it didn't do much to help people distinguish between storms. So the next year, forecasters at the National Weather Service fell into the habit of using the names of their wives, girlfriends, and mothers. For the first couple of years, theirs was a mostly internal practice, but by 1953 storm names were being issued to the public as well. The equal rights movement led to the inclusion of male names in 1978, a convention that has endured. Still, picking a storm's name is no easy endeavor. Today, storm monikers are regulated by a byzantine process housed at the World Meteorological Organization (WMO). There, five regional bodies invite nominations from their members, which committee heads then consider. What results is a series of lists that include six years' worth of names: twenty-three names for each year, listed by alternating gender. The lists pay homage to the cultures where they'll be broadcast: Pacific typhoons are given names like Akoni and Walaka; North Atlantic storms are given names like Arlene and Walter. When a storm proves particularly epic — like Katrina or Andrew — that name is retired from the list and is replaced by one of the new names approved by the committee.

The WMO's official rationale for their overall approach is that, because names are easier to remember than a random series of letters or numbers, laypeople will have an easier time keeping the storms straight. They also contend that names make it easier for the media to issue warnings and for forecasters to avoid errors. All of that is undoubtedly true. However, since time immemorial, naming has also been about our need to control — or at least to give the appearance that we can control. And when it comes to a desire for dominion, no meteorological event is more demanding than a hurricane.

In the meteorological hall of fame, hurricanes are the Muhammad Alis. Or maybe it'd be more accurate to compare them to an NFL defensive line, since a hurricane is actually a formidable collection of dozens of fierce thunderstorms swirling together. Small wonder scientists and writers often employ metaphors of Armageddon and nuclear annihilation to explain the power of these storms. And as our ability to create technologies capable of previously unimaginable destruction has grown, so has our vernacular for describing hurricanes. Along the way, we've accrued a pretty impressive list of analogies. Hurricanes detonate the power of a megaton bomb every ten minutes. Over the course of its life, a hurricane will generate as much energy as ten thousand atomic blasts. Minute for minute, a single storm can exceed the energy produced by all the world's power plants — five times over. In a single day, a hurricane can release so much water (twenty billion tons, on average) that, if desalinated, it could supply a year's worth of drinking water to a small country.

When faced with that kind of power, it's hard to feel anything other than our collective mortality — and a profound lack of control. Part of that helplessness undoubtedly comes from our lack of knowing. We are often frightened by what we don't understand — especially if that thing is barreling toward our house. Perhaps that's why indigenous tribes once saw the storms as the manifestations of vengeful deities and European explorers insisted those same hurricanes were the hand of a wrathful god. Even today, scientists know a lot less about this weather phenomenon than you might think.

Hurricanes have been around for at least tens of thousands — if not hundreds of thousands — of years, but it wasn't until humans formed a relationship with the sea that they became an issue for our species. Typhoons defeated Kublai Khan's massive navies in their two bids to take Japan. The second, in 1281, sank an estimated two hundred ships and killed tens of thousands of men. The Japanese saw it as a gift from the gods, and bestowed the name *kamikaze,* or "divine wind," upon the storms. Not everyone has been so grateful. In 1559, a hurricane thwarted Spain's attempt to create the first European settlement in North America, sinking thirteen ships and plucking another off the surface of the ocean and tossing it inland, as if it were Dorothy's house being lifted to Oz. A similar fate befell a French fleet that was attempting to colonize the entire Eastern Seaboard of North

America later that century, and also the Dutch, who were attempting to claim Cuba in 1640. As far as these explorers were concerned, hurricanes were nothing short of supernatural. Spanish explorers believed such storms were the devil's revenge — and punishment for being Catholic. British sailors were inclined to agree. And they all felt certain that no terrestrial explanation was sufficient to explain the wrath a hurricane can wreak.

That idea prevailed well into the nineteenth century, when scientists and sailors began clashing in earnest over the origin of these all-powerful storms. The dominant voice in this conversation was Henry Piddington, a British sea captain and amateur scientist. Piddington made detailed notes and observations on weather phenomena while he was at sea. These notes, coupled with reports he collected from other captains, formed the basis of his theory that tropical waters manifest a particular — and often peculiar — type of rotating storm he named *cyclone,* from the Greek *kyklon,* or "circling." He published the sum of his findings in 1848, under the cumbersome title *The Sailor's Horn-book for the Law of Storms: Being a Practical Exposition of the Theory of the Law of Storms, and Its Uses to Mariners of All Classes in All Parts of the World, Shewn by Transparent Storm Cards and Useful Lessons.* There, Piddington rehearsed the most common theories of hurricane genesis produced by his generation: Some scholars, he explained, claimed the storms were the result of electricity and magnetism in the sky; others said that whirlpools of air were formed in the upper atmosphere and then sank down to Earth. Still others contended hurricanes were prompted by volcanoes or massive forest fires on land, which in turn caused the air to rotate. They speculated about the connection between earthquakes and cyclones. Piddington gave all these theories equal attention in his *Horn-book,* but was also careful to note his own views on the subject: *Cyclones,* he proposed, "are purely electric phænomena formed in the higher regions of the atmosphere, and descending in a flattened, disk-like shape to the surface of the ocean, where they progress more or less rapidly." But, he was quick to add, this theory should, at best, be considered speculation. The only thing Piddington and his peers knew for certain was that they knew nothing about hurricanes for certain — not their causes, not their full effects, not even their courses, which even then were clearly capricious in the extreme.

The advent of satellites, radar, and computer modeling has changed a lot about how we view these storms; nevertheless, hurricanes remain frustratingly mysterious. Scientists are still unable to say with any certainty which disturbances will turn into tropical storms, let alone whether any given tropical storms will peter out or turn into Category 5 disasters. They don't know where the storm will go and why, or when it will dissipate. That, too, can create a certain helplessness.

Over the years, we've devised strategies ranging from the haplessly hopeful to the downright absurd to mitigate these sensations. The Caribs would spit bread in the air in an attempt to keep a hurricane at bay. The Aztecs would play horns and drums, hoping that a musical welcome would placate the storm. At the start of hurricane season each year, ancient Mayans would cast a virgin into the sea in an attempt to appease the storm god. To make sure she arrived at his underwater lair, they would also sacrifice a warrior to guide her. Spanish explorers regularly hung a knotted rope in doorways during hurricane season, hoping Saint Francis of Assisi might intervene on their behalf. On plantations throughout the Caribbean, African slaves draped herbs in the rafters of their quarters in an attempt to keep the air quiet and calm.

By the dawn of the twentieth century, scientists knew a little bit more about how hurricanes work, but they were no closer to controlling them. That didn't stop them from trying. In 1947 a meteorologist at General Electric named Vincent Schaefer attempted an experiment to dissipate these storms by spraying particles of dry ice into a developing hurricane. His thought was that the super-cooled ice would be enough to bring down the ambient temperature, forcing the clouds to disintegrate into heavy rain. Results from Schaefer's study were inconclusive, which was enough to make researchers at the National Weather Service want to keep trying. So began Project Cirrus, a cloud-seeding experiment. For more than a decade, B-17 bombers dropped enormous amounts of dry ice into developing hurricane systems. At this same time, the US navy was trying unsuccessfully to chart hurricane courses with seismographs stationed up and down the East Coast. There, navy scientists perched in listening stations, hoping they could triangulate a storm's location. They soon discovered they were wrong more often than they were right.

Meanwhile, Project Cirrus grew into a

full-blown assault on hurricanes dubbed Project Stormfury. The experiment, funded by the US government, was driven by a prestigious National Academy of Sciences board, which comprised meteorologists from noted universities, including MIT. The program was initiated by Robert Simpson, but soon transferred to his wife, Joanne, the first woman to hold a PhD in meteorology, and a longtime employee of NOAA and NASA. Project Stormfury became her obsession, and it had all the elements of a cold war drama: For nine days during the summer of 1965, navy pilots took off from secluded Puerto Rican runways, carrying with them sealed envelopes with top-secret instructions for dropping metal canisters from staggering heights. Once discharged, these canisters careered through hurricane clouds, releasing silver iodide — a bright yellow compound once used in film developing. Silver iodide binds with water droplets and freezes quickly, and it was the Simpsons' belief that this would be enough to depower an immense heat machine. Initial findings looked promising, and by 1978 navy airplanes known as Sky-warriors were releasing three metric tons of silver iodide into storm systems each year. The US Congress allocated $30 million to cover expenses. What they got in return turned out to be unsubstantiated at best. Project Stormfury was eventually scuttled in 1983.

But that didn't prevent researchers from attempting other plans, including pumping super-cool water up from the ocean floor in an attempt to deprive a hurricane of heat (which failed), and releasing millions of plastic beads into hurricanes, an idea that, luckily, was dismissed before it was ever actually implemented. Bob Sheets — the legendary longtime director of the National Hurricane Center — says the most common suggestion he has received from the general public is that we go nuclear: Detonate an atomic bomb right in the heart of a storm. That's a ridiculous proposal, says Sheets: Even the strongest bomb is minuscule compared to the strength of a hurricane. And there's also the undesirable side effect of massive nuclear fallout each time a bomb is detonated. Chris Landsea agrees with Sheets. Put a nuclear bomb in a hurricane, says Landsea, and at best you're going to get an angrier — and now also radioactive — storm spinning around the North Atlantic.

Try as we might, we just can't control a storm. Accepting that fact requires a level of humility many of us find hard. Certainly it's been the source of unending frustration for meteorologists, who must not only confront the fact that we can't control what a hurricane does, but must also admit we're not all that good at predicting its actions.

It's a perennial problem. And it's precisely what was nagging forecasters as Tropical Depression Sandy continued to grow.

4:45 P.M.
Miami, Florida
82°F
Barometer: 29.95 inches (rising)
Winds: 17 mph (NE)
Skies: Scattered clouds

As Rich Harter and the rest of the exhausted Hurricane Hunters made their way back to Biloxi, Richard Pasch was settling in for his shift at the National Hurricane Center. It was still miserably sticky in Miami, and the senior hurricane forecaster trundled to the hurricane operations area, glad to be inside the climate-controlled cave that is NHC headquarters. He wiped his face and sat down heavily in the executive chair at the forecasting desk. Pasch didn't care for heat. And at sixty years old, he was fairly certain he shouldn't have to. Pasch is second only to Avila in terms of years served at the National Hurricane Center. They share a love for big storms and classical music performances, but their similarities end there. Pasch calls himself an old-timer, and he reminds his colleagues that he can retire whenever he likes. He's the resident curmudgeon on staff and claims he has been a self-professed cynic since he was a kid. He's been seriously intimidated by hurricanes since then, too. Pasch was twelve when Hurricane Cleo passed over his house in 1964. He remembers wind, then the eerie calm of the eye — the way everything seemed like a perfect summer day for a few hours. But what he remembers most about that storm is what happened after the eye passed over: the way the gusts picked up and shrieked, even harder than they had before (later, meteorologists would report that those winds topped 100 miles per hour), the way his house shook like it might collapse. It was the first time he was ever terrified of weather. And that terror, says Pasch, was all it took to solidify a lifelong obsession. He began begging his parents for trips to the Weather Bureau. He pursued the National Hurricane Center's then-director, Gordon Dunn, the way most kids his age followed Hank Aaron. After getting his PhD, he tried college teaching, but felt that he lacked peers who shared his research interests. So he joined the National Hurricane Center as a forecaster in 1989 — just in time for Hurricane Hugo.

His office is a memorial to his subsequent twenty-five years on the job. Rows of dusty journals fill the bookcases, vying for space with yellowing stacks of paper and stuffed manila folders. An impressive hot-sauce collection on one bookshelf is culturally balanced with a Valhalla screensaver — a testament to his great love of Wagner and, he admits, maybe an affirmation that he has dedicated his life to working in the meteorological promised land.

However, says Pasch, it's not a place removed from uncertainty. On this particular day, he was feeling a lot more of that than he would have liked. And to make matters worse, he was now dealing with not just one tropical storm, but the possibility of a second one, also in the Atlantic. The same tropical wave that had spawned Sandy had also created this disturbance, which had been drifting slowly over the eastern portion of the Atlantic for a week or so, causing the occasional thunderstorm. But as it continued on its meandering path, the system had begun to organize, and by 6:00 P.M. that evening, Pasch saw enough organization to designate it Tropical Depression

19. Now he had two storms to toggle between. And he didn't like what he saw when he pulled up images of Sandy. Radar images revealed that thunderstorms were growing around the center of that storm, collecting on its northern front. Still, the storm seemed reluctant to do much of anything and wasn't really building — at least, not by hurricane standards. The storm wasn't really moving much, either. In fact, it had all but stalled out, and was now completing a small, reluctant loop in the southern Caribbean Sea. He began to write his official discussion for the storm.

> REMAINING NEARLY STATIONARY OVER THE WARM WATERS OF THE SOUTHWESTERN CARIBBEAN SEA IS NEVER A GOOD SIGN FOR THIS TIME OF YEAR.

Sandy was poised to get fierce. For that matter, so could the growing tropical depression. Two systems, both with the potential to become major hurricanes, and neither was giving much of a clue about what would happen next. All of this at what was supposed to be the end of tropical storm season. Pasch shook his head at what he was certain was bad, dumb luck.

"We thought we were in good shape," says Pasch. "It had been such a slow season, we were about to write off 2012. We really thought we were going to get out of there without any problems." One look at the radar, though, and Pasch soon realized otherwise. "It was like, *not so fast.* Never doubt Murphy's Law."

Pasch has spent his life trying to minimize the variables that Murphy's Law throws at him. He likes order. He hates surprises. He's a scientist and a pragmatist, and he gets frustrated when he can't accurately predict what a storm is going to do. "It's stressful," says Pasch. "I don't like it. It causes problems."

He says those problems are as much public as they are personal. Landsea is inclined to agree. "It's definitely not good. I don't like not knowing."

Pasch sent out a request for condition reports from any vessel within 300 nautical miles of the storm. He and Landsea then set to work creating probability tables: What was the likelihood that the system would remain a tropical storm? Would it build to become a hurricane? And if it did? Of what category? And where would it go?

To try to answer these sorts of questions, forecasters use a variety of computer models intended to approximate real-world data and account for the innumerable factors that affect how weather is produced. A forecasting model converts everything from temperature and humidity to wind strength and barometric pressure into variables that can then exist in a series of complex equations. For the equations to work, there has to be a lot of data — and it has to be spot-on in terms of accuracy. That's one of many reasons the work of the Hurricane Hunters is so important — without their ability to record precisely what is happening in and around a storm, models would be useless.

The National Hurricane Center employs about forty-five different computer models for hurricane forecasting. Some are simple statistical programs that square what a storm is doing against historical precedent, and then make predictions based on what storms have done in the past. This kind of work is a fairly simple task for a computer and doesn't take much more than a few minutes and a personal laptop to complete. But if hurricanes love to do anything, it's bucking trends, so forecasters tend not to put too much stock in this kind of prediction. Whenever possible, they favor more complicated programs called dynamical models, which take into account everything from air density to the effect of aerosols on a storm (scientists believe that they may accelerate circulation at the edge of a cyclone, possibly weakening it by dissipating energy from its core). The sheer amount of data and computation needed to run a dynamical model requires an advanced kind of supercomputer with the power of a V12 engine, and there aren't many of them around. The forecasters at the National Hurricane Center have five or six favorite models, which they say have consistently proven themselves reliable. Some, like the Florida State Superensemble and the ECMWF, utilize several models to create an integrated prediction. The National Weather Service's Global Forecast System (GFS) has been a time-honored ensemble model. Increasingly, forecasters are also turning to several global dynamical models housed in European agencies. But they take hours and hours to run their data, and subscriptions have a hefty price tag — sometimes as much as $100,000 a year just to access their data.

What most frustrates forecasters is the fact that even these premier models often deliver an infuriating degree of inconsistency. The same model that makes a perfect prediction for one storm can totally fail a week later.

Forecasters know this, and most of them keep track of it. At the Mt. Holly office, they even keep a notebook with tallies about what model is doing better than others. Those tallies never settle on one model as the best. That's why, when it comes to matters like a storm's track and intensity, forecasters at the National Hurricane Center often take an average of the models' predictions, but that can prove to be a dangerous game. "Sometimes, it's the outlier that proves right," says Landsea. The life-or-death question always at stake, then, is when to trust the law of averages and when to believe that one model may have gotten something so right that the others can't see it.

The hurricane specialists tend to have favorites, they say. The ECMWF is one of them because it uses fourteen highly sophisticated polar-orbiting satellites in addition to the stationary ones more commonly employed by weather forecasters. It was the collective data harvested by these eighteen satellites that led to the bizarre forecast of a hurricane smashing into the mid-Atlantic coast of the United States. Taking away even one of those satellites could have caused the ECMWF to fall in line with the other models, predicting that Sandy would spin out to sea.

But was this outlier right? Richard Pasch wasn't sure. As the afternoon progressed, he remained glued to the forecasting desk, watching impatiently as the models began to give up their best guesses. He could see some trends emerging. In the short term, all the models were in consensus that the storm would intensify over the next few days: There was just so much warm water out there, Sandy would have a nearly unlimited supply of fuel. It could easily become a full-blown hurricane in days. Just how much stronger would the storm get? And how quickly? The models couldn't say for sure. Nor could they say where it was going.

For all its power and might, a hurricane has surprisingly little propulsive force. Instead, it bobs on existing airstreams. Avila likens a tropical storm to a cork or a stick making its way down a river. Low-pressure systems offer paths with little resistance for a storm. High-pressure systems act like boulders or other obstacles, sending a storm ricocheting off the front and toward lower pressure. For days, one of those high-pressure cells had been perched atop the Leeward Islands, all but ensuring that Sandy would be forced out to sea. Now, however, that high-pressure system was weakening — greasing the path for the storm to continue its lumbering course northward with no resistance. Landfall at Jamaica — and even Cuba — seemed all but assured. After that, Pasch couldn't even begin to wager a guess: Even with all the divergence he was accustomed to seeing in weather models, the forecaster was flummoxed by just how inconsistent these results were. Several of them, including the GFS, suggested that the storm would arc out to sea — a typical trend for a hurricane at that time of year. Others sent the storm on a corkscrewing journey farther northward. And then there was the outlier — and it was way out there. The storm smashing directly into the mid-Atlantic states was a track so unlikely, it was more than five hundred miles off the historical average for storm courses.

Pasch was at a loss. The GFS and ECMWF had been running neck and neck in terms of accuracy for more than five years, and the 2012 season was no different. Now the two most reliable models available to the forecasters were at diametric odds concerning this storm.

"There's only one thing to do with all that uncertainty," says Pasch. "You have to tell the general public. At least that way, they can share in our misery."

And so the senior hurricane specialist took a deep breath and began to type:

> BY 12–24 HOURS AND CONTINUING THROUGH 72 HOURS . . . THE NHC MODEL GUIDANCE IS IN EXCELLENT AGREEMENT ON A GENERAL SLOW NORTH TO NORTH-NORTHEASTWARD MOTION TOWARD JAMAICA AND EASTERN CUBA AS A SHORTWAVE MOVES OFF THE SOUTHEASTERN US COAST AND WEAKENS THE SUBTROPICAL RIDGE THAT CURRENTLY EXTENDS ACROSS FLORIDA AND THE BAHAMAS. BY DAYS 4 AND 5 . . . HOWEVER . . . THE MODELS BEGIN TO DIVERGE SIGNIFICANTLY WITH THE NORMALLY RELIABLE ECMWF TAKING SANDY NORTH-NORTHWESTWARD CLOSER TO THE US SOUTHEAST COAST . . . WHEREAS THE GFS . . . HWRF . . . GFDL . . . AND OTHER LESS RELIABLE MODELS TAKE THE CYCLONE NORTH-NORTHEASTWARD.

6:02 P.M.
NWS Forecasting Office
Mt. Holly, New Jersey
66°F
Barometer: 30.07 inches (rising)
Winds: 4 mph (WSW)
Skies: Clear

Gary Szatkowski was already an hour late getting home when Pasch's forecast discussion appeared on his computer screen. With his slicked-back salt-and-pepper hair and an equally slick set of silk ties, Szatkowski looks as much like an NBA coach as he does a leading meteorologist. And it's only his Poindexter glasses — and his great enthusiasm for talking about storms — that give him away. His wife, Betty, says she knew she was getting involved with a weather junkie as early as their first date. She wasn't surprised that he was going to miss dinner that night. Or that he was all but oblivious to the way the fading light of evening lit up the sky.

Outside Szatkowski's office window, a bucolic autumn tableau was unfolding: A tractor made its way slowly across half-harvested fields, and the last of the maples and oaks were still beaming color under the ebbing sun. Szatkowski's blinds on his two windows are perpetually ratcheted down so that he can better see the computer screens that take up most of his enormous cherry desk. For him, there was no bending to look out the window for signs of wind or anything else. His is undeniably an executive's office, what with the red leather couch and matching chairs, the tidy anonymity that says a lot of people pass through here. And they do. The Mt. Holly forecast office serves eleven million people in an area that encompasses parts of New York, New Jersey, Pennsylvania, and Delaware. It's an area that includes not only the Philadelphia International Airport (which serves nearly 30.5 million people a year) and the city's large port, but also some of the busiest waters in North America. The surrounding geography is known for its weather extremes, from tornadoes and ice storms to forest fires and heat advisories. Still, says Szatkowski, it's one that rarely sees anything in the way of tropical storms.

"I like to joke that everyone in New Jersey should send a thank-you note to North Carolina because the state so often intercepts our big storms. It takes a very special storm and a rather limited set of circumstances for a hurricane to make landfall here."

Szatkowski is a proud new-media convert.

And so the first thing he did after reading Pasch's discussion was to log on to his Twitter account. The discussion there was already animated. Szatkowski scrolled through the feed, watching the emerging conversation concerning this new named storm. And as he did, his heart sank. There was a trend emerging in the conversations, and what they were saying made the ECMWF prediction seem like less and less of an outlier. The consensus was that this storm had a real chance of not just glancing off New York and New Jersey, but hitting the states head on.

"These weren't just armchair hobbyists," says Szatkowski. "We're talking about professionals — private-sector meteorologists and even some National Weather Service forecasters — saying the same thing. The bottom line here was that something unusual was clearly in the works with this storm — and people were starting to talk about it."

Szatkowski got up from his desk and walked into the main forecasting room. There, the two meteorologists on duty were reviewing the information streaming in from the National Hurricane Center. Szatkowski remembers thinking that the tone in the bureau had changed — all of a sudden, it felt like there was a lot at stake. Like most National Weather Service forecasting offices, Szatkowski's includes a public service desk, though "desk" is something of an understatement: At Mt. Holly, it takes up an entire corner of the forecasting floor and is packed with six enormous computer screens. At least one of those is dedicated to Facebook at all times; the site, they say, is the best place to find out what's really going on in their region. It's what cognitive scientists call "situational awareness" and the meteorologists call "taking the temperature" of their clients: knowing what is going on out in the world so that they can decide how best to act. That didn't used to be a part of weather forecasting, but catastrophic death tolls associated with storms like Katrina brought home just how important effective communication can be in saving lives.

"We can tell people the science until we're blue in the face," says Szatkowski, "but if we don't make them understand how it's going to impact them, they're just not going to get it."

That's one reason he and other meteorologists-in-charge are increasingly dedicating resources to community outreach. His office has a full-time position dedicated to staffing the public service desk. He says they could easily use another: Every day, the office gets calls from people asking everything from whether it will rain tomorrow to how climate change is going to affect the planet. A lot of times, the meteorologist on staff can answer them. But sometimes not. And that, says Szatkowski, is the irony of his business: Forecasters have gotten much better than they used to be, but sometimes the public still thinks they're better than they are.

The public service liaison answers these calls on an archaic-looking office phone — the kind with lots of lines, like you might have seen on a receptionist's desk in 1992. On an average shift, about fifteen calls will come in on that phone — mostly the general public asking what the weather will be like over the weekend, or how much rain they got the night before. During a weather event, that number will quickly climb to fifty — or beyond.

"On this particular day, the number of calls was definitely above average," says Szatkowski. Most of the people phoning were doing so to find out if what they were hearing was true: *Could this developing storm really slam into the mid-Atlantic?*

Even on the forecasting floor, the chances

seemed unlikely. Joe Miketta, the office's warning coordination meteorologist, was as uncertain as Szatkowski. And as he and Szatkowski talked about the situation, he says he found himself, somewhat inexplicably, thinking about his high school fiction class. He remembered his teacher explaining Samuel Taylor Coleridge's concept of the willing suspension of disbelief. *That's what it's going to take,* the affable Miketta thought. *That's the only way I'm going to buy that this storm is going to hit us.* If anything, he says, the fact that the models were saying that scenario was a possibility this far out made him more confident than ever that it could never happen. "Models shift around so much that a bull's-eye on you seven days out is almost always a surefire sign that the storm is going to hit elsewhere," he says. "They just don't have much skill that far out."

Miketta and Szatkowski joined a small group that was forming in front of the four big-screen TVs mounted on the wall behind the main forecasting desk. All four were on now — tuned to local stations and national news feeds and, yes, even the Weather Channel. The forecasters watched, looking for clues as to just how big a story Sandy had become. They needed to know if it was on the minds of residents in their coverage area; that would force their hand. Forecasters are, above all else, scientists; as such, they want to accumulate as much data as possible before arriving at a conclusion. Sometimes the media gets out ahead of them, and they're forced to chime in before they'd like to, lest they get scooped by armchair meteorologists and local reporters. When those sorts of personalities start talking about weather, the forecasters feel like they have to as well. And in the cavernous inner sanctum of a forecasting office, those TVs are the only window into what people are saying as close as just outside their door.

Szatkowski and his staff watched for a few minutes. News shows love to lead with stories of extreme weather, says Miketta. If Sandy was becoming an imminent concern for the country, they'd know by watching just a few minutes of TV.

"A potential storm is always the top story," says Miketta. "Always."

That fact alone, he says, has dramatically changed the way forecasters do their work. In a social psychology sense, the storm happens before the actual storm happens. Not so long ago, the average person had just two opportunities a day for a fleeting glance at a rudimentary radar screen, provided by the nightly news. And the National Weather Service very much had the corner on the market of weather information. "That meant we had the luxury of sometimes holding back a little," says Miketta. "We could take a little extra time to decide if the information we were about to convey was really consistent over time — like taking one more check before pulling the trigger."

But that, he says, is all but impossible in the era of twenty-four-hour news networks and social media. Weather, like much of the news, has become democratized — has become a citizen science where ordinary people regularly break stories in places like Twitter and Facebook, and even the smallest local news network has access to sophisticated prediction tools. Conversations about a potential weather threat tend to spin up in a heartbeat with access like this, says Miketta, and that demands a new kind of responsibility from forecasters. "People are looking to us. If we're silent while others are making predictions, we're not helping."

The question now, however, was just how many people were talking — and whether the conversations were extending beyond what Miketta calls "the weather weenies" (and he's quick to include himself in that category).

They continued to watch the screens. There was live footage of the violence in Beirut and ongoing coverage of the presidential debates . . . and no mention of the brewing storm.

"The patient didn't have a fever," says Miketta. But that didn't mean one couldn't develop at any second. As a culture, we are particularly adept at transitioning from apathetic to panicked at a moment's notice.

Szatkowski was circumspect about all that. As the meteorologist-in-charge, he had the authority to write an official storm briefing to warn the general public of an impending threat. But doing so comes with heavy consequences — and a lot of responsibility. A storm briefing, he says, interrupts people's lives. It can force evacuations and closings, can cost a staggering amount of money in lost revenue and state expense: On average, it costs about a million dollars for every square mile of coastline that is evacuated. That number is significantly higher for urban areas such as Charleston or Tampa Bay. For places like Philadelphia and New York City, it's nothing short of astronomical. Knowing that creates a real sense of responsibility for a forecaster.

"It's like jiggling people's elbows and saying, 'We know you're busy, but you need to stop what you're doing and really pay attention to this,' " says Szatkowski. "A storm briefing can very quickly become panic inducing: It's like sounding the alarm to a potential five-alarm fire."

That's why, historically, the National Weather Service has tended to take a conservative view of warnings. Szatkowski wasn't sure he wanted to buck that trend. He pulled down his glasses, looked again at the computer data.

"What do you think?" asked one of the forecasters. "Is it time for a briefing?"

"Oh, jeez," said Miketta. "We're still really far out."

Szatkowski agreed. "Let's give it another twenty-four hours," he said. "Let's see if that's enough time for this storm to tell us what it wants to do."

7:30 P.M.
Keesler Air Force Base
Biloxi, Mississippi
72°F
Barometer: 30.08 inches (rising)
Winds: 10 mph (ESE)
Skies: Clear

The sun was already slipping below the horizon when Jon Talbot stepped out onto the tarmac. The air had become cooler, drier. The meteorologist buttoned his flight suit and lingered outside the C-130 for just a moment before stepping in to prep for his flight. Thankfully, this time there was no drama, no threat of a malfunctioning plane. Just a perfect takeoff into a red sky and another long flight down into the southern Caribbean. The sun had long since set when the aircrew arrived at the outer edge of the storm. But even in the dark, they could tell Sandy was growing. Distinct bands of clouds had consolidated themselves into rings. Closer to the center, a seemingly impenetrable wall of thunderstorms surrounded what was now a well-defined eye. Everything else was black.

That was the first thing Talbot saw out his plane window: the heavy blackness of clouds, the way they surrounded the plane and blocked out even the brightest stars; the way the dark streaks of rain were illuminated by angry lightning. It was as if the storm had swallowed the entire sky.

The plane banked hard, dropping to one thousand feet. It pitched in the turbulent air, sending instruments chafing against their straps. But the hellacious din of rain pelting against the fuselage soon eclipsed even the sound of hundreds of thousands of dollars in equipment straining against a pitching plane. Even Talbot was surprised. All tropical storms have a character, he says, and Sandy's seemed to be driven by the volume of precipitation she was spewing.

He craned around the desk, hoping for a look at the sea. Winds had risen since Harter's reconnaissance flight — enough, now, to blow the tops off of waves and to turn the sea into a churning white mess. Dropsonde data registered gusts of more than 50 miles per hour.

Sandy, Talbot thought, was following all the rules of a tropical storm. And that meant the storm would continue growing, becoming more fierce by the hour as it spun up higher and higher in the troposphere and began a march toward Jamaica. In all likelihood, it'd be a full-blown hurricane by the time it arrived. Talbot asked the lodemaster to drop a few more sondes — extra data that would help the Hurricane Center get a better read on this thing. They stayed until the plane was low on fuel, and then rose to a safe cruising altitude before beginning the long ride back. As the plane leveled out, Talbot unstrapped himself long enough to warm up some leftovers in the microwave, and then returned to his desk. With a plastic container in one hand and a fork in the other, Talbot watched the new data stream across his computer, on its way to the National Hurricane Center. This storm wasn't going away anytime soon. Of that, everyone was now certain.

Talbot prepared himself for what would undoubtedly be a long week of reconnaissance flights and a constant guessing game concerning where the storm was and what it would be doing. If he had learned anything during his tenure with the 53rd, it was that tropical storms are, by their very nature, highly unpredictable: The ones that begin formidably sometimes prove all but harmless; the ones that seem like nothing will become cataclysmic Category 5 hurricanes when you least expect it. Sometimes, category doesn't even matter. Neither does size. Hurricane Katrina had been downgraded to a Category 3 when it became the costliest hurricane in history. Hurricane Floyd was much, much larger than Andrew, but it was the latter that has gone down in history as one of the most devastating storms — despite its diminutive size.

Which storm is going to do what often feels like as much a mystery to Talbot as it does to the general public — maybe even more so, since he has the data that shows just how capricious a hurricane can be.

"These storms change in intensity very quickly," says Talbot. "When they do, that changes your idea about pretty much everything: where and when you're going to evacuate, what warnings you're going to send, who the storm is going to affect and why. And that can decide who lives and who dies."

Talbot knew that he and his crew had provided critical information about the winds' speeds and directions, pressure and temperature changes, along with the overall size of the storm. That made him feel pretty good. But he was far from calm or confident that night. And that's because Jon Talbot also knew it's what he couldn't determine that would soon matter more than anything: where, when, and how this monster was going to come ashore.

TUESDAY

8:00 A.M.
National Hurricane Center
Miami, Florida
77°F
Barometer: 29.98 inches (rising)
Winds: Calm
Skies: Mostly cloudy

Richard Pasch hadn't slept well. He'd been on the forecasting desk well into the night. Now it was early morning and he was back again. He was tired. His back hurt. And the schedule was a mess: Avila was on his way to Cuba for the ballet convention; another forecaster was out on paternity leave. Chris Landsea was flitting between the marine and hurricane forecasting desks, a big smile on his tan face. "Wow," he kept saying. "This is really something." The remaining hurricane specialists kept shuffling their shifts, showing up at odd times. Pasch didn't like all the irregularity and displays of enthusiasm; it was making him grouchy.

So, too, were the two systems out in the Atlantic. Sandy's twin was still churning one thousand miles southeast of Bermuda, and had caught the forecasters unawares overnight, bursting to life with synchronized winds and quickly coalescing into a closed system. Now it, too, was a tropical storm with a name: Tony. But what was really happening inside this new tropical storm was anyone's guess. Radar and shortwave infrared imagery were both unable to locate the storm's center. If anything, they seemed to be suggesting that the storm had multiple centers. That made it hard to pinpoint the storm's location, and next to impossible to suggest where it would be heading. Pasch studied the satellite data. The system was too far from land to commission the Hurricane Hunters, and they clearly had their hands full with constant Sandy flights, anyway. Those aircrews not up in a C-130 were busy packing up their operations. Colonel Jeff Van Dootingh had decided that there was no point staying in Biloxi any longer: Every minute it took to get to the storm was that much less time they'd have to map it. They needed to get closer to Sandy's projected course, so Van Dootingh ordered the entire unit to relocate to Savannah, Georgia. Crew members said good-bye to their families; they packed for what would no doubt be days and days at an anonymous motel with bad coffee and vending-machine Danishes on some country highway. They're used to that sort of thing, says Talbot. It's part of their job.

"We go where we have to to make it work," he says.

Outside his office, a team of maintenance crews prepped all seven of the Hurricane Hunters' planes for an immediate departure. The remaining personnel loaded onto bright blue school buses for the ten-hour drive to Georgia.

Meanwhile, Talbot and Richard Pasch waited to hear what the airborne crew could tell him about Sandy. The storm had taken on a decidedly asymmetric shape, and bands of deep clouds bulged from its eastern edge like an angry tumor. As the scatterometer made its daily pass over the region, Pasch watched the ribbons of data unfold. Winds recorded there looked surprisingly light, even at the storm's center. But the forecaster couldn't tell for sure — he'd have to wait for the Hurricane Hunters to report back before he knew anything for certain. As for the storm's track, there wasn't much more agreement than the day before: A path across Jamaica, Cuba, and the Bahamas seemed assured now. After that, the spread remained — though a few other models were beginning to suggest that a westward track was increasingly likely. The problem, though, was that they could very well say the opposite a few hours later. And that makes it hard for a forecaster to predict a specific course.

The hurricane specialists tend to be pretty conservative in their decisions to change the predicted track of a storm, even when they start to see a growing disparity in the models. "We really hate to yank a forecast back and forth," says Landsea. He has a variety of ways of describing that problem — windshield-wipering, when they move the storm to the left and then to the right and back again; or tromboning, when they speed it up, only to pull it back like a brass slide. That kind of thing tends to irritate the general public, he says, and suggests that the forecasters don't really know what they're doing. That's one reason they tend not to show various model tracks in their forecasts as well: There's just too much variability and changeability there, says Pasch. The last thing they want is emergency managers making a decision based on one track, only to announce a completely different one a few hours later. That can cost the government millions of dollars. And besides, no one likes to admit they are wrong — let alone over and over again. That's bad for business.

8:40 A.M.
NWS Forecast Office
Mt. Holly, New Jersey
52°F
Barometer: 30.13 inches (rising)
Winds: Calm
Skies: Overcast

Gary Szatkowski was reconsidering. He, too, hadn't slept well that night, and when he walked into the forecasting room that morning, he could tell his staff hadn't, either. Even from his office, he could hear the ceaseless ringing of the phones at the public affairs desk. Calls to the office were increasing, and they weren't just from concerned residents anymore. Some of the state's emergency management teams had begun to phone as well, wondering if they needed to start initiating storm plans. "Something was definitely cooking," says Szatkowski. "Things were beginning to spin up."

And with that spin-up would come an inevitable pile of growing rumors that would turn into extreme or even ridiculous stories of Armageddon. That's the last thing Szatkowski wanted. But he didn't want an erroneous forecast, either. If there's anything that gets the general public distrustful, it's telling them about a storm that never manifests. Any effect Sandy might have on the mid-Atlantic was still seven days out — further than had ever been forecast before. Still, the ECMWF was remaining constant in its prediction. And the meteorologists on his listserv were inclined to believe it.

It'd be a big risk to make any kind of definitive statement so early in the game. He quizzed his staff: What did they feel confident about? What could be said in a storm briefing at this point? What was too big a risk?

"We have a way of forgetting what storms can do," says Szatkowski. And that makes him really frustrated. "People lose sight of the damage tropical systems have already done to this region." A massive hurricane hit New York in 1821, bringing with it flooding so high that the Hudson and East Rivers converged across much of lower Manhattan. Since then, a series of storms have wreaked havoc on the Big Apple. In 1954, not a single hurricane struck Florida, Georgia, or the Gulf states. But an unprecedented three hurricanes swept across New York and other North Atlantic states, collectively resulting in more than $500 million dollars in damage (about $4.8 billion dollars today) and the deaths of 229 people, most of whom drowned. Carol, the worst of the three storms to hit the New York region, brought storm tides of fifteen feet; many parts of Providence, Rhode Island, were left with ten feet of standing water. "Considering past experience, which indicates normal expectancy of only five to ten hurricanes per century in New England, two in one year is extraordinary," wrote Walter R. Davis of the Miami Weather Bureau office.

Less than a year later, Davis and other hurricane specialists watched, dumbstruck, as Hurricanes Connie and Diane battered southern New England and flooded large portions of Connecticut and New York. With just days between the two storms, the hurricanes not only called into question just how unlikely an appearance they were in northern latitudes, but also how prepared the region was to deal with them. Diane soon earned what Davis called "the unenviable distinction of 'the first billion-dollar hurricane.' " In the year-end report he authored with other meteorologists from the Weather Bureau, Davis also deemed the storm "undoubtedly the greatest natural catastrophe in the history of the United States."

It was a distinction that would soon be eclipsed by more than a dozen other storms. And, like Diane, several of them would leave a path of destruction across the North Atlantic region. In 1960, Hurricane Donna flushed New York Harbor with eleven feet of storm tide. Nearly forty years later, Tropical Storm Floyd forced massive evacuations as 60-mile-per-hour winds battered New York City, bringing with them more than a foot of rain. The Great Atlantic Storm of 1962, quite possibly the worst storm to hit the region, brought forty-foot waves off the coast of New York and New Jersey, along with torrential rain and flooding for much of the region. More than forty-five thousand homes were destroyed in New Jersey alone.

Most Americans either don't remember these storms or never heard about them in the first place. That makes it next to impossible to learn any lessons from them. And that makes the otherwise unflappable Gary Szatkowski mad.

"When it comes to dealing with risk, we need a lot of improvement as a society. I get passionate about that." True to his Midwestern upbringing, Szatkowski gets passionate by tapping his hand on his desk and smiling. That, and putting down his head and getting to work.

The best solution he had at his disposal was the creation of a storm briefing. But no one had ever made one of those for a hurricane that might make landfall seven days later.

"A week out, you can't be talking in any level of detail," says Szatkowski. "The best you can say at that point is, 'Yes, there's a storm out there. It might be impacting us.' "

Maybe, he thought, *that will be enough — enough to at least get people thinking.*

"It takes a while to get people to the right place to make the right decision," he says. And even then we tend to make the wrong decision when staring a natural disaster in the face. Szatkowski didn't want to see that happen.

An hour later, he was pretty sure he had a plan. So, sitting at his computer desk, he began to write what would soon become a historic report. "Tropical Storm Sandy is expected to reach hurricane strength on Wednesday," he began. "It will continue to move northward. This storm system will bring multiple potential threats to the region."

Szatkowski paused. This was the kind of

statement that ratcheted up panic levels. It'd be all the emergency management teams needed to shift into high gear. Yet, for all he knew, it could be totally wrong: With days to go before landfall, the storm could just as easily peter out or make a beeline for Europe. He looked at the data again. He thought about the worst-case scenario. And then he decided that he didn't want to be responsible for anyone living that scenario. He included the map of the computer model tracks — twenty of them, in fact. He pointed out that there was still an enormous spread — thousands of miles, actually — between them. But the European model, while still in the minority, was no longer alone in its prediction that Sandy was destined for the Eastern Seaboard. The effects of that track, he said, could be disastrous. The entire region could be assaulted by very strong winds. The slow, lumbering pace of the storm meant that total rainfall amounts would cause major flooding. "The takeaway message is that our region could be close to the path of a very dangerous storm. Our region is clearly at risk."

Szatkowski printed out the draft and returned to the forecast room. He handed out copies to all the meteorologists there and then sat down, waiting for his staff to read it. He watched them carefully.

"Does this make you uncomfortable?"

They shook their heads.

"Is the emphasis right?"

They said it was. So their supervisor went back into his office. But he didn't publish the briefing right away. Instead, he sat for a while, his hands resting on the keyboard. He thought again about the consequences of this briefing — the way it would undoubtedly turn the country's biggest metropolitan area into a bluster of storm preparations. *This storm could turn out to be nothing,* a voice said somewhere inside his head. And that statement of doubt held sway — but just for a few moments.

"Our job at the NWS is to make sure people know what they need to know when they need to know it," says Szatkowski. That time, he decided, was right now. He took a deep breath and hit send.

9:10 A.M.
Chesapeake Bay
59°F
Barometer: 30.14 inches (falling)
Winds: Calm
Skies: Overcast
Seas: Calm

One of the first people to read Szatkowski's

briefing was Jan Miles. The sixty-one-year-old captain of the *Pride of Baltimore* sat at his kitchen table out on Maryland's Pasadena peninsula. His iPad and a cup of coffee vied for space in front of him, and he considered both from behind a pair of well-scratched wire-rimmed glasses secured by a soft lanyard around his neck. They, along with sea-tousled red hair and matching mustache, make Miles look very much the part of a career sailor. And that makes him a career weather watcher, too. As a kid, he and his family took a passenger ship from America to England. On the first day out, they hit a big storm. Miles never forgot the feeling of that rocking liner, the sound of wind and growing waves against a hull. He was terrified and obsessed at the same time. In the years since, he's logged tens of thousands of miles at sea. He's crossed the Atlantic Ocean five times. He's voyaged across the Pacific three or four times — he can't quite remember. But while the details of each trip begin to blur together over time, the experience of setting sail never gets old. And he still approaches every voyage with some of the wariness he felt on that steamer. Miles admits that, for him, sailing is about that fine line between the known and the unknown: On one hand, there's that mystery implicit every time a ship goes over the horizon — will she, and all who are aboard, come back? On the other hand, there is the relative comfort that comes from knowability — the idea that you can minimize risk, that you can do everything in your power to get back safely. That, he says, is as exciting as the prospect of the voyage itself.

In 1981, Miles became one of three rotating captains on the *Pride of Baltimore.* He was just thirty years old. The tall-ship renaissance was in full swing, and the city of Baltimore had built a replica of its signature nineteenth-century vessel, the Baltimore clipper, as a way of getting in the game. A clipper is kind of like a windjammer on steroids; it has all of the maneuverability of a schooner, and huge fore and aft sails. But, unlike the schooner, the clipper also uses two enormous square sails on top of the foresail. This extra canvas can catch a lot more wind, and that's a good thing. The original clippers were often hired as mercenaries — private ships fighting on behalf of a navy. Later, these ships were engaged in the Chinese opium trade. During the height of the California Gold Rush, they were the fastest way from the East Coast to San Francisco. Along the way, many of them were converted into pirate vessels. So they had to be fast — really fast.

The *Pride of Baltimore* was. But nowhere near quick enough to outrun a microburst.

In 1986, after the vessel and its crew completed an extensive European tour, the *Pride* was heading back to Baltimore by way of the Caribbean. On the afternoon of May 14, the crew encountered a storm and reduced sail. They thought the worst of it was behind them. And then, without warning, the winds rose to hurricane strength. The *Pride of Baltimore* had encountered a microburst — a small, violent draft of air that charges down out of a thunderstorm, and often with more destructive force than a tornado. Armin Elsaesser, the ship's acting captain, tried to bear away from the wind to ease the strain on his vessel, but it was too late. Within seconds, the *Pride* was over on its port side, its masts and sails submerged. Water streamed inside the hull. Minutes later, the ship went down. It all happened so fast the crew was caught unawares: no time to send a distress signal, to secure ditch kits, to don survival suits. They were left with one self-deploying raft, which took the crew six exhausting hours to inflate. In the meantime, four people died, including Elsaesser. The survivors bobbed for days before being sighted by a tanker ship and eventually recovered. It took a few more before they were delivered to Puerto Rico, where they rendezvoused with Miles.

What Miles found when he arrived in the Caribbean was a group of scared, quiet, and frankly defensive people. He and the crew spent the rest of the week together, slowly unpacking what had happened. A week later, the coast guard and National Transportation Safety Board (NTSB) convened a full investigation of the accident. The mere existence of microbursts had been proven only a few years prior, when Delta Airlines flight 191 crashed just short of the Dallas–Fort Worth airport, killing 137 people. Eyewitnesses said the plane, which had begun its approach of the airfield, entered what looked like a small band of clouds (the air traffic controller at the time called it "a little rain shower" and advised the pilots to utilize their instrument landing system). Other pilots in the area said the system looked "harmless," like barely a blip on the radar. But a few seconds later, Delta 191 seemed to fall from the sky like a stone. A subsequent investigation would determine that the plane fell at a rate of five thousand feet per minute, and that the force of this crash was caused by a microburst. Nevertheless, plenty of people in the weather industry still doubted whether such a phenomenon exists. It would take decades — and millions of dollars — before the airline industry created protocols to deal with this threat.

The maritime industry has struggled to keep up. In their concluding report, the coast guard determined that there was simply no way the crew of the *Pride of Baltimore* could have anticipated the disaster nor mitigated it once it was under way. It recommended no further action in the matter. The NTSB was not quite so forgiving in its conclusions. In its report, the NTSB urged the National Weather Service to improve marine forecasts with intensified aircraft reconnaissance data and to begin predicting microburst action; both, it said, needed to be a priority action.

Meanwhile, the city of Baltimore set to work re-creating its beloved ship. But that re-creation also found itself in peril. While competing in a tall-ship race from England to Spain in 2005, the *Pride of Baltimore II* encountered an unexpected squall off the coast of France. Within minutes, winds grew to 40 knots and seas to seven feet. That's significant weather, says Jan Miles, but well within the capability of a ship like the *Pride II.* Still, it was enough to cause a bobstay iron — a metal fastener that secures the ship's standing rigging — to fail. The ship's bowsprit gave way and soon took both enormous masts — along with thousands of pounds of rigging — with it. The whole mess crashed onto the deck while the ship was under way. Miles still thinks it was somewhat miraculous that no one was killed or injured. Speaking to a reporter for Maryland's *Capital Gazette* at the time of the dismasting, he said, "This is the worst rig failure I have ever experienced." A decade later, he says that's still true — and that he is still shaken by the incident. The squall, he says, came out of nowhere. It could happen again.

That's made Miles increasingly cautious. And he's hell-bent on making sure that kind of tragedy never again occurs on any vessel he's associated with. He's developed a variety of means to try to prevent such catastrophes, from increased crew credentials and training to clear lines of hierarchy at the home office. Deckhands don't step aboard his vessel unless they've had significant experience on at least two other tall ships. But, he says, the best way to keep people safe is to always, always, always defer to the capriciousness of Mother Nature. "Risk always comes down to the boat and what you can do on that boat. When weather steps in, you can't control that boat anymore. And sooner or later, everything you do won't be enough," he says.

His habit now is to study weather. And restudy it. He's so familiar with the NOAA web pages that he can tell you from memory in what order each image appears in its daily briefings. He can read them upside down and from across the room. But more than anything, he worries about what these reports don't say. That, he says, has to be a mariner's biggest obsession. It's fine to have a plan, but you have to know that the unknowns will force you to deviate from that plan. And, says Miles, no matter how hard you prepare, there will *always* be unknowns.

The morning of October 23, Captain Miles felt more concerned than ever by what the National Weather Service wasn't saying. And he felt pretty certain Szatkowski was on to something with his unexpected storm briefing. Sitting at his kitchen table in a thick sweater and jeans, Miles squinted at the iPad screen, toggling between charts of the Gulf Stream and the NHC's tropical weather outlook. Miles thought the language in these reports seemed even more speculative than usual. Still, most of the governments in the Caribbean were taking few chances. Jamaica had already issued a hurricane warning. Cuba had called for a hurricane watch in six of its provinces, including Guantánamo, which sent the US army scrambling to make arrangements for its base there. The Bahamas had issued a tropical storm watch, even though any potential landfall there would be days away — if it happened at all.

From there, the models spread out in a massive fan of predicted routes. The ECMWF still said landfall. The National Weather Service's GFS said out to sea. They were both emphatic.

"It was like watching a tennis match," says Miles. "You're sitting there wondering who is going to give up first."

And that, he adds, can create a real problem for crews at sea. Most captains follow what is called the "Mariner's 1-2-3 Rule," which attempts to accommodate the inevitable error in long-range hurricane forecasting. The consensus in the industry is that ships and their crews ought to do everything they can to avoid winds above 35 knots (or about 40 mph). To be safe, they're encouraged to imagine a wind radius that grows by 100 nautical miles each day: If, for instance, a 35-knot wind field is 75 miles in diameter the day a vessel sets out, in three days its crew should be at least 375 miles away from the edge of the storm's track. In its official guide for mariners, the NHC recommends that "larger buffer zones can and should be established in situations of tropical cyclones with large forecast uncertainty, limited crew experience, decreased vessel handling, or other factors as determined by the vessel master. The 1-2-3 rule does not account for sudden & rapid intensification of tropical cyclones that could result in a rapid outward expansion of the 34 KT wind field. Also, the 1-2-3 rule does not account for the typical outward expansion of the wind field as a system transitions from tropical cyclone to extratropical gale or storm in the North Atlantic." In other words, if you have a young crew, or equipment that you're not comfortable with, or a storm that has meteorologists scratching their heads, you want to be as far away from that storm as possible.

Jan Miles lives his life by principles like the 1-2-3 Rule. And he expects that everyone else associated with the *Pride II* will as well. This would be the first time the vessel had been in port during a hurricane. They needed options, depending upon what the storm would do. Miles wanted the vessel docked and his crew secure. The question would be what harbor would offer them the safest berth during the storm. If it wasn't Baltimore, he was prepared to relocate. But first he'd have to get his ship and crew out of harm's way.

Miles pulled up a website that tracks vessels in real time, using their AIS, or Automatic Identification System. Already it seemed like ships of significant size were making a beeline away from the southeastern coast of the United States. Miles zoomed in on the *Pride of Baltimore II* — nothing more than a tiny pink diamond in the southern basin of the Chesapeake Bay. The ship was on its way back from Virginia under the leadership of Jamie Trost, Miles's co-captain. The two men, says Miles, are a whole lot like an old married couple who have to share one car. They tend to check in on each other — and that car — a lot. Trost is a licensed captain with more than a decade of experience. He served under Miles as first mate of the *Pride II* before assuming the role of master of the ship. Miles trusted in Trost's command. But the senior captain had nearly thirty years of experience on him and, at the time, was also serving as acting director of the entire Pride of Baltimore organization. Both, Miles says, gave him permission to worry. He texted

Trost to confirm their plans for beating the storm. Trost responded right away. As planned, the ship was on its way to a tall-ship festival in Chestertown, a little village across the bay from Baltimore. Everything was great on board; the crew was in good spirits and the weather was beautiful. Miles relaxed. Chestertown was an easy six-hour sail to Baltimore.

"She was coming home," says Miles. "She was almost in our own backyard." Once the ship got there, it'd be easy to tend to her, no matter the conditions. Until then, Trost knew every port and hiding hole in the bay — he and the crew could duck in just about anywhere if they needed to ride out the wind and the waves. Miles relaxed further, lulled by what he says was "a kind of hubristic confidence." Managing risk, he says, is one constantly shifting feasibility study. On that day, feasibility looked all but assured. *How marvelous is this?* he thought to himself. *We don't have to run around and shout and panic. We can sail now and prepare for the wind this weekend.*

Dan Moreland, captain of the *Picton Castle,* had no such luxuries ahead of him. He and his crew were due to sail from their home port of Lunenburg, Nova Scotia, to the South Pacific, by way of Bermuda,

Grenada, and, eventually, the Panama Canal. It was to be a formidable trip, even by the standards of the well-traveled *Picton Castle:* more than eight thousand miles, and much of it in storm-prone waters. Moreland had planned to depart on Monday, October 15 — a full two weeks earlier than has been traditionally considered safe with regard to hurricane season. But those notions have changed in recent years, says Moreland, thanks to advances in weather forecasting and warnings. So the captain felt good about his decision in the months leading up to their departure. But as the fifteenth approached, Moreland began having second thoughts. Forecast models were predicting a series of gales in the North Atlantic. Moreland didn't like the looks of them. So he postponed the trip for a couple of days. And then a couple more. As early as the nineteenth, he and his mates saw what they call a "hotspot cooking in the central Caribbean." There was nothing overtly threatening in the system at the time, but Moreland had a hunch it could develop into a real threat. He just didn't know where. "That disturbance could have gone anywhere at that point," says Moreland. "So I put the sailing day back again just to see what might develop in the forecasts."

There were grumblings on board about his decision.

"The *Picton Castle* was ready for sea," says Moreland. "We were ready for autumn on the North Atlantic. The ship was stowed, the crew was drilled up. After weeks of preparation, our gang aboard was quite keen to get under way."

But Moreland kept delaying, and by the twenty-third, he was beginning to side firmly with Szatkowski. He was cautious. He and his wife had a brand-new baby. He had a crew of young sailors. And like Miles, Moreland was no stranger to tragedies at sea.

In December 2006, the *Picton Castle* encountered a late-season storm about five hundred miles southeast of Cape Cod. Seas grew to twenty-five feet. The wind howled. The crew worked for hours trying to keep the ship on course. Among them was Laura Gainey, the twenty-five-year-old daughter of Bob Gainey, longtime star of the Montreal Canadiens. For most of her life, Laura Gainey had wandered in much the same way Claudene Christian had, and her life took a scary turn with the help of some drug addictions. But tall-ship sailing gave her the same welcome structure it provided Christian, and Gainey had fallen in love with her new role as an unpaid trainee aboard the ship. Just before the *Picton Castle,* under the direction of relief captain Michael Vogelgesang, departed for this fateful voyage, Gainey had been promoted to paid deckhand. She was, by all accounts, deliriously happy. And as the storm raged on, she worked ceaselessly, taking only an hour or two break — just long enough to record the deteriorating conditions in her journal: "Very rough out, I've been up a lot, 6 p.m. to 4 a.m., then 6 a.m. to now 3 p.m. or 4'ish. People are sick, scared, falling, etc." Her supervisor advised her to get some rest. But rather than stay below, Gainey returned to the deck, where she and the crew continued to battle the storm. No one was wearing a life jacket, which is not unusual on a tall ship — later, Vogelgesang would argue that personal flotation devices (or PFDs) would only have inhibited the crew's ability to work. Some were wearing climbing harnesses, but without jacklines strung about, there really wasn't anywhere to clip in. And so, when an enormous wave swamped the stern of the boat, at least three strong men — including the captain — were knocked from their feet and sent crashing in the ship's bulwark. Laura Gainey wasn't nearly so lucky. That same wave swept her overboard. The crew last saw her trying to tread water and screaming for help. Her body was never recovered, and that final image of her flailing in the sea continues to haunt all those associated with the accident.

It doesn't matter to Dan Moreland that he wasn't on the ship when this accident occurred. It was still a tragic loss, he says, and one that demonstrated yet again how often we lose when we fight Mother Nature.

He says he's always been cautious, but Gainey's death made him even more so. He'd weathered three or four hurricanes while in port. He'd been out in a hurricane once or twice. This was the first time a planned departure would coincide with one.

It was no surprise, then, that he spent October 23 watching the weather dispatches with the same intensity as Jan Miles. What had looked like a hot spot a few days earlier was now clearly a formidable storm. And unlike the *Pride of Baltimore II,* the *Picton Castle* was leaving her home turf; where she was heading, there wouldn't be much in the way of safe harbor.

Moreland says three facts were becoming abundantly obvious to him and his officers: "This was going to be a big, broad storm covering a whole lot of ocean; we could not hope to dodge it; and we would not want to try to dodge anyway."

Delaying would set their trip back two additional weeks. It would disappoint — and put on edge — trainees more than keen to get sailing. Neither consideration mattered to him at all. "Schedules are flexible," he says. "Ships are not. Hurricanes are not, either."

Moreland called his crew together and gave them the news: Nobody was going anywhere anytime soon. He told them to settle in and make peace with being dockside; they all had a lot of heavy-weather preparation ahead of them. "I told them to get used to Lunenburg for a spell, 'cause we are hanging out for a while." The North Atlantic, he told them, "can stay a pretty uncomfortable place for a while after a big storm."

It was, Moreland would later say, the easiest weather call he has ever made as master of a vessel. "This ship is steel, of a powerful latter-day, square-rig design, and still, that was an exceedingly easy decision to make. I saw no chance of sailing around or dodging this hurricane, or anything to be gained by considering such a maneuver."

But if his friend Robin Walbridge was having any such thoughts, he certainly didn't let on to his crew. Nor did he seem at all concerned about the status of the ship. If anything, he seemed a little more sentimental than usual. As the ship approached New London, Walbridge waxed aloud about love and a life at sea. It had been a month since Walbridge had seen his wife, Claudia — and that had just been for a quick weekend while the ship was in Boothbay. The two had spent their only full day together ducking in and out of museums in their hometown of St. Petersburg. They spent extra time at the Dalí Museum — Claudia says it has always been Walbridge's favorite.

That evening, they rendezvoused with Ralph McCutcheon, an eccentric guy in his late sixties and one of Walbridge's closest buddies. Their mutual acquaintances like to joke that the two men were separated at birth: Both are a little heavyset, and both wear their thin hair in a ponytail and thick glasses. They both favor oversize Hawaiian shirts and sandals, no matter the weather (though, as Ralph is quick to point out, he knows better than to wear socks with his). Ask McCutcheon to say more about his connection with Robin Walbridge, and he'll tell you it's because they're both Scorpios and they're both jacks-of-all-trades. For his part, McCutcheon came to tall ships by way of technical theater and window displays for upscale clothing stores (he was once asked to help Diana Ross pick out a dress for a comeback concert). He's worked as a tour guide; he attended boat-building school. The sum of all these stints led him to find his calling as a cook on the USS *Constitution,* which is where he met Walbridge. The *Bounty* captain invited him to come aboard, and McCutcheon said yes. He was tasked with working as a mess mate, but McCutcheon had a feeling he'd soon be working in the thick of repairing the crumbling ship. He showed up on his first day of work carrying a chainsaw, and it was at that moment that a deep friendship was born.

Over the years, Robin had begun to lean on Ralph and trust his judgment, particularly where technical aspects of the ship were concerned. The captain would call any time of day or night whenever he was in a jam or couldn't troubleshoot on his own. Ralph became a fixture on the ship. He hosted parties for the crew whenever they were in town; he became their unofficial historian — and historical guru. He made the ship's bosun, Laura Groves, a set of caulking mallets and a whistle, the traditional way someone in her position summons a crew. He says she cried like a baby when she opened the box. While back in St. Petersburg, Walbridge reminisced about those days with Ralph and Claudia as the three of them sat at the Thunderbird, a throwback beach resort on the Gulf with a tiki bar and a sound system that plays vintage samba and bossa nova. They sat at one of the small beach tables there, shared an order of buffalo wings, and drank some beers. As the sun set, Robin asked Ralph to take a photo of him and Claudia. Ralph spent some time posing the couple, whose faces were beaming with the kind of youth that only love can create. Ralph wanted to make sure he got both wedding rings in the photo. The resulting picture is as sweet as you can imagine: Robin has his left arm around Claudia, his hand resting comfortably on her bare shoulder. She has her left hand placed firmly over his heart. Their smiles are immense. It's hard not to feel anything other than really sentimental about that image.

Robin and Claudia had had next to no contact since that night at the Thunderbird, which was unusual for a couple that usually spent a small fortune keeping in touch by satellite e-mail. Claudia wasn't worried, though. She had left for an Italian tour with some girlfriends. Robin would be home in November. She'd been waiting for him for much of the two decades they'd been together; another month or so wasn't going to make a difference. Besides, his birthday was just two days away. They'd catch up then. Claudia didn't know that Walbridge had spent much of the season wondering how it would end. He hadn't told her about the cough that wouldn't go away, or the chest pain earlier in the year, or the premonition he'd had as a kid that he wouldn't make it past his sixty-second year. And he certainly didn't tell his crew any of that. Instead, says the crew, he teased them with more rhymes and watched with a quiet smirk as they struggled to remember how to sail their ship. That, they say, was exactly what they had come to expect from their captain: This was a guy, after all, who read books on Buddhism for fun; he was a disciple of Tony Robbins, and had even walked on fire at one of the self-help guru's conventions.

Later that day, after the seas began to increase, Walbridge called one of his standard meetings at the ship's capstan — an enormous, four-foot winch near the stern of the vessel and the traditional site of a ship's daily captain's briefings. Walbridge leaned his elbows on the top of the capstan. He smiled at his crew, most of whom were looking pretty green. Half of them were downright seasick. He asked them how high the waves were. Somebody said they thought about eight feet. Walbridge agreed. It was enough motion to send the ship on a kind of corkscrewing motion a lot of inner ears can't take. People were throwing up. Walbridge assured his crew it was no big deal — everybody was feeling a little rusty. It'd take a while to get their groove back.

Walbridge always emphasized self-sufficiency on his vessel. He wanted his crew to feel confident in their own skills. "He was the type of person who always made sure you're okay," says Katie DePrato, who sailed under Walbridge aboard the *Bounty*. "He always wanted to make sure we were very safe. He turned every captain's meeting into a lesson." She says they had been through plenty of nasty weather, especially off Cape Hatteras, which everyone on the boat knew by its historic nickname, "the Graveyard of the Atlantic." That didn't stop them from sailing through it. When they did hit weather, Walbridge stayed calm. He let the crew try to figure stuff out by themselves. He called them the *"future captains of America."* When they made mistakes, he forgave them. When someone really messed up, he'd send that person home to think for a month or two, rather than fire him or her outright. That didn't work for everyone — some crew members stepped off the ship almost as soon as they arrived, saying that conditions were way too lax for them to feel safe. But those who remained developed a fierce loyalty to their captain. They called him a genius — a badass. When an engineer couldn't figure out the engine, Robin would go down and get the job done. When yard workers couldn't cut off part of the mast, he'd climb up with a torch and do it himself. When rigging snapped in a storm, Walbridge would fix it. It didn't matter to the crew that snapping yards and masts isn't typical on tall ships. Their captain always had the solution, which meant few things really felt like problems to the crew. Walbridge let them think through solutions on their own. This captain, everyone agreed, was old-school. He'd send seventy-five-year-old women up into the rigging without harnesses. When Claudia questioned him about it, worrying that it might be a bad idea, he'd shrug. *They'd lived that long, hadn't they? Besides, a little fear has a way of making sure people hold on really tight.* People learn best by doing, Walbridge always said, and by doing things the traditional way. He liked to turn off the navigation equipment out in the middle of the ocean so the crew could learn to steer by stars. And they did.

When it came to the *Bounty,* Walbridge was always a glass-is-half-full kind of guy. And everybody in the industry agreed: Robin Walbridge was single-handedly responsible for the ship's constant improvement. When his crew wanted to experiment — try a new cheaper sealant on the hull, for instance — Walbridge encouraged that, too. He trusted their growing expertise. That kind of thing mattered. And the fifteen people sailing with him on that trip were the best crew he'd ever had.

So, that afternoon at sea, when Walbridge let them off with some gentle teasing, the crew lightened up. They joked that they had lost their sea legs after the month in dry dock, though there wasn't much time to wallow. Doug Faunt, who was even tetchier than usual, spent the day rewiring the crew cabins. He wanted to get to the temporary lights in the tank room, too, but it didn't look like there'd be time. The crew quarters were still in the process of being painted as well, so people were sleeping in the tween decks or the great cabin — kind of a collective slumber party on shifts, with blankets strung up over the glass windows on the stern to keep out the light. Down below, second mate Matt Sanders led a crew who were working to finish the new fuel lines. Chris Barksdale, the new engineer, was among them. And he admits he was struggling to find his footing. Water, he said, poured into the ship through the deck every time it rained. Jess Hewitt had warned him to keep all of his electronics in Ziploc bags, but that didn't seem like much of a solution to Barksdale. No one had gotten around to his safety training, either, so he was feeling a little lost — and definitely pretty queasy. He was also having a hard time getting used to just how much noise the ship made belowdecks — the creaking of timbers bending and rubbing up against one another, the way they seemed to moan and shudder. He kept asking: *Is that normal?* The more seasoned mates told him it was fine.

Meanwhile, up on deck, the rest of the crew worked their way through watches, half of them still fighting seasickness and the rolling waves. But Claudene Christian, at least, seemed impervious. She was as chipper as ever and sung her way through cleanup: finding new places for the survival suits, Shop-Vaccing, and just generally being her cheerful self. She and Sanders had become an item; they'd plan dates in between shifts. Everything seemed perfect.

Christian didn't know it, but some of her boat mates were worried. While the ship was in dry dock in Boothbay, a couple of the *Bounty* officers, along with some of the yard workers, had found a lot of rot on the ship. Walbridge was worried, but he didn't let on to the crew. Nor did he seem concerned that the ship's bilge pumps were not working all that well. It was a familiar position for the captain of a ship that never had enough resources. In 2007, a coast guard inspector came for a routine dockside attraction-vessel inspection. He wasn't supposed to be looking for structural integrity, but he did find notable areas of soft wood, which he indicated as "problemsome." In 2010, during the vessel's mandatory hull exam, a ten-foot plank on the starboard side had to be replaced because of worm damage. Rot was found in a deck beam in the parlor, too. But the ship had been fine those seasons, and Walbridge was sure it would be for the rest of this one, too. He told the ship's owner to try to sell it as fast as he could, and then he got back to business; they just didn't have the time or money to do a major repair. The yard manager says he wanted to keep the ship there — that he even thought about chaining it to the dock or taking off the rudder so the *Bounty* would have to stay. But, in the end, he knew it was up to the captain. He told Walbridge to avoid heavy weather and wished them well. He and Walbridge were friends. They had a lot of respect for each other. But as the media began to grab hold of the Sandy story, the manager began to have second thoughts. *Should he — could he — have kept them from going anywhere?*

4:23 P.M.
Atlantic Ocean
Latitude 18° 9'35.11"N
Longitude 64° 4'23.07"W
77°F
Barometer: 29.98 inches
Winds: 9 mph
Skies: Mostly cloudy
Seas: 1–2 feet

Jamie McNamara knew they'd be going out in hurricane season when she and her husband booked a family cruise on Disney's *Fantasy.* But, she reasoned, that storm season goes on for six months — that's a full half of the year, and a lot longer than most seasons actually see hurricanes. Besides, no self-respecting captain would drive her and her family through a major storm.

The McNamaras had been saving up for this trip for years. Their kids were six, eight, and eleven: the perfect ages for a Disney adventure. And what better place than a ship especially built to entertain kids? At 128,000 gross tons and a length of more than 1,100 feet, the Disney *Fantasy* didn't even make the list of the top twenty largest cruise ships in the world. But with fourteen decks and room to accommodate fifty-four hundred people, the ship was plenty formidable when it came to confronting wave and surf. It was safe, thought Jamie. It was quality. It was Disney. Brochures advertised character meet-and-greets throughout the day, films and live musicals, boutiques for princesses, and arcades for everybody. Five pools and three water parks promised endless outside fun. In short, says McNamara, her whole family was certain that a cruise on the *Fantasy* was going to be the vacation of a lifetime.

Certainly it had started out that way. The family of five flew from their home in the suburbs of Denver, then boarded the ship in Port Canaveral. For the first three days at sea, everything seemed to be going as planned: The kids were totally enraptured with the water slides, the shows, and the fact that they could reach out and hug their favorite characters. Yes, the seas felt choppy, but McNamara was sure it was nothing to be concerned about. Their first port of call was St. Maarten, on the twenty-second. It had been a long, great day, followed by a late-night pirate party back on the ship. Everybody dressed up. There were fireworks that went on late into the night. The kids were exhausted.

By the time the McNamaras returned to their state room, Everett, their six-year-old, had gone from feeling pretty low to sporting a low-grade fever. Thursday was the scheduled highlight of the cruise — an entire day at Castaway Cay, Disney's private island in the Bahamas. The McNamaras wanted to be rested. So at about 10:00 P.M., while Brian stayed with the kids, Jamie made her way down to the guest services desk, hoping she could get a refund on what had been a sizable excursion fee for the St. Thomas port adventure scheduled for the next day. The rep asked McNamara if Everett needed a doctor, but McNamara declined: *He's probably just had too much sun,* said the stay-at-home mom with big blue eyes and a fantastic Texas accent. But, she explained, the family had paid almost $500 for the next day's activities and would love it if they could get a refund. The rep said she'd have to check on that. So McNamara waited at the desk and listened with increasing curiosity as the couple next to her began interrogating another Disney employee about whether or not the *Fantasy* — and its passengers — may soon be in danger.

The couple explained that they had been watching Fox News, where it was being reported that Tropical Storm Sandy was about to be upgraded to hurricane status as it moved across Jamaica, about nine hundred miles due west of the *Fantasy.* From there, according to Fox, the hurricane was projected to continue its march northeastward, perhaps making landfall in the United States as early as Saturday. Jamie McNamara was stunned. "We were all totally in the dark about the storm up until that point."

She listened intently to the couple as they expressed their concern to the guest relations representative. They wanted to know if and how the storm was going to affect their cruise — if they were okay out in the ocean with a hurricane brewing. "Don't worry," said the rep. "The captain gets plenty of warning for serious weather, and we haven't received any word about the storm. We're far away; it's not going to impact us at all; we haven't heard anything about it; we're on top of it." The contradiction in the representative's statement didn't strike McNamara as noteworthy at the time. Instead, she says she mostly just felt reassured: *Of course,* she thought to herself. *They have weather satellites and all that technology. The captain will know so far in advance, the storm will never be a problem. This is Disney, after all.*

McNamara had never been on a cruise before — she says she just never really thought she was that type. But everything about the trip so far had made her feel secure. She placed her confidence in the brand, in the idea that the master of a ship stands steward over his passengers. A Disney captain wouldn't steer her anywhere dangerous, right? "You assume you're safe," she says. "They're telling you you're safe, so you assume it's true."

But back in her cabin — and for the first time that entire trip — she turned on CNN. Most of the coverage was still about the presidential debate from the night before — foreign-policy stuff, and who would take Florida in the election. Sandwiched between all that discussion was a quick check on the weather. A photo of a rain-smeared Jamaican flag standing at attention appeared on the screen; everything else in the shot was blurred by the pounding rain. "Things are about to get very interesting in the Atlantic," warned the CNN host by way of introduction. "Just how interesting?" she asked meteorologist Rob Marciano.

"Well," he said with uncharacteristic hesitation, "there are a lot of different options right now."

Jamie McNamara watched as he showed radar images of Sandy, its color-enhanced bands swirling tentacle-like over much of the Caribbean. It was hard to tell just how far those bands spiraled out, and Marciano was standing directly in front of the Virgin Islands on the map. McNamara wiggled around, hoping she could get a better view. She wanted — she needed — to know if the storm was going to hit the *Fantasy*. But Marciano's attention was squarely on Jamaica and points immediately north. Tropical storm watches, he said, were now being issued for much of Florida. What would happen next was anyone's guess. Computer models, admitted Marciano, were still at odds over where the storm would go from there. The only thing he could say with relative confidence was that a "serious storm" was about to strike Kingston. As for what would happen as Sandy approached the United States, Marciano was loath to speculate. "Could be a hybrid storm; could be just a piece of energy," he said. "Either way, it's going to be a high-impact storm up and down the coastline. It's just a matter of how close it comes."

That was enough to send cruise discussion boards into high gear. Scott Sanders, author of the *Disney Cruise Line Blog,* began posting the same NOAA weather charts Jan Miles was studying, along with predictions for storm impact near some of Disney's destinations. He reported that tropical storm winds were extending outward from the center up to ninety miles. Both the Disney *Fantasy* and *Dream,* he added, were likely to experience heavy wind and rain. What would happen beyond then was getting awfully confusing. Forecast models were changing — suggesting that this storm, once predicted to barrel into the open ocean after crossing Cuba, was now on course to hit the Bahamas. The possibility of tropical storm winds pummeling Disney's private island was now 60 percent. But Sanders was siding with the conservative models beyond that: Once the storm passed over Castaway Cay, he predicted, it would most likely turn east and head out to sea.

Readers about to board the ships responded to news of the storm with dread and concern. *Please cancel, Disney!,* beseeched several commenters. *Impossible,* wrote others. *Don't worry,* wrote a veteran cruiser, *Captain Henry will steer us clear of any rough weather.* But other readers weren't so sure. Dave, a first-time cruiser, logged on to say his house was in a panic. *My wife is terrified,* he wrote. *Almost like she's being held hostage!* Others shared his sentiment. *Why would you put so many people at risk?* a mother of four asked Disney.

The company didn't reply.

WEDNESDAY

10:30 A.M.
National Hurricane Center
Miami, Florida
83°F
Barometer: 29.94 inches (steady)
Winds: 19 mph (ENE)
Precipitation: Rain
Seas: 5–8 feet

Out in the Atlantic Ocean, Tropical Storm Tony was changing. As the storm bumped across cooler ocean water, Tony's ability to fuel itself became irregular. And as the storm's core began to cool, its engine began to sputter, losing its tight convection and orderly cloud formation as it did. The system was beginning to crumble, sending its winds and clouds outward and upward, propelled by their own instability. Seas directly below the storm were at nineteen feet and beginning to drop. The storm's strongest winds, once located near the ocean surface, were now found high up in the troposphere, where they registered temperatures as low as −70 degrees Fahrenheit.

Tony was now in the throes of what meteorologists call extratropical transition, and the resulting instability is rarely a welcome image on a forecasting desk. Extratropical cyclones are difficult to predict: Their irregularity means they defy most modeling systems, sometimes leaving forecasters helpless when it comes to predicting their intensity or track. They're notorious for turning on a dime or erupting with newfound ferocity in what can seem like the blink of an eye, and often in the most unlikely of places. In 1954, extratropical remnants of Hurricane Hazel killed eighty-one people in and around Toronto, Canada. An extratropical remnant of Tropical Storm Janis left dozens dead and twenty-two thousand people homeless in Korea.

Part of the unpredictability of an extratropical cyclone stems from its generation and locomotion. Unlike a hurricane, extratropical systems derive their energy from a complex interaction between differing conditions in the atmosphere. Where two extreme temperature differentials and systems of atmospheric pressure meet, a powerful instability known as a barclonic system occurs. Those conditions drive an extratropical system, increasing its size as its core weakens. Along the way, that system will also become distorted and asymmetrical as it joins other fronts in the atmosphere.

These factors were expected to come to bear on Tony over the next twenty-four hours. Until then, all forecasters could do was hold their breath. That, and check on the storm's growing twin down in the southern Caribbean Sea. There, Sandy was forming a ragged eye as warm air continued to spiral up, up, up, feeding the storm and creating tightly spun winds. The storm was feeding itself, building denser clouds and stronger winds that now stretched out across a hundred miles. Inside the storm, pressure continued to drop, creating a vacuum capable of raising sea level as it sucked in more wet air. As the storm passed over the ocean, it pulled with enough force to create an enormous bubble of water — a kind of low-slung mountain of water that moved with the storm.

Forecasters were still at a loss as to what the storm would do next. "I have rarely seen such a perfect case for chaos theory so willingly showing its ugly face," wrote the forecaster at the Upton, New York, NWS office.

For most scientists, chaos theory can be a ton of fun to study. It feels like a fun house for theorists: It's the pursuit of surprise, of accounting for the unaccountable. It's about delighting in disorder, whether that disorder appears in stock markets or the behavior of your neighbor. Chaos theory is about accepting the fact that tiny, imperceptible effects can have gargantuan consequences that we won't even know about until they are practically on top of us. The theory was first proposed by Edward Lorenz, a meteorologist at MIT. Lorenz was, like most in his profession, utterly baffled by just how often weather forecasts failed. He wanted to know why. And, after a great deal of study, he came to a conclusion as elegant as it is simple: Because we can never know the origins of an event in absolute detail, we also cannot predict its conclusion in perfect detail. Any error we make in initial calculations will grow exponentially as the event progresses, ultimately making prediction impossible. Lorenz presented his findings in a 1972 lecture for the American Association for the Advancement of Science titled, "Predictability: Does the Flap of a Butterfly's Wings in Brazil Set Off a Tornado in

Texas?" The theory he postulated there (namely, that yes, a butterfly may very well spur a tornado in Texas or a hurricane in the North Atlantic) sparked a revolution that impacted all of science. Certainty, we now knew, was impossible.

That idea makes for fantastic conversation at academic conferences. It makes meteorologists crazy. The recognition that weather can be impossible to predict perfectly doesn't mean it can't be predicted in terms of probabilities. But we don't have an intuitive grasp of probabilities, which makes weather forecasting that much more difficult. In the case of Sandy, the limits of predictability were starting to make pinning down the storm seem like a wild-goose chase. Even the best models, wrote the Upton meteorologist, were producing extremely divergent outcomes:

> ALTHOUGH THERE ARE INFINITE SOLUTIONS TO THE CURRENTLY EVOLVING PATTERN . . . IN GENERAL IT SHOULD BE QUITE CLEAR THAT THERE WILL BE AN IMPRESSIVE-TO-EXTREME TROPICAL-TO-EXTRATROPICAL SYSTEM DEVELOPING OFF THE EAST COAST THIS WEEKEND AND INTO EARLY NEXT WEEK . . . ONE THAT

WILL HAVE PAPERS WRITTEN ABOUT IT IN YEARS TO COME. IT IS IMPOSSIBLE TO COVER EACH OF THE VARYING SOLUTIONS . . . BUT WE CAN ROUGHLY BREAK IT DOWN INTO THREE POSSIBLE OUTCOMES:

1 — SANDY MOVES INLAND . . . BECOMES EXTRATROPICAL WHILE ITS REMNANT CONTINUES TO MOVE WESTWARD INTO SOMEWHERE WITHIN NYS. THIS PRODUCES A WHOLE BUNCH OF RARE FORECAST ISSUES . . . WITH HEAVY RAIN . . . HIGHER ELEVATION SNOW . . . AND A NE WIND MONDAY INTO TUESDAY.

2 — SANDY MOVES INTO NEW ENGLAND . . . BECOMES EXTRATROPICAL BEFORE OR AFTER LANDFALL . . . BUT A SECONDARY SYSTEM FORCES NEW LOW DEVELOPMENT INLAND WITH COLD AIR MOVING IN FROM THE WEST AND A SURGE OF TROPICAL MOISTURE WRAPPING AROUND THE DYING EXTRA-TROPICAL SYSTEM. THIS TOO WOULD PRODUCE AN ELEVATION SNOW EVENT . . . WITH LOTS OF RAIN AND POSSIBLY SOME WIND TOO MONDAY AND TUESDAY.

3 — SANDY MOVES HARMLESSLY

OUT TO SEA AND BECOMES A FANTASTIC FISH STORM. ANOTHER SYSTEM EVOLVES AND SPREADS PRECIPITATION ACROSS THE REGION . . . OR MAYBE THIS SYSTEM DOES NOT EVEN EXIST.

WITH SUCH WILDLY VARYING SOLUTIONS . . . WE HAVE NO CHOICE BUT TO FORECAST A CHANCE OF RAIN . . . AND HIGHER ELEVATION SNOW SUNDAY NIGHT THROUGH MONDAY NIGHT.

It was an unimpressive forecast for a most unusual situation, and the forecasters knew it: *A chance of rain, when a record-breaking hurricane might be on its way?*

Senior Hurricane Specialist Mike Brennan was at the forecasting desk at the NHC that morning. He was a brand-new dad; his eyes were bleary on a good day. And on this day, they were even more so. Sandy had grown to hurricane strength: The latest data from the Hurricane Hunters confirmed it. Their dropsondes were registering winds as high as 99 miles per hour; the SFMR was recording sustained winds of 80 miles per hour. Inside the storm, pressure was dropping, creating an even stronger vacuum capable of sucking up still more energy-producing moisture. Sandy was going to keep growing. And the forecaster at Upton was right: What would happen a few days out was, Brennan wrote in his 11:00 A.M. update, "highly uncertain."

The Caribbean, on the other hand, was confronting very different odds. Sandy was on the move, trudging northward, and there was no other weather system that could stop it. In Haiti, the National Meteorological Center and the Department of Civil Protection were issuing a series of press releases urging vigilance across the country. The nation's health institutions were also on red alert. In the Bahamas, Prime Minister Perry Christie activated both the National Emergency Operations Centre and the National Disaster Committee, then took to the airwaves in a national press conference, where he announced the shutdown of schools and banks.

That's good, thought Brennan. *They've got it.*

The forecaster's real concern, however, was Jamaica. Sandy was just one hundred miles south of the island and on an unstoppable collision course. Brennan picked up a landline and called the Meteorological Service of Jamaica. He wanted to make sure they knew what they were in for.

Richard Pasch says that was the first sign

this storm was getting serious.

"Making that call is the biggest decision we make in any given year, and usually the lives of thousands are at stake. That requires a lot of trust on both ends of the line."

Over the years, forecasters in the NHC have formed strong friendships with their peers in Caribbean offices. And the tone on the phone is often light. Chris Landsea does a pretty good imitation of a Jamaican accent — enough to get a few appreciative laughs from his colleagues in Kingston. But on this particular morning, he stood by quietly as Brennan spoke to his Jamaican counterpart. New data from the Hurricane Hunters was streaming in: The SFMR had measured winds of 100 miles per hour in the storm, more than enough to make it a proper hurricane. And conditions surrounding the storm were only going to make it stronger. Landsea could feel the dread on both ends of the line.

"You never want to make that kind of call," he says. "Living in Miami, we know all too well what it's like to be bracing for a storm of that magnitude."

A few minutes later, Brennan's morning storm discussion was posted on the NHC website: Based on the forecast, a tropical storm watch was now in effect for the eastern Florida coast. Landsea sucked in his breath. *All too well indeed,* he thought, staring with newfound intensity at the pictures of the growing storm.

Noon
Kingston, Jamaica
78°F
Barometer: 29.15 inches (falling)
Winds: 43 mph
Precipitation: Heavy rain

Jamaica hadn't seen a direct hurricane hit in nearly twenty-five years — not since Gilbert plowed across the island in 1988, wreaking $4 billion (US) in damages and killing an estimated forty-five people. The storm had been a titanic disaster for many reasons, not the least of which was the tepid response to forecasted warnings: It'd been so long since the previous hurricane strike that few Jamaicans could say they had experienced such a storm firsthand. For most of the island's residents, a hurricane was just an idea — difficult to imagine beyond what they'd seen in pictures or on TV. Further complicating the situation was the fact that the nation's emergency alert system was slow to issue a hurricane warning for Gilbert, giving residents just three daylight hours to prepare. Most people took a leisurely approach to storm preparations, even after the warning was issued: They just assumed they'd have time to resume their work the following morning, but they learned the hard way that preparing for a hurricane is virtually impossible in 70-mile-per-hour winds, capable of ripping away plywood and tarps faster than you can secure them to windows and leaky shanties. By the end of the next day, Gilbert had wiped out the island's entire banana and poultry industries; it tore the roofs off an estimated 80 percent of all homes. A full four hundred thousand people — a quarter of the island's population — were left homeless. Surveying the damage in the wake of Gilbert, Edward Seaga, then prime minister, said that Jamaica looked an awful lot "like Hiroshima after the atom bomb."

Scars from the storm can still be seen across the struggling island. So, as Sandy bore down, few residents were willing to take their chances again. In Kingston, residents woke up to a stern government-issued hurricane warning: The Office of Disaster Preparedness and Emergency Management had already issued a mandatory evacuation for low-lying areas. Across the country, 140 shelters had been opened. Red Cross staff and more than one hundred volunteers were in the process of prepositioning emergency supplies: hygiene kits and blankets, jerrycans of water and fuel, tins of mackerel and beans. Prime Minister Portia Simpson-Miller, who had been visiting Canada to commemorate years of successful tourist relations between the two nations, aborted her trip and sped home. Meanwhile, Acting Prime Minister Peter Phillips took to the airwaves, announcing that "all Jamaicans must take the threat of this storm seriously." To demonstrate just how serious he was, he then promptly issued a mandatory curfew.

This time around, most residents heeded the warning, using the remaining daylight hours to prepare for the storm. Mobs formed at the island's gas stations, pumping many of them dry. Workers rallied together to board up medical clinics and stores. Wealthier residents attempted to shore up their gated homes, hoping to barricade themselves from possible storm surge. Those in the poorer neighborhoods roamed vacant lots and dumps, looking for anything that might reinforce already leaky roofs.

Within hours, all schools and governmental offices had closed. So had both of Jamaica's international airports, along with Kingston's massive port. There, fishermen toiled to secure their boats, covering outboards with old T-shirts and lashing hulls to whatever they could find. On the northern coast, all three piers at Montego Bay's enormous cruise-ship terminal stood ominously empty: The forecast was enough for both Royal Caribbean and Carnival cruise lines to cancel their scheduled itineraries, diverting more than eight thousand passengers out to sea and away from the storm.

As the day progressed, the rains became a steady downpour. They sheeted down over the mountains, creating first ugly brown waterfalls and then full-blown mudslides. They loosened trees and boulders, sending them plummeting down toward villages. One struck a seventy-four-year-old man as he struggled to get inside his home, killing him instantly.

The Jamaica Constabulary Force, clad in bulletproof vests and riot helmets, patrolled the streets looking for looters. The rain continued to pour, but there was still no wind. Everyone on the island, though, hunkered down, waiting, as the growing storm lumbered northward at 10 miles per hour. Residents of Kingston's shantytowns — people who lived in the hundreds of ramshackle abodes built of tarp and pallets and splintered plywood — would soon be the most vulnerable. And they knew it.

"Everybody's worried about it here," Philip Salmon, a dreadlocked laborer living in a shanty near the American Embassy, told the Associated Press. "This storm is no small thing."

The storm was still eighty miles south of Kingston, though its pace was increasing — as was its rate of development.

The Caribbean Sea, normally a dulcet, clear blue, first heralded the storm, churning alternately white and brown, as it picked up sand and sediment. The waves grew with no direction — no organization — as they raged with froth and marched closer and closer to shore. They overtook beaches and seawalls, knifed through harbors, then inundated the streets, where they collided with mountain runoff, creating a chaos of thick, confused water. It poured through gates surrounding upscale homes where, inside, residents sat crowded around candles, listening to the winds howling. In the few international hotels located in Kingston's financial district, tourists hunkered down in their bathrooms, afraid the windows in their rooms would implode. Below them, metal roofs spun off homes and careened into parked cars.

Nearby, the storm flooded mangroves,

where fishermen had relocated their boats in a desperate attempt to save them. As the water poured through, it carried with it many of the other mangrove occupants, including at least a dozen crocodiles, who — dazed — were relocated in streets and front yards as far away as the city of Portmore, itself a reclaimed swamp. There, the animals quickly regained their senses and began roaming the neighborhoods, impervious to the wind, rain, and human sensibilities.

The temperature began to drop. By 2:00 P.M., thermometers read 74 degrees — a new record low for the normally balmy nation. At 3:00 P.M., Sandy's eye made landfall just south of Kingston. The storm brought with it winds of 116 miles per hour and no sign they would diminish as it swept across the island toward Cuba. In Kingston's shanty-towns, roofs continued to take flight. Tree branches crushed those shanties that remained, exposing mattresses and microwaves. Outside the city, entire banana plantations were decimated, in some cases leaving not even a single tree standing. More than seventy-four hundred acres of farmland were destroyed. An estimated one hundred schools and thirty-six hundred houses were, too. Nearly twenty inches of rain fell in Kingston alone. Portions of the nearby Portland Parish reported rainfall of twenty-eight inches. The water kept rolling, flooding. It tried to escape through drains and canals, but most of the public works in the impoverished city had long since become clogged with trash and overgrown vegetation. So instead, brown rivers flooded roads, making many impassable. Those not completely flooded were soon inundated with streams of curious residents. Throughout the capital and surrounding towns, police attempted to maintain the imposed curfew, but that didn't prevent scores of people from stepping outside, some wearing bright yellow slickers, others sporting trash bags with crudely cut holes for arms and heads. They carried tattered golf umbrellas or, in some cases, broken boards that they shook in front of camera crews, as if defying the storm. At night, the police patrolled by the dozens, still wearing heavy bulletproof vests, and now carrying even heavier guns. But that didn't stop the looters, one of whom shot and seriously injured an officer.

By the end of the day, officials were already estimating storm damage upwards of $100 million. Nearly two thousand Jamaicans were stranded in shelters. And, despite what forecasters had hoped and even predicted, Sandy was still showing no signs of weakening.

"We started to catch on pretty quickly that something was up with this storm," says Pasch. "It was starting to act outside the box."

The storm continued to metastasize, intensifying rapidly as it crossed the Cayman Trench. The tight mass of thunderheads forming its eyewall now rose fifty thousand feet in the air — nearly scraping the ceiling of the troposphere. Down at the base of the clouds, the spinning winds sucked up moisture from the ocean, only to send it gushing back down as angry brown rain. In Puerto Rico, a man was swept away by a swollen river just outside the town of Juana Díaz. Two people also drowned while trying to cross surging rivers in the Dominican Republic, where thirty thousand residents were forced to evacuate after their homes and neighborhoods flooded. At least three people died there, and the government estimates that damage to the nation's agricultural sector was more than $30 million. But it was neighboring Haiti that perhaps suffered the worst, even though it was not in the direct path of Hurricane Sandy.

Initial reports gave conflicting accounts of the casualties there, but the number soon found a grim — and growing — consistency. People drowned trying to cross overflowing streams. Their shanties were crushed beneath the weight of hills sliding into the sea. A forty-year-old mother and her four children were buried when one such mudslide destroyed their home.

"If the rain continues, for sure we'll have more people die," morgue deputy Joseph Franck Laporte told an AP reporter. "The earth cannot hold the rain." And Haiti, already compromised by the 2010 earthquake, could not hold its refugees. More than seventeen thousand people poured into the nation's temporary shelters, some packed in so tightly they could not sit or lie down.

Haitians are familiar with hurricanes and the havoc they wreak. They have an expression there: *lapli ap tonbe,* which means things are going really badly, but literally translates as "the rain is falling." And when the rain falls in Haiti, so does much of the landscape. The island underwent severe deforestation as a result of Hurricane Hazel in 1954. In the years that followed, agriculture and industry continued the process until, by the turn of the millennium, less than 2 percent of the island's trees remained. More than fifteen thousand acres of topsoil are washed away by rain each year. When those rains are as heavy as they potentially can be in tropical systems, it can seem as if the entire country is streaming into the ocean. It is a country with few hospitals, one in which years of political instability have resulted in crumbling infrastructure, no building codes, and an emergency management plan described as "fledgling" by scholars. When Hurricane Flora struck in 1963, the storm killed five thousand people in Haiti. Neighboring Dominican Republic lost just four hundred. In 1994, Hurricane Gordon claimed the lives of more than eleven hundred Haitians. The six other nations in the storm's path lost a combined twenty-four lives.

As Sandy approached, the Haitian government issued a red alert, which activated the National Risk Management and Disaster Plan and warned residents that the hurricane was imminent.

Lines of people, many carrying their worldly possessions on their heads, made their way toward safer ground. However, for many of Haiti's residents, there was little they could do. Tens of thousands still resided in temporary tent encampments, having lost their homes in the 2010 earthquake and then again when Tropical Storm

Isaac struck just two months before Sandy. That storm killed twenty-four and left thousands homeless. It also caused more than $200 million in damage to Haiti's agricultural economy. In the intervening months, many Haitian people were already on the precipice of starvation and disease, as they struggled to stay one step ahead of malnutrition and cholera.

Many tried to find safety in firehouses and emergency shelters, but discovered they were already filled well beyond capacity. With few wastewater treatment facilities, hospitals, or residents able to store multiple days of food and water, Haiti's miseries are far from over once a storm passes overhead. Conditions deteriorated rapidly. One woman, a twenty-eight-year-old mother of three, told the Associated Press that she and her family had no choice but to remain in their home, fashioned from crudely hung tarps; the shelters, she said, were simply "unlivable."

As the rains fell there, rivers leapt their banks, flooding neighborhoods and shutting down water-treatment facilities. Houses crumbled as if made entirely of sand. At the Port-au-Prince market, vendors caught in the storm struggled to build impromptu rafts out of pallets, tires, and produce boxes.

They trudged their way through muddy water as high as their chests, hoping to ferry their carrots and parsley, their pork and eggs, to safety. And, just as in Jamaica, the rain continued to fall, turning streets into raging white water. It swept away cars and shacks, and drowned livestock — cows, chickens, pigs, and goats, mostly — by the thousands. The government estimates that more than sixty-four thousand livestock animals were lost. So, too, were entire plantations: acres of corn and beans, bananas and peanuts, cassava and rice.

Speaking to an aid worker, one man described his experience in the kind of plain speak only a person who has already endured profound hardship can muster: "When Sandy hit there was heavy rain and sudden gusts of wind. After three hours my house began to crack. My wife and I began to pray as our children cried. We wanted to call for help but we didn't have a mobile phone. At the end of the night, a big part of our house collapsed and we lost five children and some animals."

By the end of the day, more than two hundred thousand Haitians were homeless. But for many, that was just the start of the horror that awaited them. As the rains continued, reports of cholera erupted; just a few cases here and there at first, but soon it was clear an epidemic was at hand. Before long, the number of confirmed cases would reach twelve thousand — with at least fifty-four dead. That figure, too, would keep rising.

That, says Senior Hurricane Specialist Eric Blake, was one of the hardest facts he'd ever had to confront in more than ten years at the National Hurricane Center. Surveying news of the devastation in Haiti, he felt sick. Powerless. Haitians heeded the evacuation calls. They tried to make it to shelters. Those who couldn't get into town made their way to higher ground or built makeshift bunkers in their homes. None of that, concluded Blake, was enough to save them from the growing storm. That terrified him. "People did exactly what they were supposed to do. And they still died."

4:15 P.M.
Atlantic Ocean
83°F
Barometer: 29.86 inches (falling)
Winds: 15 mph (ESE)
Skies: Overcast
Seas: 1–2 Feet (building)

The Disney *Fantasy* was still docked in St. Thomas when the McNamaras heard about the updated forecast. Everett was feeling better, but the family was lying low and was hunkered down in the ship's movie theater. The film paused, and Captain Tom Forberg came over the intercom, announcing that the ship would not be departing for Castaway Cay, Disney's private island in the Bahamas. Instead, they would be heading out to sea in an attempt to avoid the worst of the storm. The kids groaned. Jamie's heart sank. As they made their way back to their room, they watched as families began returning to the ship, flushed from the sun and their time onshore. She began rethinking her decision to stay on board that day. But mostly, she says, she was just really bummed. A few hours later, she watched as the ship pulled away from the dock. Three or four enormous cruise ships remained in the port. Clouds were building on the horizon. McNamara remembers having a sense that maybe they should stay — that the other cruise lines might be on to something. At dinner, she began hearing rumors from some of the other passengers that this was a test. They told her Disney wanted to put the *Fantasy* through its paces on its inaugural voyage across the Atlantic, but that the ship hadn't encountered the kind of extreme weather the crew had hoped for.

Maybe, speculated some of the people at the McNamaras' table, *they were driving into the storm so the captain could really assess the ship in rough seas.* That idea terrified the mother of three. Disney reps assured her nothing could be further from the truth — that they were, instead, monitoring the storm closely in an attempt to avoid the worst of it. The press release issued by the company that evening echoed the sentiment: "The safety and security of our guests is always our top priority. If necessary, our captains are always prepared to alter the ships' courses or itineraries to navigate away from inclement weather."

Why, then, wondered McNamara, *are we traveling toward the storm?*

Millicent Frick, also a first-time cruise-ship passenger, was wondering the exact same thing. Earlier in the day, Frick and her husband had departed Miami aboard the *Norwegian Sky,* a seventy-seven-thousand-ton ship capable of carrying more than two thousand passengers. Frick, the mother of three and a Christian life coach, had boarded the ship with other participants in the Grace & Strength Lifestyle, a biblically based weight-loss group, for a reunion of sorts. The twenty-five women had met online while they were participants in the program. Two years later, they were still in regular contact as coaches, but few had met in person. So there had been a lot of screaming and hugging in the airport two days earlier, along with a little crying. And that outpouring of emotional celebrating had continued through the night at their Miami hotel. The cruise, says Frick, was a chance for them all to finally come together and commemorate the work they had done — and the relationships they had formed along the way. But the sense of revelry dampened somewhat when Frick and the other life coaches received word that their cruise ship was about to hurl headlong into the hurricane.

By 9:00 A.M. that day, a tropical storm watch had been issued for Miami and the surrounding area. By noon, most of the Bahamas — less than one hundred miles due east of Florida — were under a tropical storm warning. That afternoon, the weather alert would quickly morph, first into a hurricane watch and then a hurricane warning. Sandy was approaching — and fast. The cruise line contacted Frick and the other passengers of the *Norwegian Sky* and informed them that the massive ship would be departing early that day in an attempt to get out of port before Sandy struck. It wasn't news the first-time cruise passenger wanted to hear. Still, Frick and her fellow group members decided they'd try to make the best of it.

The seas grew rough almost as soon as the ship left its Miami berth. Frick remembers a lot of swaying and rocking that afternoon. The ship stopped for a scheduled afternoon at Grand Bahama, but the damp and dreary weather left few passengers interested in a beach day. Back on board, the movement of the ship continued to intensify. "It was like trying to walk on a waterbed," Frick says. The crew began handing out free doses of Dramamine. By dinner, there were as many people lining up for the little white tablets as there were people queuing for banquet tables. As dinner approached, the seas began to build. Captain Ron Chrastina was now making regular weather announcements about the storm over the ship's PA system. He assured passengers that the crew was tracking the storm and its path. They hadn't quite decided what they were going to do, but they were going to do their best to stay out of the worst of the hurricane.

"At that point, I was pretty much hoping and praying we weren't going to hit it," says Frick.

People began having trouble staying upright. Even seasoned cruise passengers were talking about how bad the conditions were. At dinner that night, Frick had the sensation that the ship was cresting each wave only to slam down hard on the other side, filling the interior with the sounds of hundreds of thousands of tons of crashing metal. "It was difficult to get used to how noisy it was," she said. "It was just so loud in there." Still, throughout most of the dinner service the passengers seemed at ease, and they laughed at one another as drinks wobbled away from their hands and forks missed their intended targets. But by the close of the meal, many of those same people were growing ill, including Frick's husband, Ben. "It wasn't pretty," she admits. So the Fricks turned in early that night, retiring to their cabin, where they could flip through television channels and try to ignore the ceaseless rocking of the ship. As they made their way through the dial, they stopped on Fox News, which had dedicated its entire coverage that night to the very storm now overtaking them. That, says Frick, felt a whole lot like watching your own made-for-TV movie, and one in which you really wish you didn't have the starring role. "It was bizarre. Really bizarre. I kept asking myself, 'Is this really happening?' "

Radar images showed a fully formed hurricane — angry swirls of red pulsing out from a distinct eye twenty miles wide and hovering just south of Cuba. Hurricane Hunter data revealed that the storm's peak winds were mounting — and accelerating at a rate no one, not even the National Hurricane Center, had expected. That intensity, warned the NHC, was based on an amalgamation of data points. "And this could be conservative," insisted the published discussions.

> IT SHOULD BE NOTED THAT SUBJECTIVE SATELLITE INTENSITY ESTIMATES . . . ARE AT OR ABOVE 100 KT. THIS SUGGESTS THAT SANDY IS LIKELY TO STRENGTHEN FURTHER BEFORE LANDFALL IN CUBA IN A FEW HOURS.

Frick worried about what her kids were thinking, knowing that they were probably watching the same news — maybe scared to death about their parents' plight. "Growing up in Mississippi, I had been in plenty of hurricanes before. But there isn't anything like being out at sea in one." While Ben tried to sleep, Millicent watched the rain pelt their cabin windows and the caps of waves as they slammed into the ship. As she looked out through the blurry portholes, she was certain she spied the light of another ship somewhere off in the distance. *Thank God,* she thought. *At least we're not alone.*

9:45 P.M.
New London, Connecticut
50°F
Barometer: 30.21 inches (rising)
Winds: Calm
Skies: Scattered clouds
Seas: Calm

The TV was on at Hanafin's Irish Pub, but few people were paying attention. Instead, a little cluster had formed around the bar: a few guys with long beards and flannel shirts rolled up to reveal strong forearms. A couple of young women, lithe and tan. They were the *Bounty* crew, and they were doing what they did best on land: charming everyone in the bar they had chosen as their clubhouse for the night. They chased pints with top-label whiskey. They laughed a lot. They even persuaded the bartender to stick around long after her shift had ended. But by 10:00 P.M., people had started to peel off. Jessica Black, the new cook, was about to arrive on a late train from Hartford, and the crew agreed a delegation should meet her, help her with her luggage, show her they're a family. So they made their way to the train station — an unusually elegant two-and-a-half-story building with deep red brick and a dramatic sloping roof. From there, you could see all three of the *Bounty*'s enormous masts.

Hanafin's was just a block up or so — an easy walk. So Claudene and a couple of the other crew members stayed a little bit longer — long enough to see Brad Field, the local NBC station's chief meteorologist, standing in front of a large radar screen with an angry swirl of color spiraling over much of the Caribbean. But Claudene and the other crew didn't notice: Who went to a pub to watch the news?

Bars were Christian's element. She felt at home there. Back in Hermosa Beach, she'd show up at one or another wearing roller skates and cornrows. When she was super poor, she kept track of which dives had the cheapest happy hours, which bands would let her sit in for a song or two. When she was flush, she'd buy everyone enormous fishbowls filled with blue cocktails and plastic sharks. Guys loved it — this tiny, sexy woman on skates, nibbling on the tail of a plastic shark. She hardly ever went home alone.

That night, she had a rare moment of solitude as she stood outside Hanafin's, watching as the 11:31 P.M. train pulled into the station. The day's unexpected heat had lingered, and she didn't need a jacket. It felt comfortable just to stand, a cigarette in her hand. Amanda Sherer, Hanafin's bartender, was just about to leave. She found Claudene outside the door, looking out at the approaching train and humming Janis Joplin. Christian loved songs that were a little broody and raspy — songs with a lot of soul. Something about Joplin's voice — sweet and gravelly at the same time — always got her. She tried to emulate it in her own recorded songs. You can hear it, the rasp of cigarette smoke, the way she could go deep and sultry or belt it out high like the gospel singer she could have been. "Me and Bobby McGee" was her favorite. She told Sherer that, and the two of them worked their way through a few verses, no one else around, just watching the night get darker as lights went out across town. It was late and very still when she got back to the ship. And it seemed like the whole world had gone to bed.

11:45 P.M.
Havana, Cuba
69°F
Barometer: 29.77 inches (steady)
Winds: 19 mph (NE)
Skies: Cloudy
Seas: 10–12 feet

At the Hotel Roc Presidente in Havana, Lixion Avila sat on a low-slung bed, his laptop open in front of him. It was late, but the forecaster couldn't sleep. Outside, he could hear waves crashing against Malecón, a seawall and promenade on the city's north side. The surf was growing. The sound dug deep into Avila's consciousness, sparking memories of a boyhood spent fascinated by storm swell.

Every meteorologist has a pivotal storm — a defining moment when they saw just how forceful weather can be, when they stood, dumbstruck and captivated, and said, *I want to dedicate my life to this strange power.* For Avila, that storm was Hurricane Flora. He was twelve when the Category 3 storm swept across the Caribbean, killing an estimated seventy-two hundred people. The hurricane pummeled Cuba with 124-mile-per-hour winds and forced the evacuation of more than forty thousand people on that island alone. The historic town of

Santiago de Cuba recorded one hundred inches of rain as the storm passed overhead; it swept away homes, bridges, and entire fields of crops, and left people stranded for days on rooftops. It was, says then–Miami Weather Bureau Chief Gordon Dunn, "the most damaging hurricane to Haiti and Cuba since the days of Columbus." Because of its magnitude, the storm prompted the retirement of the name Flora. "Fern" was the moniker given in its place.

Avila remembers everything about that storm — including the way the sea looked. As the hurricane approached, he grabbed his fishing pole, told his mom he was casting for snapper, and then spent hours standing at the water's edge, watching the big gray swells grow. This was a power like nothing else on Earth. He was fascinated. And he knew the direction of his life had been forever changed. By the time he moved to Miami to attend graduate school, he had long since committed to a post at the National Hurricane Center.

For Avila, it was the start of a lifelong vocation. Hurricanes define him. *"Ellos son parte de mi alma,"* he says. *They are a part of my soul.*

That was a large part of why Avila couldn't sleep that night. It didn't help that the world's best ballet dancers were assembling all around him. Here were his two great loves, his two great obsessions, vying for his attention. Sandy and ballet. He hopped websites, alternating between the Weather Channel and Met Cuba radar (free to the world, and accessible with even *Sesame Street* Spanish) on the one hand, and Facebook and the schedule for the ballet festival on the other. He couldn't settle on a site — he was feeling torn. This was no small deal for the senior hurricane specialist. When he's not at the forecasting desk, Avila lives in the inner circle of the international ballet world. Prima ballerinas from around the world regularly call him with questions about weather when they're embarking on tours or planning family vacations. "I like ballet. They like hurricanes. It's a perfect relationship," says Avila. His office is a testament to this long-standing relationship: Pictures of the forecaster and superstars of the dance world hang on bulletin boards and his office door, the women small and demurely dressed in draping clothes and coiled scarves, Avila all but towering over them in well-pressed slacks and smart shirts. The locations vary — New York, Havana, Miami — but the smiles and genuine affection are always the same. Avila is more than eligible for retirement, but he likes to joke that he intends to keep his position until he sees a job posting for senior luggage carrier to ballerinas.

That night, those same ballerinas were messaging him, asking if he thought their planes would make it. Some of the dancers from the American Ballet Theatre were worried their costumes might be held up. And then there was the unmistakable allure of watching the storm's approach and the continued divergence of the hurricane models, ten of which still predicted the storm would move harmlessly out to sea. Or would it?

He checked the Cuban radar, looking for clues. And what he didn't find worried him. Normally, a wide swath of high pressure sits over a patch of the Atlantic Ocean near Bermuda. Whether they've known it or not, sailors and coastal residents alike have depended upon the swath for centuries. It doesn't do all that much, but it's as dense as a wall, and storms tend to ricochet off of it, preserving trade routes and cities up and down the Eastern Seaboard.

For the first time in decades, that high had shifted to the east just as a hurricane approached, effectively destroying the last best barrier preventing the storm from making landfall. A similar shift is what allowed the 1938 hurricane to make its way as far north as Massachusetts. Unless another high swept in to thwart the storm's advance, Sandy now appeared prepared to follow suit.

Avila wanted to see more. But his cell phone was ringing, too. The dancers were worried.

"It was like *Swan Lake,*" says Avila. "The black swan — the witch — was pulling me toward the storm. The white swan was pulling me toward the dancers. I was being yanked in both ways, toward both of my passions."

And then an e-mail notification flashed on his screen. A NOAA address. Important. Work trumps even ballet, says Avila. He opened it. The Hurricane Hunters were trying to get into the storm, and that meant they needed to get into Cuban airspace. They're the only American plane regularly allowed there, but they still need authorization to enter. Cuban air traffic controllers, it seemed, had other things going on, what with a major hurricane bearing down on their country. So the Hurricane Hunters were in a holding pattern. And that meant the NHC forecasters were paralyzed. Without new data, there'd be no new forecast. Could Avila help?

He picked up his phone, called a friend at the Instituto de Meteorología de Cuba. "Hey, Jose," Avila said in perfectly accented Spanish. "Those guys really need to get in there." An hour later, the C-130 was overhead.

Thursday

3:00 A.M.
Cuban National Air Space
78°F
Barometer: 28.77 inches (falling)
Winds: 102 mph (ESE)
Skies: Heavy rain
Seas: 30 feet (building)

Sandy was mere miles from Cuba's western provinces when the Hurricane Hunters' C-130 slipped into the storm's core. The hurricane was about to make landfall just west of Santiago de Cuba, a port city bedecked with baroque architecture and home to half a million people. Rich Harter, always animated on a flight, was even more so this time.

"I think we all get an extra charge out of these big storms," he said. "We love being up there."

Harter had spent the previous day pacing around the temporary station in Savannah, trying to get the more mundane parts of his job done — scheduling flights, crunching numbers from the data streaming into the base. He'd been trying to give himself a break from the constant radar-checking he'd been doing earlier in the week, but that was proving difficult. "Being a weather guy, I'm pretty interested. Sometimes I can't help myself, so I start peeking." He'd combed online weather sites during his off hours, and logged on to the Hurricane Hunter aircraft data stream from his personal computer. "It's the next best thing to being on the airplane," he says.

Still, the meteorologist had been getting impatient with next best things. He wanted to see what the storm was doing. When he finally did, even he was impressed.

As they approached the storm, the pilot dropped the plane down to one thousand feet. They were now completely shrouded in clouds, rendering the sea surface — and everything else — largely invisible. Those few moments when Harter could catch a peek of the ocean below, he saw a mess. "It was chaotic," he said. "Large rolling waves moving through a carpet of white foam, mixed with the green of the sea. I was very glad I wasn't down there."

The plane banked into the center of the

storm, aiming for its eyewall, where winds were now maxing out at 124 miles per hour. Harter strapped himself in. Tight. "I've been in a couple of hurricanes where it felt like the bottom was dropping out from under you — like the Tower of Terror at Disney World," he said. When that happens, anything not strapped down — dropsondes, coolers, meteorologists, gumbo — takes flight, ricocheting off of walls and passengers alike. When things get really bad, heavy equipment can break its straps and become deadly. Weather Underground Director of Meteorology Jeff Masters was on one such hurricane flight. As the plane jolted through turbulence, their two-hundred-pound life raft broke free and smashed through the cabin. Toolboxes broke open, turning wrenches and screwdrivers into potentially deadly shrapnel. They collided midair with errant soft drink cans, which then exploded on impact and blanketed the entire fuselage with sticky liquid and shredded metal. That was just the beginning. Soon, the charged air of the cabin was also filled with computers and briefcases, disks and barometers, water bottles and headsets. They split open chairs and fabric; they bruised the arms of people shielding themselves from blows. All that chaos began to feel trivial, however, when Masters looked out the window and saw that one of the plane's engines had burst into flames. Another looked like it had been in a major collision and trailed debris behind. Masters sincerely thought he might die that day.

His was an extreme flight, but there are plenty in which the safety of the crew seems in jeopardy. It's not uncommon for radar to fail in the kind of conditions a Hurricane Hunter plane encounters. Lightning strikes happen more than you might expect, too. And sometimes they are strong enough to knock out a plane's electrical system for a few seconds or more. That's plenty of time to scare even a seasoned crew member.

You can't fully prepare for conditions like that, but the Hurricane Hunters do the best they can. They are required to train in altitude chambers and complete extensive survival-school certification — including four days of backcountry training in the Cascades and deep-sea survival training in Florida, along with a three-day course that culminates, oddly enough, with a parasail. Still, he says, all that training feels a little artificial once you're actually in the center of a major storm. It's an experience no simulator can really mimic. "The older you get, it seems like the worse it is," says Harter. "I can't take it as much as I used to."

With little more than the radar to assist him, Harter directed the pilot through the feeder rainbands, which spiral out from the center of the storm, bringing with them all the energy the hurricane can no longer contain — now made manifest in torrential downpours and even tornadoes. Beyond these bands loomed the eyewall — now rising up to sixty thousand feet and into the stratosphere. The storm was a monster, and it was about to swallow the plane. The C-130 struggled to break through. Harter's station went dark.

A hurricane eyewall is a vertical wall of tightly packed clouds where the convergence of wind and energy is so strong that they become a megastorm themselves: a storm inside a storm, with its own identity and patterns. Often, says Harter, that megastorm clobbers their plane with hail, lightning, and winds of more than two hundred miles per hour. Sandy's eyewall, however, seemed to be of a more mild sort — heavy wind and mostly rain.

"It was like being in a shaky car wash," Harter says.

That perplexed him. He became even more interested than usual in what the dropsondes had to say and spent the majority of the trip strapped to his desk, poring over the numbers coming in. He forgot to drink. His Subway sandwich — ham, this time — went untouched.

"You're all charged up, got a lot of adrenaline going, so it doesn't seem like you're getting tired or dehydrated, says Harter. "We were pretty busy up there."

And what he saw had him concerned: wind gusts first of 90 knots, then 95. A few minutes later, those figures leapt up again: 110 knots; then 120; 126. By the time the pilots turned the C-130 around, Harter had registered gusts over 140 knots. Hurricane Sandy was now a Category 3 storm. In total, the full strength of Sandy would batter the island nation for more than five hours, destroying 17,000 homes and damaging another 226,000. The winds were relentless: One resident of Santiago de Cuba described them as "the roar of lions." They and the rains they brought decimated coffee and cane plantations, tearing down mills and processing plants as they went by. They blew out the windows of schools and airports. In one small agricultural community, 250 homes — a full 80 percent of all the residential structures there — lost their roofs. Nine people were killed in Santiago de Cuba, including a four-month-old baby boy and an eighty-four-year-old man. In Guantánamo, where the storm forced the US military to suspend its trial of one of the USS *Cole* bombing suspects, two men were killed after being crushed by uprooted trees. By the time Sandy passed over the island, it had caused $2 billion in damage, making it one of the most damaging hurricanes in Cuba's history.

And no one, not even the National Hurricane Center, had predicted that. Instead, the models had been consistent in their estimates that the storm was unlikely to surpass a Category 1 status, which means winds should not have exceeded 82 knots, or 95 miles per hour.

Lixion Avila says he was as surprised as anyone by the unexpected intensity of the storm, but not by the fact that the NHC got it wrong. If he's learned anything during his years as a meteorologist, it's that there are always as many unknowns as there are knowns.

"Don't be fooled by people who say they know," he warns. "Good meteorologists become very humble very quickly in this business."

Back in Miami, his colleague Richard Pasch took a critical view. "People think we're a lot better than we are," says Pasch. "But the truth of the matter is, we're just not very good at forecasting. We say it all the time: We've got to get a lot better at this."

Criticism over storm forecasting has been a time-honored tradition, going back millennia to Aristotle, who first attempted to explain storm phenomena in his *Meteorology,* and Aratus of Soli, a third-century Greek poet and author of *Phaenomena,* arguably the first formal how-to guide for the amateur weather forecaster. There, Aratus advised readers to look for signs of storms — things like mice throwing straw into the air, ashes that form in the shape of millet seeds, and she-goats rapidly mating with the same male. The horns of the moon, he added, could be equally accurate harbingers: A slender and ruddy moon, he insisted, would herald stiffening winds. The position of the horns, he believed, could predict the intensity of the storm sure to develop.

Not surprisingly, the error rate in forecasting continued unabated under the Aristotelian and Aratus schools of storm prediction. It might have continued to do so, were it not for the invention of an ingenious little device known as the hygrometer, first conceived of by Nicholas of Cusa in 1450 and built by Leonardo da Vinci in 1481. The idea was a simple one: Water has weight. The more humid the air, the more water one ought to be able to collect. And so, based on Nicholas's drawing, Leonardo crafted a simple scale: On one side, he set a large wad of cotton; on the other, a series of removable stones. As the cotton became increasingly saturated, he would add additional stones to maintain equilibrium. The more stones, the more humid the air had become. That, contended Leonardo, was the surest way to predict rain. The hygrometer grew in sophistication over the next several centuries, eventually resembling a kind of lyre, often made of human hair, which contracts and expands in response to moisture in the air. It was joined by the invention of the mercury barometer in 1644, which was the first reliable account of air pressure available to scientists. Scientists soon began to extrapolate a correlation between high pressure and clear, fair days on the one hand, and low pressure with stormy weather on the other. Significant falls in pressure often heralded extreme weather conditions. Barometers, though, were in seriously short supply. And even if you had the means to own one, it would really only tell you what was happening right where you were. That didn't offer much time in terms of planning or storm preparation.

Well into the nineteenth century, meteorological reporting remained capricious at best — particularly where hurricanes were concerned. The first person to predict them with any real accuracy was Father Benito Viñes, a priest and physics professor forced to leave Spain during the Jesuit expulsion. Viñes found safe harbor in Cuba, where he assumed the directorship of the Magnetical and Meteorological Observatory at Belen College, a Jesuit preparatory school founded by Queen Isabella II. There, Viñes and his staff initiated a rigorous and heavily codified system of weather observations, taken ten times a day from Havana. They coupled these with extensive record-keeping — newspaper stories about previous storms, eyewitness accounts, investigations of hurricane-struck regions — and a growing network of regional reporting stations.

The Cuban observatory's model soon became a best practice in the world of storm prediction, and one that the United States was keen to emulate. Each year, tropical storms were responsible for untold loss of lives and fortunes, particularly at sea. It seemed a senseless waste to Dr. Increase A. Lapham, a natural scientist in Milwaukee, who began clipping newspaper articles about maritime casualties and sending them to his congressmen. *Surely,* he wrote, *these disasters could be averted.* Lapham made a persuasive case, and his argument was soon championed not only by the representatives of Wisconsin, but also by politicians from New York and other key ports. Together, they crafted a resolution that would empower the secretary of war to take weather readings at military stations in an effort to predict the appearance of storms on the Great Lakes, the Atlantic Ocean, and the Gulf coasts. President Ulysses S. Grant signed the resolution in 1870. With it, the signal service — America's first official meteorology branch — was born.

A post in the signal service was not for the faint of heart. While it asked its employees to be meteorologists foremost, they were also very much members of the military. The signal service existed as a cavalry division of the Department of War, and recruits were sent to Fort Myers to endure the paces of basic training, including horsemanship and saber-handling. Many of the recruits, recalled the legendary Isaac Cline, were ill-equipped for this kind of work and soon became "badly frightened" by the exercises. Life off the training field was no more pleasant. Bed bugs at the base were common; so were humiliating punishments. Each recruit was given an agonizingly thorough physical exam, including the mapping of their moles — so that they would be easily identifiable if and when they deserted. Once graduated, they were dispatched to yellow fever–ridden Gulf towns and frontier outposts. They weathered oppressive heat and deadly storms and enormous rattlesnakes and locust clouds so thick they darkened the sky.

Even worse was the criticism they endured. Early signal service forecasts were notoriously, miserably wrong. Proverbs that they published (including "Hark! I hear the asses bray, We shall have some rain today" and "Clear moon, Frost soon") resulted in as much public ridicule as weather awareness. And, in truth, they were not much of an improvement on the prophesies of Aratus of Soli.

Neither was their work ethic. Some of the forecasters were no more than dilettantes when it came to their jobs; some pushed the moral bounds considerably further. One famously pawned his federally issued equipment to pay off gambling debts; another turned his office into a boudoir. The head of the agency was found guilty of embezzlement.

To the forecasters' credit, many were doing the very best — and in some cases, heroically great — jobs with incredibly limited information. To predict the future of a storm, you need to know its history, and that required an extensive system of reporting from around the region. Father Viñes attempted that kind of reporting with his network of scientists, and he was assisted in his efforts not only by ship captains willing to take readings, but also by the imperial predilections of Great Britain and France, who had begun to lay a massive network of underwater telegraph lines throughout the Caribbean (Britain's similar efforts in Hong Kong would offer the same benefit to meteorologists studying typhoons there). Soon, Viñes had a robust community of weather reporters in Jamaica and Puerto Rico, along with islands from Barbados to Antigua. Each day, scientists at these stations would send Viñes an account of what they saw: the direction in which clouds were moving, what the barometer was doing, how fast or slow the wind was blowing. Based on this data, Viñes was able to forecast where and how a storm was traveling. In September

1875, he issued his first formal hurricane warning, correctly predicting when and where the storm would make landfall several days before it hit Cuba.

The United States had no such network in the Caribbean, and the high cost of wiring information to Washington soon proved so prohibitive that the forecasters were left to rely upon spotty reports from ships at sea and land-based signal offices. This data included information about wind direction and temperature, along with changes in barometric pressure. That allowed them to form hypotheses about the development of storms and their tracks. The United States issued its first official hurricane warning in August 1873, when forecasters predicted severe storm damage from New Jersey to Connecticut. To warn residents there, the signal service raised special storm flags up and down the coast. Forecasters missed the mark on the storm's track — it made landfall in Newfoundland, and killed more than two hundred people along the way — but the first use of the warning system was considered a success nevertheless.

Its efficacy, however, would prove controversial in subsequent years. In 1875, US forecasters failed to sound a warning as a major hurricane approached Indianola,

Texas. The already busy port city was packed with spectators for a high-profile trial resulting from the long-standing Sutton-Taylor feud, the bloodiest in the state's history. The storm leveled the town, including the signal service building and the courthouse, which allowed Bill Taylor, who was on trial for murder and other crimes, to escape. Forecasters were not so lucky. The chief signal officer in Washington, D.C., had predicted that the hurricane would make landfall in Alabama and ordered warnings issued for that coast. No such precautions were taken for Texas until it was too late. The botched forecast prompted a flurry of accusations ranging from neglect to utter incompetence. Eleven years later, a storm would again assault the city. Again, no signal flag was raised: According to forecasters in Washington, the storm was sure to stay well east of Texas. It didn't. As winds and rain pummeled Indianola, Isaac Reed, a captain in the signal service, remained in his office, telegraphing conditions back to Washington. The building began to seize and ripple around him. Still he remained. By the time he relented and attempted to make his escape, it was too late: The building collapsed, pinning Reed underwater. The rubble soon caught fire, making what was already an unlikely rescue impossible.

In the decades that followed, several catastrophically bad forecasts continued to sully the reputation of meteorologists nationwide. In 1893, US forecasters correctly predicted landfall of a hurricane in New York City. But later that season, they missed a major storm that swept across Louisiana, taking with it the lives of thousands. Amid sharp criticism of their failure to notify residents around New Orleans, forecasters argued that there hadn't been any time: The hurricane, they said, had formed just a couple of days before hitting land. Subsequent investigation would reveal that it had been nearly a week in the making and had moved across the entire Yucatán Peninsula before setting its sights on the Gulf Coast.

Even the venerated Viñes had his share of difficulty in forecasting. The Jesuit scholar advanced a theory of hurricane tracks based on seasonal trends: Early-season storms, he hypothesized, tend to stay well to the south of the Caribbean Sea; mid-season storms curve west-northwest; late-season storms cross the southern United States and then head northeast. There was a certain wisdom to his theory and, indeed, storm trends today tend to bear it out in broad brushstrokes. But such broadness is never enough for accuracy: Hurricanes love to prove exceptions to the rule. In September 1889, Viñes began issuing advisories for a storm "of great intensity and magnitude," which the forecaster predicted would follow a west-northwest path north of Puerto Rico, eventually spinning out into the Atlantic somewhere east of Florida. Instead, the storm surged northward, stalling just off the coast of New Jersey. Caught unawares, the signal service there rushed to issue warnings, but it was too late: Vicious winds had already torn down telegraph lines and disabled railroads, making communication impossible.

The inability to forecast this storm effectively was a particularly hard blow for a meteorological organization already suffering from a compromised reputation. A year later, Congress wrested control of the signal service from the military and, instead, created a civilian organization called the Weather Bureau — the new locus of storm prediction, run by the Department of Agriculture and with a centralized headquarters in Washington.

That did little to quell criticism — or improve forecasting. In 1898, Cuban hurricane prediction suffered a massive setback when the United States severed telegraph lines around Cuba in one of its first acts of aggression in the Spanish-American War. Meanwhile, American forecasters — some of whom were holdovers from the signal service days — continued to suffer from highly variable work ethics. In 1934, as a tropical storm bore down on Galveston, Texas, officials there contacted the federal warning office in Washington, asking for news. The response was as short as it was telling: "Forecaster on golf course — unable to contact."

Even had that forecaster been available, says David Longshore, author of the *Encyclopedia of Hurricanes, Typhoons, and Cyclones,* he would have had a hard time saying with any certainty what that storm was going to do. Year after year, catastrophic and unpredictable storms "revealed that only improvements in storm tracking, coupled with an updated warning network, could lessen the nation's hurricane problem." At best, forecasters were able to deduce that a hurricane was out there, but not necessarily where it would hit. So when they were able to issue warnings at all, it was often for immense swaths of land, sometimes as wide as the entire Eastern Seaboard. Sometimes, they weren't able to issue warnings at all —

or at least not until it was too late. The worst of these storms was by far the Great Hurricane of 1938, which assaulted Long Island and surrounding areas with a ferocity that surprised even the most seasoned of storm scientists. By the time the storm dissipated, more than six hundred people were dead. Storm damage topped $400 million (about $6.5 billion today).

Storm forecasting got a big boost in the decade that followed the Great Hurricane of 1938, thanks largely to the British Air Ministry. There, Robert Watson-Watt, a Scottish scientist, demonstrated that a radio detection device could indicate the presence of objects in the air. His initial thought was that this would help pilots plot thunderstorms nearby, but the device soon proved most useful for identifying German bombers. After the war, meteorologists continued to use the imaging technology to identify the locations of storms. Weather-specific radar emerged in 1959, but it, too, was slow to evolve over the next several decades — a source of unending frustration for meteorologists, says Mike Smith, founder of AccuWeather. "During the period when America was putting a man on the moon and demonstrating its scientific powers to the world," writes Smith in *Warnings: The*

True Story of How Science Tamed the Weather, "weather radar technology hardly changed at all." Indeed, says Smith, by 1980, forecasters were hard-pressed even to find replacement parts for their radar systems. The only place that still used the outmoded vacuum-tube technology was the Soviet Union. The deployment of the first weather satellite in 1960 and the first hurricane-specific satellite in 1975 helped some, but forecasting still remained an exceptionally imprecise science.

More than anything, says Smith, it was computer modeling that presented the first real improvements to storm forecasting. This is not an entirely new concept: Meteorologists have been using statistics to compute their forecasts since long before Benito Viñes issued his first hurricane warning. But as Viñes himself learned time and time again, a law of averages will really give you only information about what ought to happen on a particular day — not what really will. That kind of information can only come from complex formulas capable of representing mathematically the various weather systems and conditions happening around the world. That's just too much information. To manage it effectively, meteorologists devised a grid system that would allow them to focus on a particular area. However, a single grid box still represented an almost unfathomable amount of data — far too many numbers for even a team of forecasters to crunch in their poor human heads.

In 1950, a team of scientists at Princeton tested the first computerized forecast model. Their computer was a lumbering conglomeration of ugly boxes and tangled wires that took up the better part of a large lab room at an army research station in Maryland, and it was considered state of the art for the time — capable of making about three hundred thousand calculations each minute. Still, it proved no match for the intricacies of weather data. Because the computer lacked internal memory, scientists had to constantly feed and refeed data into its system using paper punch cards — about twenty-five thousand of them for a single forecast. And even with its rate of computation, the model still took an entire day to generate even a simple forecast — and one with only a 50 percent chance of accuracy.

Historically speaking, their lack of success may not have been such a bad thing. The Princeton team was led by John von Neumann, a key proponent of cold war–era tactics to eradicate communism. For von

Neumann, weather modeling was ultimately about weather control: His hope was that, if he could determine what the weather would do and why, he would ultimately be able to harness it as a weapon of war — one capable of destroying crops across Russia or raising seas capable of sinking a navy. But a generation of scientists soon learned once again that not only were they unable to control the weather, they couldn't even say with any certainty what it would do. A model — no matter how good — can never accurately reflect what is actually happening in the world.

"Even twenty years ago," says Gary Szatkowski, "betting against the weather forecast could almost always earn you a little money."

Since then, computer sophistication has evolved by leaps and bounds — by 2012, a single NOAA supercomputer was capable of making more than seventy-seven trillion calculations each second. This kind of modeling cut forecast error in half and made betting against a forecast an increasingly ill-advised risk. But hurricanes remained enigmatic. Why are they one of the most scientifically mysterious, seemingly unknowable natural phenomena?

The answer, says Chris Landsea, has as

much to do with the elusiveness of the storms as it does the limits of science. Computer models require massive amounts of real-time data and observations to run, and this kind of information is expensive and arduous to acquire on land, where forecasters rely on weather stations at airports and forecasting offices. There are about five hundred of the observation systems in operation at any given time, but that still leaves massive geographic gaps where we just don't know what's happening. It's even more difficult to say for certain what is going on in the upper atmosphere. For that, the Weather Service relies on weather balloons. Seventy-five stations currently deploy them twice a day. But, again, 150 readings isn't much when spread out over nearly four million square miles. That kind of knowledge gap is exponentially worse when it comes to divining conditions at sea. That's bad news for cyclone predictions. Tropical cyclones spend their genesis — and most of their life — far out at sea, where data-collection capabilities are sparse. The advent of the Hurricane Hunters was a huge help where data was concerned, and their reconnaissance flights have dropped hurricane prediction errors by 20 percent. That's particularly helpful when it comes to predicting hurricane tracks. But they're still a serious concern. Track errors grow on average forty to fifty miles a day; that can be the difference between predicting landfall in southern Florida or North Carolina, or it can be the difference between a storm that slams into a major metropolitan area and one that spirals out to sea. On any given day, the average forecasting error regarding where a hurricane will land is almost one hundred miles. In fact, many experts say there is only a one in five chance that a hurricane will land within the predicted warning area. When there is an error, it's mostly because a storm strikes farther westward than predictions anticipated. Those errors are even worse when it comes to predicting tropical storm–force winds: Most computer models forecast only storms of hurricane strength, which means that forecasters have to rely on satellites, buoy data, and a whole lot of luck to anticipate those systems.

For that reason, the National Hurricane Center issued only three-day forecasts up until 2001, and still doesn't go beyond five-day predictions (which is why Szatkowski's seven-day briefing on Sandy was so extraordinary). Today, the best five-day hurricane forecast still comes with an average error of 250 miles. And even that number is highly variable. In 2012, Tropical Storm Debby more than tripled the long-term forecast error, and early model predictions showed her taking tracks that spanned from Texas to Pennsylvania. Hurricane Kirk proved equally problematic. On the other hand, track forecasts for Beryl and Michael were nearly perfect.

In general, says Landsea, the National Hurricane Center is pretty happy with its average track forecast. There's still a strong human element to it — one that includes not just computer models but other data forecasters glean, including changing weather conditions and, sometimes, their own past experience with storms. Landsea thinks that combination of information is working pretty well. But he says they're still a long way away from assuredness where other aspects of a storm are concerned.

"We're still really terrible at predicting more complicated factors like wind speed, size, and intensity."

The equations in the prediction models are what scientists call "nonlinear partial differential equations," which means they cannot be solved exactly, or the same way every time. And if that sounds to you like a maddening attribute in a tool used to forecast the weather, you're not alone. It's the kind of thing that drives the otherwise unflappable Chris Landsea absolutely crazy.

"You need to know precisely how warm the water is. How deep it is. Everything that's happening in the atmosphere around and over the hurricane. And then you have to know how those conditions are going to change the storm in the future. We can't get at that kind of data right now. So we really stink at that kind of prediction," says Landsea. "And the kind of equations required to compute all that data are more than even our best computers can handle right now. The tools aren't great, and we're not great, either."

James Franklin, branch chief of the Hurricane Specialist Unit at the NHC, agrees. "Track forecasting has improved because the models have. Right now, forecasters can beat models that predict a hurricane's intensity more times than not. That's a limit of science. We're not any smarter now than we have been when it comes to intensity. And we're not going to see any improvement until better models start beating us on a regular basis."

That goes double, he says, for predicting storm surge — the rapid rise of coastal waters that often causes deadly flooding. Storm surge kills more people and is responsible for more damage than hurricane winds.

"We're really cognizant of the limits of science," says Franklin. That, he adds, is why they are particularly quick to say they can't do something, like issue predictions about hurricane winds more than thirty-six hours out — the technology, he says, just isn't dependable enough for something like that.

It doesn't help that some of the tools available to the National Hurricane Center may very well disappear — at least for a while. The United States' polar-orbiting satellite program — the system of sophisticated, moving satellites that allows leading models like the ECMWF to do their work — is falling apart. In addition to the scatterometer that failed in 2009, the United States also owns a series of rapidly aging polar-orbiting satellites, which are expected to fail at pretty much any moment. The first replacement isn't scheduled to be launched until 2017 (and many insiders say that date is optimistic). To make matters worse, an on-time launch is contingent upon a significant budget increase, which seems unlikely. All of this means that chances are good that the United States could very well be without this technology for a year or more. That will make accurate computer modeling — and hurricane forecasting — even more difficult than it is now. It is such a mess that a top-level review team deemed it "dysfunctional" at best. Less than a month before the formation of Tropical Storm Sandy, Jane Lubchenco, Under Secretary of Commerce for Oceans and Atmosphere, called the situation "a national embarrassment due to chronic management problems."

Without these tools, says James Franklin, forecasters have a hard time determining just how organized a storm is — or where its eye is located. That's particularly serious if a storm is out of the reach of the Hurricane Hunters. Without either their data or the help of an orbiting satellite, the forecasters are thrust back forty years in terms of their capabilities. It'll take a miracle of funding, says Franklin, to make sure that doesn't happen.

Funding is also in short supply for research and development, a budget line at the National Hurricane Center that has endured reductions in recent years. In 2006, while NOAA's two P-3 Orion Hurricane Hunter jets sat unused on the tarmac because of a lack of cash, Congress killed the National Hurricane Research Initiative Act, a bill that would have created a multi-agency organization with representatives from NOAA, NASA, and the US Army Corps of Engineers, along with FEMA, the Environmental Protection Agency, and the Department of Energy. Had it passed, the newly formed initiative would have subsidized infrastructure assessment, disaster response, evacuation protocols, and advances in tropical storm forecasting.

Meanwhile, the Joint Hurricane Testbed, an initiative to develop better hurricane modeling and prediction that is overseen by Chris Landsea, has struggled with funding since its inception in 2001. In 2005, more than $300,000 was diverted from the program. Other years, it looked like it might be canned altogether. Even in its best years, the relatively small amount of money (about $100,000 per project, on average) allocated to chosen research proposals means that the testbed has difficulty competing with organizations like the National Science Foundation, which grants researchers as much as twice the funds for similar projects. Even if they did get more proposals, administrators at the NHC say they lack the staffing they would need to grow the program — and maintain it during hurricane season, when staff members like Landsea are pinch-hitting on the forecasting floor.

That's just another example of a more endemic problem of staffing shortages at the NHC. It's one they've been suffering from for years — and that's particularly true in its technology and science branch.

"The staff we do have there can barely keep the trains running," says Franklin. "They don't have time for anything else."

He believes his forecasters are on the cusp of being able to issue reliable seven-day forecasts, but the NHC lacks the IT staff needed to develop the software packages that will get those new forecasts out to the public. They'd like to offer forecasts based on Global Information Systems, a sophisticated computer system that processes geographic data, for surge, but they don't have the resources to do that, either. During the off-season, some of his younger hurricane specialists are often reassigned to IT duties, which means they have less time to improve their forecasting skills — that delicate place where data meets a combination of scientific method and gut instinct. That combination of knowledge and instinct, says Avila, takes years to hone.

So, too, does the ability to convey storm information to the general public in a compelling way — something the NHC has struggled with for years.

In the days following Hurricane Audrey's 1957 assault on Louisiana, politicians and reporters spared few words in their dissatisfaction with the brand-new National Hurricane Center, claiming that the NHC had done little to warn people. Some went so far as to say that the NHC was directly responsible for the lives of the hundreds of people who died in the Category 4 storm. Subsequent investigations into the center's handling of the storm found that they had issued adequate warnings, but that towns and organizations at the local level had no idea what to do with these warnings once they were issued. Similar debate arose in 1995, when Hurricane Erin trapped tens of thousands of people on Florida's barrier islands. Later, they would claim it happened because no warnings were issued. But the NHC shot back in its official report, accusing residents of not taking its forecasts seriously: Because the NHC didn't show the eye of the storm passing directly over the region, individuals assumed they weren't in danger; they either forgot, or never knew, that hurricane winds — and surge — can spiral out for well over a hundred miles from the center of the storm.

The NHC attempted to compensate for what it called this "critical misuse" of its forecasts by depicting a storm's path not with a straight line but, instead, an ever-widening funnel-shaped path it calls "the error cone" or "the cone of uncertainty," which it introduced as part of its formal forecast package in 2002. The cone was an attempt to make transparent prediction uncertainty by focusing not on a single path but, rather, on a spectrum of possible directions based on average forecasting errors over a ten-year period. It did little to allay public confusion. The cone of uncertainty shows only the predicted path of the eye of a storm; it doesn't take into account the total size of that storm, or how strong it is. Most people don't know this. Instead, they tend to assume either that the cone is the actual breadth of a storm's reach, or that if they live outside the cone they're safe from harm. Given that at least one out of three storms lands outside the cone of uncertainty, relying solely on it when making decisions about your safety and that of your loved ones is a very dangerous game.

Florida learned that the hard way in 2004, when Hurricane Charley wobbled its way toward the state's west coast. Despite NOAA's recommendation that officials and private citizens use all of its products when making decisions about how to remain safe during a storm, most people in the region relied almost exclusively on the error cone when judging what (if any) action to take. Not only that, but they assumed the cone was a certain prediction of the storm's reach.

Richard Pasch was on the forecasting desk for much of the storm. He says the track models shifted significantly as the storm moved toward land, befuddling meteorologists. Forecasters attempted to alert the general public to the uncertainty in their forecasts. One such briefing during Charley read: "It is unusually difficult to pinpoint Charley's landfall . . . as small errors in the track forecast would correspond to large errors in the location and timing of landfall." Maybe, said the forecasts, the storm would hit Tampa. Maybe not. When the storm tracked one hundred miles farther south and made landfall at the small city of Punta Gorda, criticism of the NHC was fierce. The head of emergency management for Lee County insisted that it was the track line that left people confused about where the storm was heading, that when the line deviated away from their county and toward Tampa Bay, they assumed they were safe. Even local meteorologists criticized the NHC, saying their track forecast made it difficult for them to do their jobs. The national media picked up on the storm and began questioning the efficacy of the National Hurricane Center.

Robbie Berg, a hurricane specialist who was working the forecast desk with Pasch, shot back in an AP interview, saying forecasters had given Floridians ample warning. But when pressed, he acknowledged that there were gaps in their knowledge. "Sometimes our models just aren't good enough to get everything that happens in the atmosphere," Berg was quoted as saying the day after the storm. "It's chaotic."

That's particularly true, he says, where issues of intensity and storm surge are concerned. And he has plenty of examples, from Hurricane Andrew to Hurricane Katrina, to prove his case. It's a case Richard Pasch hates having to make. The only solution, he says, is to report uncertainty.

But if forecasters agree about anything, it's that the general public has been slow to catch on to their difficulties. The planet, says Mike Smith, suffers a "hurricane disconnect problem," which he describes as a "debate between meteorologists and those outside the profession about the potential threats of hurricanes." Part of that disconnect stems from where people go to get their weather information. The National Hurricane Center issues six-hour advisories, along with cone maps and marine charts, but most Americans go elsewhere to get information about tropical storms: to places like the Weather Channel, their local TV station, or online sites like Weather Underground. These media outlets, in turn, use the information provided by the National Hurricane Center to very different degrees. Some depict the NHC advisories and charts verbatim; others include their own meteorological interpretations. In the case of Hurricane Charley, several local forecasters say they deviated significantly from what the National Hurricane Center was predicting. Confusion over the track of that particular storm caused some weather outlets to stop showing the cone altogether; they felt that it gave a sense of certainty where there was none. Others maintained the cone, and a handful maintained the thin black line in their graphics. Even nomenclature changes from source to source: While the NHC is rigid in calling the predicted hurricane path "the cone of uncertainty," meteorologists in the private sector refer to it as simply "the cone," "the cone of error," or, in some cases, "the cone of death." But it's the moniker "cone of probability" that most disturbs

James Franklin and his staff. "People hear 'probability' and they think 'probable,' " says Franklin. "That loses sight of the real ambiguity involved."

That ambiguity has created a kind of image problem for the National Weather Service. And it didn't help forecasters' cause much when, in 2010, the National Center for Public Policy Research, a think tank based in Washington, D.C., created a media firestorm when it commissioned a chimpanzee to beat the NHC's predictions for the year. (The chimpanzee, named Dr. Hansimian, ended up falling short of the NHC's predictions, though that failed to attract even a fraction of the media attention his initial challenge garnered. And the next year, the NCPPR commissioned a team of fifth graders in Dr. Hansimian's stead. The media loved that, too.)

That kind of stunt is right up James Franklin's alley. The bureau chief loves a good joke (the signature line for his e-mail reads, *Damn it, Jim — I'm a meteorologist, not a doctor!*), and he's thrilled when anyone or anything pokes holes in the legitimacy of the seasonal forecast.

"I hate that forecast," he says. "It's not useful and it doesn't help anyone. If anything, the forecast of a quiet year tells people they can put their guard down. I'm delighted whenever it's wrong."

Before he was a bureau chief, before he flew missions in the NOAA Hurricane Hunters' jet, James Franklin was a hurricane specialist at the NHC. And he spent many days sitting on the forecast desk. He received a lot of calls from people in Miami then, who wanted to know if the seasonal forecast meant they had to get ready for storms. One woman in particular called him almost weekly, miffed that she needed to buy storm shutters for her house. *Why bother,* she asked, *if it's going to be a light year?* Franklin reminded her that 1992 was one of the quietest tropical storm seasons in history — or at least it had been, until Hurricane Andrew slammed into Miami with all the deadly force of a Category 5 storm.

That wasn't good enough for the caller. And it isn't good enough for plenty of other people, either. Their lack of concern worries Franklin.

"The chance of a hurricane hitting any coastal resident every year is small, but that doesn't mean it won't happen. And when it does, it can be catastrophic. We want people to be ready."

And that, says Franklin, means they need to get better at forecasting, too. Chris Landsea agrees. And the thing that terrifies him the most — the realization that keeps him up at night — is that meteorologists are soon going to reach a ceiling of error from which they will not be able to escape. It's called "the limit of predictability," and it's the place where models bump up against their own ability to compensate for unknowns and other variables. Landsea says we're almost there — he estimates we'll reach that limit in about ten years, just in time to confront what promises to be not only a particularly active era in hurricane activity, but an era complicated by a changing climate. Nothing infuriates a forecaster more than that, and it's one of the few subjects that will cause Landsea to throw up his hands in real frustration. "We've made precious little progress there in the last twenty-five years," says Landsea. "And pretty soon we won't be able to make any more. It's terrible. Incredibly terrible."

Statements like that one tend to get a lot of climate-change watchers really concerned when they consider the future of hurricane activity. After Katrina pummeled the Gulf Coast, media outlets from *USA Today* to *National Geographic* predicted that that caliber of storm could begin making regular appearances on our coasts. After Hurricane

Irene, the Natural Resources Defense Council, along with environmental writer and climate-change activist Bill McKibben, drew even more dire connections: "Irene's got a middle name, and it's Global Warming," wrote McKibben. That same year, *Newsweek* called "horrific hurricanes" the "new normal."

Landsea and other hurricane specialists remain divided with regard to the effect of climate change on hurricanes and the limits of prediction. In 2004, Landsea withdrew his participation from the composition of an intergovernmental panel report on climate change after the lead author of the report convened a press conference in which he contended that global warming was likely to cause more outbreaks of intense hurricane activity. Landsea saw that conclusion as premature at best and, at worst, part of a preconceived political agenda (this has earned him the reputation of being a climate-change skeptic in some academic circles). As far as he's concerned, any effect of climate change on hurricanes will be quite small. NOAA's official position is that it's too early to tell to what degree climate change has affected — or will affect — the nature of hurricanes. They cite the butterfly effect in their position paper: that our activities may have already caused changes to hurricane activity without our even realizing it. Probably, they say, hurricanes will grow more intense on average as a result of ocean warming: More heat equates to more fuel for a storm. The number of intense storms may also increase over the next fifty years; so, too, may the amount of rain each storm produces. But to what degree climate change will cause these intensifications remains anyone's guess. The WMO agrees. In a 2010 paper, they argued that over the last forty years, there has been no discernible increase in hurricane activity beyond what they call "the variability expected through natural causes." In other words, there is no evidence that humanity's contribution to increased atmospheric carbon levels has affected hurricane trends. Whenever the subject comes up (and it often does), Chris Landsea is quick to point out a phenomenon known as the Atlantic Multidecadal Oscillation (or AMO). It's a swing in hurricane activity that occurs every forty years or so, as we move from a period of above-active hurricane seasons to one of below-active hurricane seasons. The last swing into an active period occurred from about 1920 to 1960: the years responsible for not only the Great Hurricane of 1938, but also for the storms that did so much damage to the mid- and north-Atlantic states. Landsea estimates that we're about twenty years into another active cycle, which means we probably have another twenty to twenty-five years of above-active seasons to go.

"To what degree is this activity the result of the AMO versus man-made warming? I don't know," says Landsea. "The climate models are a great tool. But the thing is, the Earth-ocean-atmosphere system is so complex that we can't get all of that into a computer model. Our computer models are so simple compared to reality. They could be showing too much global warming, or not enough — we just don't know. What I've learned as a meteorologist and a climatologist is that you're always surprised, that we know a lot less than we think we do. We have to be prepared for surprises."

5:23 A.M.
Miami, Florida
75°F
Barometer: 29.76 inches (steady)
Winds: 13 mph (NNE)
Precipitation: Rain
Seas: 8–10 feet (building)

Hernán Zini hadn't slept for two days now.

The fleet captain for Royal Caribbean International had been watching Sandy develop, and now things were looking serious. Zini is a smiley, funny guy. He likes to crack a joke, and he has a million-dollar smile. There's a casualness — a lightness — to him that surprises most people: They expect someone dour, arrogant even. Zini has never needed that kind of affectation. At thirty-four, he became the youngest captain in the Royal Caribbean fleet. Now forty-five, he has a little gray in his hair, but his face is youthful and utterly handsome: big, dark eyes, full lips, and enthusiastic gestures. He waves his hands when he talks. He jumps up and down and laughs. A lot. His jokes somehow sound even funnier with his Argentinean accent and frenetic delivery, so he gets a lot of laughs when he tells them. He likes to yuk it up — especially when he's on camera.

But this wasn't one of those times. It was still dark in Miami when Zini settled behind a large computer monitor that showed the locations of and conditions encountered by each of the twenty-one ships in his fleet. Clicking on each one, he could see everything about the conditions they were experiencing: wind, wave height, weather. His captains have sovereignty over their ships —

that's maritime law — but whenever those masters anticipate encountering waves higher than twenty feet and winds greater than 45 knots, he wants to hear from them.

"I want no surprises," he says. "I don't want a ship in ten-meter waves without me knowing about it."

Zini requires his captains to report any potentially severe weather five days before it arrives. During a tropical storm, he wants to know a week out. And so, that morning, he was getting calls and e-mails from pretty much every captain in his fleet. The biggest concern of all was coming from the Caribbean: Seas were getting bad out there.

Zini grew up sailing in Argentina. He attended a naval high school and graduated a reserve officer at the age of seventeen. He received his master's license nine years later. If pressed, he'll admit he has fantasized about being Christopher Columbus — about exploring the Caribbean before any other westerner had laid eyes on it. Sometimes, he dreams about heading down to Antarctica to experience the brutal conditions there. It takes a lot to impress him, weather-wise, mostly because he's seen a lot of it. And already, he was blown away by this storm. It wasn't that Sandy was the biggest or most powerful storm he'd ever seen, but it was definitely the most complex. Cruise ship captains assess risk based on three degrees: Conditions are green, yellow, or red. Low visibility or heavy traffic is enough for a code red, which requires every officer to man the bridge. They'd long since passed that level, and captains were getting concerned.

"We mariners are always aware of the weather," says Zini. "We have a lot of respect for Mother Nature."

In 1965, the US Naval Institute published its *Heavy Weather Guide,* a kind of bible for blue-water sailors. In it, the authors outline the twelve basic tracks for hurricanes and tropical storms. They are defined by names as absurd as they are descriptive: names like *the straightshooter* and *the longboozer, the lazy looper* and *the big blooper.* Their paths knot themselves up, double back, run tracks that would never pass muster at a police roadblock. All, that is, except for one: the textbooker, a late-season storm that makes a deliberate, unwavering arc out to sea. This late in the season, more than 90 percent of all hurricanes follow the textbooker path. Those rare storms that make it past the Bermuda high are usually whisked out to sea by the jet stream, a powerful band of wind that occurs high up in the troposphere.

The planet has several of these bands, and they are particularly strong in places with a lot of temperature differential. One can typically be found around 30°N (right above Baja and Florida); another usually hovers around 55°N (which encompasses parts of Alaska and Quebec). Jet streams are exceptionally strong currents of winds that regularly blow at speeds more than 275 miles per hour. The motion of the planet usually keeps them flowing from west to east; however, a whole host of factors, ranging from pressure systems to extreme temperatures to the time of year, can cause them to take a more meandering path. As they do, that powerful air current will take a twist or turn, moving to the north or south for a time before returning to its more typical east-west route. The strength of the jet stream is such that just about everything within it will take that twist or turn as well. That's why a quick veer to the east is such a textbook track for a North Atlantic hurricane in the fall: The jet stream almost always scoops it up and sends it out to sea.

Already, Zini could tell that Sandy was showing signs of bucking textbook trends. And it was about to get plenty of support from the jet stream, which was showing unexpectedly large wave patterns across

North America. Climatologists suspect that these large dips were being caused by abnormally warm temperatures in the Arctic. Zini says he'll leave the science to them, but he does know that he was dealing with an abnormally strong stream of air that was going to keep rocketing Sandy northward, along with ocean temperatures registering an average of five degrees above normal. That was going to create even more fuel for the storm. He had a hunch it was going to hit the mid-Atlantic — and hard. A tropical storm watch was now in place for northeastern Florida. The rest of the east coast of the state was now under a tropical storm warning. Much of the Bahamas were under a full-fledged hurricane warning. Anyone with interests along the entire southeastern coast of the United States was being instructed by the National Hurricane Center to monitor the storm closely.

Hernán Zini had more interest than most people. Royal Caribbean has twenty-one ships in its fleet. At any given time, he is responsible for the lives of more than forty thousand passengers. And that's what had Zini worried. As far as the fleet captain could tell, the storm was planning a colossal assault on his entire fleet — and it wasn't going to stop until it had affected every major port on the Eastern Seaboard.

Historically, ship captains haven't had a lot of opportunity to get out of the way of a hurricane: By the time they had seen the signs, it was too late to move a heavy ship under sail away from danger. So they took to coping with hurricanes by thinking about where they would find the least amount of danger (since every part of a storm is, of course, dangerous). What emerged was a theory known as the "navigable semicircle" — the idea that one side of a storm would be less taxing for a ship than another. The winds inside a hurricane rotate counter-clockwise, so depending upon where you are in a storm, you may be experiencing winds from any cardinal direction. If a storm is moving from south to north, for instance, and you are on the eastern or right-hand side of the storm, you will experience southerly winds. If you're on the western or left-hand side, your winds will come from the north. At first glance, it might seem as if there's no significant difference in strength there. But what complicates things is the fact that the storm is moving as well. So in that scenario, where the hurricane is moving northward, the winds on the right-hand side are actually accelerating, since they are driven not only by the circulating wind speed inside the hurricane, but also the hurricane's movement north. Conversely, on the left-hand side of the storm, those winds are being arrested, since they are blowing in the opposite direction to the hurricane's path. This shift can have effects on wave action as well. A cubic yard of water weighs almost a ton (which is about the same that a compact car weighs). A single wave, then, can easily pack the punch of thousands of tons. If you're sitting on top of that force, it can feel like an exhilarating ride. If it's slamming into the side of your vessel, it can spell disaster (and, if your vessel is wood, a shattered hull). In a hurricane, waves tend to emanate from the center outward. They also move in the direction of the wind. Sometimes that's the same direction. Sometimes it's not. Confused waves (waves crashing into one another from different directions) and breaking waves (the ones that tumble over on themselves) are much harder on a vessel than garden-variety swell.

So, if you have to pick a side of the hurricane to be on, sailors will tell you to stay to the left — that the wind and waves there are less damaging, particularly to a wooden ship.

We've made tremendous advances in hull

construction and prediction equipment, so sailors now have a lot more choices about if and when they want to encounter a storm. But that doesn't necessarily change the comfort level of people on board those ships.

"Pretty much all of our ships can go through a hurricane and come out on the other side," says Zini, "but that doesn't make it a favorable experience for the people on them. So we have to ask what is safe for the ship as a whole, and what is safe and appropriate for who and what is on the ship. Guests have a much lower threshold for comfort than the ship itself. Because of that, we've never approached the threshold of the first. These ships can go through pretty much any weather on this planet, but that doesn't make it a good idea."

Clearly, Sandy was creating conditions well beyond the comfort level of most of his passengers. Zini's captains needed to get their ships out of there. The question, though, was where to put them? And how? Any course change requires a new voyage plan created by each individual captain, approved by his officers, and then sent to Zini for review.

"If we pass those weather thresholds, we're going to deviate from a voyage plan," says Zini. "In extreme cases, we're going to change itineraries. A hurricane is always an extreme case."

He checked the NHC discussion. Sandy now had a well-defined eye that sprawled out over 20 nautical miles in diameter. And, inexplicably, the storm was still intensifying.

"That's the kind of thing that terrifies forecasters the most," says NHC's Richard Pasch. "It happens quickly and often without warning. It's our biggest nightmare. It's what tends to get a lot of people killed."

Zini wasn't ready to let that happen to anyone aboard one of his ships.

Minutes after seeing the NHC update, he sent four of his ships out into deeper waters, including *Allure of the Seas,* the world's largest cruise ship. Roughly the size and displacement of an aircraft carrier, the vessel would remain at sea rather than risk an encounter with the growing hurricane. Carnival's *Valor* and *Magic* both made a beeline for Costa Maya, Mexico, rather than the intended destination of Montego Bay. Norwegian Cruise Line also sent several of its ships to the Gulf of Mexico, rather than risk Caribbean Islands.

The storm was changing — about to merge with a large trough of air over the eastern United States. The forecasters and ships alike were entering unknown territory, and they knew it.

5:45 A.M.
Boulder, Colorado
30°F
Barometer: 30.15 (steady)
Winds: Calm
Precipitation: Light snow

It was still early in the Rockies, but Chris Landsea felt wide awake. He was at the University of Colorado to give a talk on hurricanes and climate change, where he'd say the same thing he does whenever the subject is raised: that he believes humans have affected the climate through the emission of greenhouse gases, and that this may affect hurricanes, but if it does, it's not in a significant way. Familiar territory for him. There would be questions from the audience — people who wanted him to say more, to speak out on the harmful effects of climate change. It wasn't that Landsea didn't want to do that; it's that he didn't want hurricanes used as the poster child for that project.

He'd think all those thoughts later, when he was patiently taking questions and rehearsing his position. But for now his mind was focused on the storm in the Atlantic.

Miami felt a long way away, and he pulled up the latest forecast information from the National Hurricane Center, focusing on an image overlaid on the predicted tracks of the storm. A layperson might see only a tangle of different paths, but Landsea saw a reassuring certainty. *These tracks are as close as close can be,* he remembers thinking. *There's no question where the storm is going to go.*

That may have been true. But it's not what the early forecast said:

> THE INITIAL MOTION IS 005/16 KT. AFTER A SLIGHT JOG TO THE NORTH-NORTHEAST VERY EARLY THIS MORNING . . . SANDY APPEARS TO HAVE RESUMED A NORTHWARD MOTION . . . AND THIS GENERAL MOTION IS EXPECTED TO CONTINUE FOR THE NEXT 24 HOURS OR SO. AFTER THAT . . . A DEEP-LAYER TROUGH OVER THE NORTHERN U.S. AND A SIMILAR DEEP-LAYER TROUGH OVER THE NORTH ATLANTIC EAST OF NEWFOUNDLAND ARE FORECAST TO AMPLIFY . . . WHICH WILL INDUCE MID-LEVEL RIDGING NEAR THE NORTHEAST U.S. COAST BETWEEN THOSE TWO SYSTEMS. THAT RIDGE IS EXPECTED TO

CAUSE SANDY TO SLOW DOWN AND TURN TOWARD THE NORTH-NORTHWEST IN 24–36 HOURS. AFTER THAT . . . THE RIDGE TO THE NORTH OF SANDY IS FORECAST TO WEAKEN AS AN APPROACHING DEEP MID-LATITUDE TROUGH MOVES OVER THE EASTERN HALF OF THE UNITED STATES BY 72 HOURS AND BEGINS TO ACCELERATE SANDY TO THE NORTH-EAST. THE NHC MODEL GUIDANCE IS IN EXCELLENT AGREEMENT ON THIS DEVELOPING SCENARIO. AFTER THAT . . . HOWEVER . . . THE GUID-ANCE DIVERGES SIGNIFICANTLY WITH THE ECMWF . . . GFDL . . . AND NOGAPS TAKING SANDY NORTHWESTWARD AND INLAND OVER THE DELMARVA PENINSULA BY 120 HOURS . . . WHEREAS THE GFS MODEL KEEPS SANDY MOVING NORTHEASTWARD AWAY FROM THE U.S. AND OVER THE OPEN NORTH ATLANTIC.

The difference, Landsea says, has to do with how we all make sense of probability. Say, for instance, that a weather forecast calls for a 20 percent chance of rain. Most laypeople will hear that as an 80 percent chance it won't rain. Probably, they won't bring an umbrella with them. Whether consciously or unconsciously, their minds will do a quick mental calculation: Chances are four times greater that the weather will be fine. And even if it's not, the worst thing that will happen is I'll get a little wet. It's the last part of that reasoning that really interests forecasters. When they consider risk, it's as an equation in which probability is multiplied by possible loss. What is the threat of the stimulus and the full scope of its consequences? The end result is a total account of risk.

Landsea says that forecasters still couldn't say with any certainty what, specifically, was going to happen when and where. But there were lots of possibilities that were going to cause lots of problems for residents. Even a 20 percent chance that a storm was going to hit a major metropolitan area was a significant risk in his mind. And the chance that this storm would do so was much, much higher.

Further complicating things for him and people like Captain Zini was the fact that this storm was beginning to deviate from the typical cyclone pattern. Like its twin farther east in the Atlantic, Sandy was changing into an extratropical system. As with Tony, the forecasters were about to enter into the period of heightened uncertainty that comes with those sorts of systems. Would the storm fade away or continue to grow? The models were still showing significant rainfall amounts, along with the kind of warm-core structure present in tropical systems.

Hurricanes do one of a few things when they head north out of the tropics. Normally, they dissipate, enlarged but weakened by the cold air. Sometimes, in the case of an extratropical storm like Tony, they can intensify and become dangerously erratic. And every once in a while — say, every century or so — these systems become a megastorm: They merge with another system and become a hybrid monster that possesses the very worst characteristics of both. That would force the forecasters into uncharted territory. Landsea was eager to get home. His forecasters were eager to have him back, too.

"We all knew and acknowledged that it didn't look like a typical hurricane by this point," says Richard Pasch. "We had to drive the point home that we're dealing with something very dangerous — something much more than a single point on a map. This one was going to be bad. People didn't understand that it was already massively more powerful than we had expected. It's not very often that we venture this far out of the box."

Americans awoke on Thursday morning to a flurry of sensational headlines and news reports. On CNN, Rob Marciano was predicting that weather for most of the Eastern Seaboard was clearly going downhill. "You're going to feel huge waves," he said, pointing toward Virginia and the Carolinas. "Then look what happens," he said, with the kind of excitement a scientist saves for the curious and unexpected. Sandy, he predicted, would get to Cape Hatteras, and then turn to the left. "Retrograding," he said, swirling his arms with uncharacteristic enthusiasm. "Kind of putting its gears in reverse." Most interesting, he said, was the way that the computer models had come together overnight. The storm, they all now seemed to be predicting, would soon be making a beeline for the Northeast, and along the way it was going to become a "wintry hybrid." His host scrunched up her nose. "Ewwwww," she said with disgust. "Uh-huh," agreed Marciano.

And that was just the beginning. Hurricane Sandy "experienced a stunning increase in size and intensity," reported *The*

Washington Post that Thursday morning. It is "barreling towards New York," said England's *Guardian* newspaper. Forecasters fear "a historic and potentially devastating storm for a large swath of the Northeast and mid-Atlantic early next week," read *The New York Times.* "A massive storm is expected to slam into the Northeast early next week," promised Fox News. "With each passing hour, the Garden State is under an increasing threat of taking a direct hit from a powerful — and perhaps unprecedented — hybrid storm government officials have dubbed a 'Frankenstorm,' " led New Jersey's *Star-Ledger.* "Mother Nature is not saying 'trick-or-treat.' It's just going to give tricks," said Jeff Masters, the meteorological director for Weather Underground.

Reuters and the Associated Press announced that it was meteorologists, not government officials, who had dubbed Sandy "Frankenstorm," though no forecaster remembers saying as much. One AP story called it "The pre-Halloween hybrid weather monster." Conspiracy theorists took to blogs, arguing that the storm was proof of the US military's project of weather domination: "The government has dubbed this storm 'Frankenstorm,' " quipped one Libertarian website. "Sure connotes a 'man-made monster,' doesn't it?" Even the otherwise understated NPR jumped into the melee: Expect "Halloween Horror," they predicted, as "the perfect storm . . . batters Cape Hatteras to Cape Cod."

9:00 A.M.
Mt. Holly, New Jersey
59°F
Barometer: 30.25 inches (falling)
Winds: Calm
Skies: Overcast

The tweets made Gary Szatkowski smile. By the time he got to his office, his colleagues at the Upton, New York, NWS office had already issued a hazardous weather outlook for their area, stating that they had "increasing confidence" that the entire tristate area would soon feel the impacts of a major storm. They'd been tweeting the notice ever since, and from the look of the Twitterverse, the message was getting through. As far as he and his staff were concerned, that notification seemed like the only prudent thing to do. Like Landsea, they had seen the models line up. Szatkowski says that whenever he and his staff start to see that kind of congruence, they know they're looking at something significant.

Joe Miketta agrees. "We know the performance of the models; we study them every day," he says. "And now they were all saying the same thing: This damn thing is going to get pushed onto our coast. We were now beyond the realm of disbelief."

Outside the building, workers were tuning up the building's generator and topping off its fuel tank. Szatkowski was thinking through accommodations for his staff and the reinforcements sent from New Orleans — he didn't want anyone traveling in the middle of the storm. Meanwhile, Joe Miketta was studying the new model data. And his first thought — his defining thought — was *storm surge.*

It's one of those concepts that meteorologists really, really want us to understand, and that few of us actually do. Simply defined, surge is water pushed onto shore by a storm. In a hurricane, that happens because a set of complex forces begin at the storm's eye, and the water bulges up around that center. Winds push the bulge along the hurricane track and create downward circulation. So long as that bulge and the surrounding storm reside in deep waters, there is little noticeable effect: The water simply spins along, with energy dissipating as it spirals down. But as the surge nears the coast, the rising ocean floor prevents the energy from dissipating and the water from pushing downward. Instead, the water has nowhere to go but up, and it is heaved upon the land.

What most people don't realize is that storm surge exists in addition to any normal tide in a region. Take Manhattan, where high tide is five feet. Say a storm has a predicted surge of four feet. If that storm arrives at dead low tide, four feet of water will be pushed onto the shore. If it arrives at high tide, nine feet of water will be pushed onto the shore (that total amount is referred to as the storm tide). Further increasing this level are any local waves kicked up by the storm. Factor those in, and what you have is a third category, called total water levels for an area. These can be significantly higher than any predicted surge. During Hurricane Katrina, Biloxi, Mississippi, was hit with a twenty-two-foot surge that occurred while the tide was at one foot. The storm was generating eleven-foot waves at the time. And so the total water level that inundated the region was thirty-four feet.

In September 2008, Hurricane Ike made landfall around Galveston, Texas, as a Category 2 storm. It brought with it storm surge as high as twenty feet in some places. The National Weather Service issued a warning stating that those people who did not evacuate in advance of the storm would face "certain death." Still, as many as forty thousand people resisted the evacuation order. Seventy-four of them died. According to Jamie Rhome, the storm surge team leader at the National Hurricane Center, that's when they really realized just how big of a problem they had. "The forecast was accurate, but people still didn't understand. That screams a communication challenge." He says they've been working on it ever since.

It doesn't take nearly as much water as Ike's surge to make life dangerous for coastal residents. Just six inches of surge is enough to knock a grown man off his feet; a foot of water can sweep away a full-size car. The Saffir-Simpson Scale, which rates hurricanes from 1 to 5, used to attach a surge prediction to that rating (a Category 1 storm would come with a prediction for a much smaller surge than a Category 4 storm, for instance). But scientists quickly discovered that there's a lot more at work in determining an actual surge forecast — everything from the shape of the continental shelf to a hurricane's size to the angl which a storm hits land. Scholars estimate that the worst-case scenario for all of these factors puts the highest theoretical storm surge in New Bedford, Massachusetts. With a perfect set of circumstances, it could witness a surge of 38.5 feet. New York City could see more than 32 feet. Factor in surf and tide, and that could easily result in more than 50 feet of water. (As a point of comparison, consider that the 2004 tsunami, which devastated much of Indonesia, had waves that averaged between 50–100 feet.)

How all of these factors add up may well determine whether you live or die. Meteorological historians contend that surge has killed far more people than wind or any other aspect of a hurricane. The entire National Weather Service employs just one person who specializes in storm surge: Jamie Rhome. Rhome's title of team leader is something of a misnomer — he's a team of one — though he does oversee some subcontractors, who help him crunch data. He says there are certain generalizations that you can make about surge: A slow-moving storm is more likely to create surge problems inland, and in protected waterways, higher winds create higher surge. But more than anything, local features like topography and the shape of a coastline determine a storm surge's impact. For him to do his job, he relies heavily on people like Joe Miketta to tell him about their regions.

The communities on the New Jersey coast are at sea level. Much of Manhattan is just a few feet above that. Miketta estimates that there are about twenty thousand buildings — commercial and residential — around him situated firmly in the floodplain. In New York alone, approximately two hundred thousand people live within a few feet of high-tide levels. New Orleans is the only American city to have more. And unlike New Orleans, New York doesn't own a single levee. It wouldn't take a lot to swamp much of the city. And the surge already being predicted could easily inundate the residences of more than a million people.

Miketta walked over to the calendar hanging near the forecast desk. Every year, on January 1, one of the meteorologists in the office circles every new and full moon: The astronomical high tide is really high on a full moon; it's higher still on a new moon. The next full moon was just four days away. If the storm struck as predicted, on the twenty-ninth, much of the mid-Atlantic could be flooded with more water than it had seen in two hundred years. Miketta's second concern was temperature. The thermometer would be dipping down into the forties the following week, and there would undoubtedly be millions of people without power and heat. "I was like, *oh, nooooo,*" he says. "This is bad. This is really, really bad."

Already, it seemed like people weren't getting it. Speaking at a press conference that afternoon, New York City Mayor Michael Bloomberg told reporters: "If this storm merges with another storm coming from the Ohio Valley, it has the potential to give you real weird weather, like snow, and a lot of rain and high winds. On the other hand, it might just go out to sea, and they just don't know. What we are doing is we are taking the kind of precautions you'd expect us to do, and I don't think anybody should panic."

Joseph Lhota, the head of the city's Metropolitan Transportation Authority, told a reporter that he was prepared to move the city's thousands of buses to higher ground if need be. When asked if he had considered shutting down the subways, as he had done a year earlier for Tropical Storm Irene, Lhota said he thought that unlikely. "I don't think we're looking at anything like that for what's happening next week," Mr. Lhota said.

At the National Weather Service Eastern Region Headquarters in Bohemia, New York, acting director Mickey Brown disagreed. He'd spent twenty-five years working for the National Weather Service, and had begun his career at the Tropical Analysis and Forecast Branch at the National Hurricane Center. Hurricane forecasting is very much a niche enterprise, and the scientists involved are small in number. Brown knows Landsea and the others at the National Hurricane Center. During a storm, he's on the phone with them a lot. And he's the supervisor of Szatkowski and all the other meteorologists in charge of local NWS offices in his region, so he spends a lot of time with them as well. It's his job to think about what those offices need to succeed.

The forecast discussion emanating from the National Hurricane Center was enough for Brown to see how dire a situation he now faced. The models weren't just showing that Sandy may well slam into the mid-Atlantic. They were also saying that the storm wasn't going to stay a simple hurricane for long. Instead, as Sandy moved northward, the storm was predicted to merge with an enormous upper-level trough already responsible for major snowfall as far west as the Rockies. No one was certain what would occur if that merge happened. But the closest antecedent they could find wasn't pretty: Hurricane Grace, which in 1991 merged with a massive nor'easter, quickly becoming what writers and meteorologists dubbed the perfect storm. That monstrous hybrid had the teeth of a hurricane and the heart of a nor'easter: Instead of dying out as it moved across cooler ocean temperatures, the perfect storm accelerated, gaining in power as it crossed the open ocean. If a scenario similar to the perfect storm occurred with Sandy, the results would be much, much worse: They would pummel not the Atlantic, but the nation's most populated region, with everything from blizzard conditions to fifty-foot waves.

Worst of all, people might not know it was coming. And Brown might not be able to tell them.

For good reason, everything at the National Weather Service is codified by procedure and policy. Every potential scenario has a strict and specific set of rules governing how forecasters should respond. That makes good sense in a lot of cases: It ensures synthesis between forecast offices, and it gives both media partners and the general public the kind of consistency they need to make important decisions. These procedures almost always work to everyone's advantage. But they were about to implode in spectacular fashion. And Brown knew it.

On the subject of hurricane advisories, that policy was resolute: The National Hurricane Center issues only tropical watches and warnings. Once a system becomes something else, it's out of their purview. And that meant that, should Sandy morph as predicted, responsibility for issuing storm warnings would land squarely in Brown's lap.

That presented a whole host of problems. They were exacerbated by the fact that, like the National Hurricane Center, some of Brown's local forecasting offices were understaffed — the meteorologist-in-charge position at the Buffalo office and both the systems analyst and information technology officer positions at the Upton, Long Island, branch were vacant. Without those key officers, getting critical, accurate, and detailed briefing information to places like the New York City Office of Emergency Management was going to be difficult.

Even Brown's fully staffed offices were already working hard — harder than Brown had any right to expect them to, he knew. He is a meteorologist, yes. But he's also a manager. And he was worried about his people.

"With a full staff, you have to make hard decisions. With a short staff, you really, really have to make decisions," says Brown. "If you don't have to add a level of challenge into an already busy office, then why do it? I don't want to throw them a curveball if I don't have to," he says. That goes for his forecasters as well as his customers.

Brown called the Mt. Holly office. The phone there was now ringing nonstop. Even Eastern Region Headquarters had a hard time getting through. And when Brown finally did, he found the meteorologist-in-charge as resolute as he had ever heard him.

"We're humans," said Szatkowski. "We do human things. That's what really scares me."

Chief on Szatkowski's mind was what had happened during Irene the year before. The hurricane was downgraded to a tropical storm just before making landfall. Residents assumed they no longer had to evacuate, so they didn't. That spurred Governor Chris Christie to exclaim, "Get the hell off the beach!" during a press conference. The clip went viral, but people still stayed. Those who'd left returned to undamaged homes and an intact coastline. They complained that the media had overhyped the storm — that they had been persuaded to leave unnecessarily. Those who went inland had different complaints. The flooding there trapped many for days. They would have been better off staying put, they said. It was hard to argue.

"Irene set us all up for failure," said Szatkowski. To make matters worse, he says, Irene "was a well-behaved hurricane." She did what she was supposed to. Sandy was showing no such compliance.

"The last thing I wanted people thinking was 'hurricane,' " said Szatkowski. "I didn't want Hurricane Irene on the brain. I wanted people thinking 'worst coastal flood on record.' We are a highly populated area with very little hurricane experience. It takes a lot to get people out of here."

Brown asked if he had any ideas how to do that.

"Don't change horses in midstream," said Szatkowski. "Don't change warnings. People are just going to get confused. We've got to keep everyone together and on message."

That made sense to Brown. He knew what he would say, and he didn't have to wait long to say it.

The National Hurricane Center maintains

a special tropical storm hotline. It's an actual landline phone with a handset and cord. It's remarkably unmodern in its appearance. But that doesn't matter, because this phone is the lifeline that connects the NHC to Brown and forecasters at the NWS branch offices (there are twenty-three in his region alone), along with weather and ocean prediction offices and governmental branches like the navy. Big decisions get made on the calls that come across these lines, and during a major storm event, there will be as many as four conference calls a day. Everyone on the call that afternoon knew it had even more gravity than most.

At the National Hurricane Center, James Franklin was discussing options with Chris Landsea and the hurricane specialists.

"We are faced with three bad options," said Chris Landsea. "And each one is worse than the others."

The first lousy option would be to continue calling Sandy a hurricane until it completed its transition, and then switch to post-tropical warnings — the changing-horses-in-midstream analogy Szatkowski wanted to avoid. Franklin wanted to avoid that, too.

"If we take down hurricane warnings twelve hours before a storm hits, all people are going to think is 'canceled warnings,' even if we replace them with something different. That's a horrible idea."

Brown agreed. "You're going to put my staff in a really tough spot if they have to switch gears," he said. "Besides, it's not what emergency managers want."

Gary Szatkowski was quick to agree. "This is not public service the way we want it," he remembers saying. "Not when we're changing labels while a storm is having tremendous effects and negative impacts. Whatever we're going to be doing, we ain't going to be swapping headlines, particularly during the most hectic time of the storm."

"We know that," said Franklin. He sounded a little testy.

The second idea would be for the Hurricane Center to begin issuing non-tropical watches and warnings before the storm transitioned.

"That's risky," said Franklin.

"I don't even know if our computers can do that," agreed Landsea. "We could literally break our software packages."

Franklin agreed. He tried to picture what would happen to their partners — private organizations like the Weather Channel that regularly plug NHC data into their own software packages. *What would happen if that information included non-tropical warnings?* Franklin didn't know.

"Trying to wing it without testing a package first could be a disaster," he said. "I'm not confident."

The third lousy option would be to immediately hand over control of the watches and warnings to the local NWS offices. They could forecast non-tropical weather events from the start. But that, too, came with problems. There were Brown's staffing issues. Moreover, everyone agreed that a warning from a local office doesn't make nearly the splash that one from the National Hurricane Center makes. People could miss it.

That seemed unlikely to Franklin. He'd never seen a storm more hyped than Sandy. *You could hardly not know this storm is coming,* he thought.

Someone from the National Weather Service spoke up. "Couldn't you continue to call it a hurricane? Even after it's transitioned?" A few other voices on the line agreed. That, at least, would convey the right level of danger to the public.

Franklin thought about that. He has always agreed that there could be a little play involved wherever science meets operations. And he even believes that, in instances when the science could go either way, it's okay to tip a scale in the direction of life and safety.

"We could stretch it a little bit," he said. "Maybe for a few hours. But we can only go so far."

He felt like the voices on the phone wanted him to do more.

Things were getting heated. Franklin felt like the consensus from National Weather Service voices on the call was clear: They wanted him to fudge. That annoyed him. What they were suggesting didn't sit well with him. At all. He wanted to call things what they were. And besides, it was the National Hurricane Center's credibility on the line, not the branch offices of the National Weather Service. *I can understand why they wouldn't care about our credibility,* he thought. And he considered saying that. But he didn't.

"Look, I recognize we have a problem," he began instead. "But we can't perpetrate fraud on the American public."

That ground the conversation to a screeching halt. But it's a conviction Franklin holds more dear than just about any other. He's proud of the reputations of the National Weather Service and the Hurricane Center; he feels they've worked hard to become the most respected governmental agency in the country. *Hell,* he says, *they even have a web page that lists every single forecasting mistake they've made since 1970. And he dares you to find another governmental agency that does that.*

Don't bother looking, though.

"No other organization is so up front about the limitations in what we do. I want to keep it that way."

As Franklin pushed back, he felt that the initial resistance he encountered was dissipating. They were back to three lousy options. And they still didn't have a solution.

"We've never had such a challenging scenario," Franklin said to no one in particular. The silence on the other lines was all the confirmation he needed. They were stuck, and agreed on only one thing: They would be consistent. Once a type of warning had been issued, they weren't going back.

As the conference call ended, Senior Hurricane Specialist Mike Brennan was finishing up his afternoon storm discussion:

> SIGNIFICANT IMPACTS WILL BE FELT OVER PORTIONS OF THE US EAST COAST THROUGHOUT THE WEEKEND AND INTO EARLY NEXT WEEK,

he began. Though just how significant remained to be seen:

NOTE THAT THE TROPICAL CYCLONE WIND SPEED PROBABILITIES ARE NOT DESIGNED TO HANDLE THE TYPE OF STRUCTURAL CHANGES ANTICIPATED WITH SANDY DURING THE FORECAST PERIOD. AS A RESULT . . . THESE PROBABILITIES WILL UNDERESTIMATE THE ACTUAL RISK OF STRONG WINDS AWAY FROM THE CENTER OF SANDY.

Brennan didn't like typing that. The advisory didn't sit well with Gary Szatkowski, either. He got off the phone and walked out into the forecasting room.

"How sure are you about this storm?"

"Pretty damn sure," said Dean Iovino, one of the branch's meteorologists. "I think everybody agrees something really bad is going to happen."

That was enough for Szatkowski. He returned to his office and began to type. "The likelihood of the storm affecting our region has once again increased over the past twenty-four hours." That didn't seem very emphatic to him. So he kept writing:

This storm, if it moves toward us, will bring

multiple threats to the region:

- Strong damaging wind gusts
- Extremely heavy rainfall
- Major flooding along streams and rivers
- Major coastal flooding (full moon occurs on October 29).

He thought about it again, then added another line. "This is a very dangerous scenario," he typed. He signed his name, and included the office contact information. And then, just to be sure, he typed in his cell phone number, too. He knew he was asking for a flood of calls at all times of the day. Once he hit send, there wouldn't be much rest for him or his wife until this thing was over. But he was already putting in twelve-hour days at the office. Betty knew what they were forecasting — she knew this threat wasn't going to go away. It was the right thing to do.

He hit send.

9:45 A.M.
Coast Guard Air Station Elizabeth City, North Carolina
70°F
Barometer: 30.19 inches (falling)
Winds: 3 mph (NNE)
Skies: Overcast

As Szatkowski e-mailed his briefing, Lieutenant Aaron Cmiel walked to a hangar at the edge of Air Station Elizabeth City. Situated on North Carolina's Pasquotank River, the air station looks like a strange amalgamation of a KOA campground and high-test military base: Near the river, a pod of RVs and drive-up cabins share their waterfront access with a family beach area and outdoor volleyball courts. A few pleasure boats dock alongside, most with fishing poles or a wakeboard inside. Once a day, though, a Jayhawk helicopter — the coast guard's version of the Blackhawk — will descend in a hover near those boats and drop one of the planet's most highly trained rescuers into the propeller-chopped water below. It's all part of the swimmer's continuous training. And it's a reminder that Elizabeth City is the epicenter for the coast guard's search-and-rescue program. If you've seen the film *The Guardian,* you have a pretty good idea of the scene at Elizabeth City. The movie about a coast guard trainer and his star trainee was filmed here, and in the years since its release, the school has become even more high-tech: It now boasts pools capable of simulating five-foot waves and choppy surf, and helicopter frames that simulate aborted missions by crashing into the pools, flipping upside down, and dropping to the bottom of the pool with trainees strapped inside.

Life at this base is full of dichotomies. The pilots, the swimmers, and their crews are capable of heading out into the worst conditions the planet can muster. When not scheduled for actual flight, the crews work what the coast guard calls collateral jobs: doing everything from staffing the base's public relations desk and scheduling visits from TV crews to conducting daily maintenance and, if needed, entire electrical or mechanical overhauls on the aircraft. Those scheduled as on-duty flyers during the day have learned to pace themselves. A watch schedule is twelve hours, which is taxing enough, but if they are called out on a search-and-rescue (SAR) case, their day will undoubtedly get longer and a lot more strenuous. So the rescuers have perfected the posture of engaged loafing. The crew lounge is decorated with a semicircle of leather recliners, all focused on a big-screen TV that alternates between Will Ferrell movies and football games. Large Rubbermaid containers stacked on the tiny kitchenette counter contain snack-size bags of potato chips and every possible flavor of miniature candy bar. Empty helicopter hangars double as floor hockey rinks on slow days, and office computers have well-worn paths beaten to Facebook and game sites.

The crews themselves are merciless in both their self-deprecation and their teasing of one another. They're honest-to-god heroes, but the first lesson they learned was not to act that way. Walk in with aviator sunglasses and the *Top Gun* taunts will come out — allusions to shirtless beach volleyball games featuring jacked-up fighter pilots. Risk your life saving someone, and they'll spend hours deciding who will play you in a movie (and it's rarely a flattering choice). They taunt one another relentlessly about their rock-star status — particularly when one of them is quoted saying something cliché in the news, or tries to affect a tough-guy swagger in a TV special. After one rescuer made the mistake of bragging about one of his Clearwater, Florida, rescues on an episode of the Weather Channel's reality-TV show *Coast Guard Alaska,* others began betting a case of beer for every time someone managed to mention the bucolic coastal city in conjunction with treacherous danger.

That kind of thing may make the Florida tourism industry sick to its collective stomach. And it may seem like these rescuers don't take their jobs seriously. But the truth of the matter is that their joking is a way of coping with the salient reality of their jobs. On any given day, these people may very well be asked to risk their lives in order to save ours: to fly their aircraft into some of the worst weather imaginable; to tend to everyone from hypothermic sailors to HIV-positive cruise-ship passengers; to push their own physical limits as they embark upon missions that may take them hundreds of miles out over open, teeming ocean, knowing perfectly well that they may never come back.

To do this sort of thing, a person has to go one of two ways: megalomaniacal hyper-masculinity (again, think *Top Gun*) or graveyard humor. To a person, the coast guard rescuers at Elizabeth City opt for the latter. It's what gets them through calls where they spend hours looking for a merchant mariner who disappeared off her ship during a night watch, or a father and son who capsized their kayak on a blustery day. It's what allows them to come to terms with repeated rescues where far more people are lost than found and grim casualties are commonplace.

Everything about the lives of these crews is based on forecasting and minimizing risk. Every mission, every training flight, every time a plane is moved from one side of the base to another, the crews undertake a lengthy operational risk-management protocol: *How much sleep did you get last night? Any personal issues? What's the mission? The weather? What are the limitations on this aircraft?* Their commander and operations chief are constantly asking the same questions, trying to pair up the best teams before they go out. It's okay, they say, to have an inexperienced pilot or copilot, but you don't want both of them on the same flight. Ditto for a helicopter mechanic and rescue swimmer — one of them needs to know the ropes.

At twenty-eight, Aaron Cmiel was one of the youngest rescuers stationed here. He was also the most junior pilot as far as hours in an aircraft go. In October 2012, Cmiel was less than a year out of flight school, and he says his primary job at the base was to get as many hours in his C-130 as possible. Cmiel says he knew from the start the C-130 was his aircraft: Helicopters, he says, tend to fall out of the sky, so he feels better with two wings and four engines surrounding him. Elizabeth City is the only coast guard base that flies the C-130J — the same plane the Hurricane Hunters trust inside a major storm — and Cmiel says he likes that, too.

The coast guard's C-130 has all the power of the Hurricane Hunter plane and goes on many of the same types of missions. It contains the most advanced in avionics and navigation, along with engines and deicing capabilities strong enough to plow through any kind of weather. It can be a taxing plane to fly, and the Elizabeth City base proudly boasts that it has one of the only runways long enough to handle takeoffs and landings.

The primary task of a C-130 crew is long-range search and rescues. They can fly hundreds of miles out over the open ocean, where they can establish radio contact, drop rafts and survival kits, and be the eyes on the scene needed to initiate a rescue. When schedules allow, these same planes and crews will undertake fishery law enforcement, stage counter-drug operations, and chart icebergs in North Atlantic shipping channels. Because the plane has such outstanding range and electronics, it can also serve as a highly effective long-range radio, broadcasting announcements and warnings to mariners for hundreds of miles. Doing so is part of a partnership with the National Weather Service that is more than seventy-five years old — dating back to when the coast guard was the only reliable source of weather reporting and in possession of the only ships powerful enough to get out into the storm.

On October 25, Cmiel still had fewer than one hundred hours in the cockpit of the C-130 — and most of that time had been spent tracking the local fishing fleet — so he was pretty excited when he got the call saying he was going up that day. The coast guard regularly broadcasts weather forecasts on a high-speed radio format and using a synthesized voice. For years, that voice was known as "Perfect Paul." His perfection lies, at least in theory, in his distinctiveness. But those in the industry disliked him and gave him nicknames that ranged from "Imperfect Paul" to "Mr. Roboto." So in 2003, Paul's voice was replaced by one the NWS named Tom, who was said to have more nuance, and his female counterpart, Donna.

(Weather forecasters jokingly call her "Misty Dawn" and, if pushed, will sheepishly admit they like the underlying stripper connotation of the moniker.)

When a C-130 crew gets called in to broadcast weather live, it's a sure sign things are getting serious. On the twenty-fifth, Cmiel's mission was to fly what the coast guard calls a search-and-rescue patrol (or SARPAT): a long transect up and down the path of a storm, while warning mariners that dangerous weather is approaching. The C-130 took off from Elizabeth City and banked south toward Wilmington, then headed out two hundred miles to sea, at just about noon — the same time Harter and the rest of the Hurricane Hunter crew were on their way back to Savannah. The two C-130s were now on either end of a growing network of storm communication, which began with Harter's data. That same information, which had been sent to the NHC for calculations and forecasting, which had then been crafted into an advisory by the NOAA forecasters, had then been delivered to coast guard district headquarters. What resulted was a script that would be read by one of the C-130 crew members every fifteen minutes:

> Mariners are encouraged to make preparations for heavy weather and smaller vessels are encouraged to return to safe port. All vessels should keep abreast of this weather pattern by monitoring the National Weather Service broadcasts. Synopsis: A powerful hurricane will impact coastal and offshore waters of the mid-Atlantic Ocean over the next 48 hours. Heavy winds and seas are expected to accompany the storm. There is a tropical storm warning with storm force winds in effect through Sunday evening. For Saturday: NE winds increasing to 30kts, seas building to 09 to 16ft.

"Basically," says Cmiel, "it's a way of saying, 'Just in case you haven't heard, a gigantic hurricane is coming. You might want to get the hell out of here.' "

The upper reach of their flight on that day was New York's Long Island, and it would take them about seven hours to make the roundtrip flight. That meant the crew would read this script about twenty-eight times, never deviating from the district's language. As they took off late that morning, Cmiel had a hard time believing a hurricane was barreling toward them. All of the mid-Atlantic, it seemed, was enjoying an unexpectedly perfect late-autumn day: Temperatures were in the upper seventies, winds were light and out of the northeast, and only the smallest and most unassuming white clouds dotted the sky. Cmiel watched below as scores of recreational boaters and fishing vessels zipped out for one last day on the water. The scene reminded him of rush-hour traffic on the interstate, but without the organizing principles of lanes and off-ramps. Instead, it seemed the kind of barely contained chaos that only a late-season gorgeous day can inspire.

As the plane made its way farther out to sea, Cmiel began to see evidence of heavy weather. The C-130 was approaching the most easterly point on its transect — about one hundred miles offshore. There they found abandoned fishing grounds and not a single vessel in need of a hail. Nearby, the normally crowded shipping lanes — where tankers and cargo ships, along with navy destroyers and carriers, chug along with all the structured order lacking farther inland — were vacant. Cmiel could count on his hands the number of ships he saw out there, and the few that he did count looked like they were hightailing it back to shore or port. That seemed pretty noteworthy to the young pilot — eerie, almost.

The C-130 crew slipped into an easy rhythm, continuing with their broadcast and watching the late-season exuberance below them. It seemed like the mission would err on the side of the mundane — if not the outright boring. But then the radio lit up with a call from the command center at sector, the shore-based operation unit responsible for coordinating and overseeing all missions. A communications specialist there charged with monitoring emergency frequencies reported that an EPIRB, an Emergency Position Indicating Radio Beacon, had gone off about sixty miles off the coast. No one at district headquarters could be certain of what that meant. Depending upon the specific EPIRB device, the distress signal can be emitted once a sailor deploys his or her EPIRB manually, or automatically when the device is submerged in water (as is the case on a sinking ship). Each year, there are dozens of false alarms, the result mostly of mariners forgetting that their EPIRBs are on board when they scrub their boats or when a dinghy gets swamped with rain.

Even with these snafus, the coast guard handles every EPIRB deployment with grave seriousness. Not even a hurricane-watch patrol trumps the idea that mariners might be in trouble, so Cmiel's C-130 was promptly diverted to the last known location of the EPIRB. Below them, the throng of boaters was still strong, and the crew was having a difficult time determining if any of those boats were in trouble. They began calling around on the radio, trying to locate a beleaguered vessel. Ten minutes passed, then twenty. Finally, a fishing boat answered the call: The crew had been in the vicinity of the sinking boat and had picked up all those on board. They were holding them now for safekeeping. The C-130 radioed for a rescue craft, remained on the scene until it arrived, then resumed their SARPAT. "Those boaters were really lucky it was a busy day," says Cmiel. "Otherwise, they might not have been found in time."

Not finding people in time is the unfortunate reality of the rescuer's job. Oceans are immense, and people are tiny — particularly if they are in a swell. It could take hours for the crew of a container ship to realize a merchant mariner has fallen overboard, and by then the search pattern needed to find him or her covers hundreds of square miles. Ditto for drunken revelers on cruise ships, who are never wearing life preservers and also have an irritating habit of falling overboard in the middle of the night. Often, even seasoned sailors and fishing crew aren't wearing protective clothing and gear like PFDs. Even those who do unwittingly pick colors — like blue or gray — that make them virtually invisible from the air. If you want to be found, say Cmiel and his fellow rescuers, throw any fashion sense to the wind and drape yourself in red, yellow, or — even better — bright orange. And when you're done, cover every inch of it in reflective tape. Then maybe, just maybe, they'll be able to find you. Maybe.

11:00 A.M.
New London, Connecticut
60°F
Barometer: 30.29 inches (steady)
Winds: 5 mph (E)
Skies: Partly cloudy

Robin Walbridge knew more about coast guard intervention than he ever wanted or intended to. In the fall of 1998, while en route from Massachusetts to St. Petersburg, the *Bounty* encountered a storm and began taking on water. Within minutes, the main bilge pump failed after losing an oil seal and rod bearing. The ship's backup trash pump — they called it the "Green Monster" — failed, too. Soon, enough water entered the vessel to short out the remaining pumps.

What followed was a harrowing rescue involving a coast guard helicopter, two cutters, a tugboat, and two naval vessels. When the navy damage-control team arrived on the scene, they found the crew of the *Bounty* moments away from abandoning ship. The resulting coast guard inquiry found that the incident was caused by master misjudgment. The report also expressed concern regarding the amount of dry rot on the vessel, along with the location of its pumps and issues with "general housekeeping on board." Walbridge was ordered to stay in port until he could demonstrate the leaks had subsided. In 2003, Walbridge received a citation from the coast guard after he misjudged the height of a drawbridge on Lake Shore Drive. The resulting collision sheared off the top foregallant yards of all three masts. No one was injured, but Walbridge was given a written warning for negligence.

The *Bounty* was investigated again when the vessel attempted to take on paying passengers in Europe. That soon led to official inquiries by both the MCA (the UK Maritime and Coastguard Agency) and the US coast guard. In the end, the coast guard upheld its previous decision: The vessel was licensed as a pleasure yacht. As such, it was welcome to carry nonpaying guests, either while it was under way or on the dock. But the vessel was not allowed to charge for the opportunity to sail aboard.

The *Bounty* also had a reputation within the tall ship industry to contend with. Adam Prokosh, a shipmate of Claudene Christian's, says that, before he got on the ship, he had heard through the grapevine that the ship wasn't safe — that it wasn't a place to work if you took your safety or your job seriously. More than that, he would later testify under oath, it had the reputation of being "a death trap."

"I heard terrible things about the *Bounty;* one of the jokes I heard a lot was that everybody who worked on the *Bounty* had a story where they almost died, and you never heard the same story twice." But, he was quick to add, those rumors seemed out of date — the *Bounty* organization had been making real strides to improve both the vessel and its reputation. Safety, he says, was always a priority.

On the morning of the twenty-fifth, Prokosh was feeling pretty good about all that. The crew was busy. Some of them were feeling hungover from their night at Hanafin's. But they had a sailing gig that day, and that made them excited. The ship's owner had arranged to take the crew of the USS *Mississippi* on a day sail, which seemed like a good time. What tall-ship sailor doesn't love the opportunity to show off his ship — especially to the crew of a nuclear submarine? The attack sub had been commissioned just a few months earlier. It was one of the newest in the navy — and the most sophisticated. The thing had laser range finders and fiber-optic signal processors and crazy pump propulsions that made it all but invisible. It was a $2 billion boat overstuffed with every possible state-of-the-art everything. The *Bounty* crew wanted to show the *Mississippi*'s crew how to kick it old style.

Tracie Simonin, the *Bounty*'s shoreside manager, would soon be arriving with potential buyers. There was still housekeeping to do. The crew washed down the decks. The pumps still didn't seem to be working quite right, but no one stopped to work on them. It didn't occur to them to check on the backups, either. Besides, there was plenty else to do. They needed to finish work from the refit and refuel — get ready for the long trip down the coast.

Simonin arrived later that morning. Forty years old, with an ample figure, ankle bracelets, and a big Long Island laugh, Simonin was a force. The crew friended her on Facebook, where she posted lots of pictures of her daughters and her dogs and videos of people doing all kinds of stupid things. Robin Walbridge called her Miss Tracie. Jessica Black didn't have much time to get to know her before she and Simonin headed off to a grocery store to do the provisioning for the trip. If the new cook had any apprehensions at that point, she didn't express them. Later, her dad would tell his cousin he thought it was "rather strange" that his daughter's new ship was about to set sail when a storm was coming up the coast. Black had never worked on a tall ship, but she had plenty of experience on motor yachts. She'd learned to trust captains.

Things were rushed as she and Simonin returned from the provisioning trip. The new stoves had arrived and needed to be installed. The galley was a mess and needed cleaning. And now they had more than two weeks' worth of food to contend with. While Black and the departing cook started stowing food, the *Bounty* crew finished their sub sandwiches and sodas, remarked on what a total luxury it was to eat on the dock on a sunny October afternoon, and prepared to entertain the navy. Then, says crew member Jess Hewitt, it was time to go. And they were glad about that, too: "Robin was like, 'We're going,' and we were like, 'All right!' "

While they were out, some of the navy guys asked about the hurricane — if they were really going to sail into it. The *Bounty* crew didn't know for sure. But they said they thought so. The crew of the *Mississippi* gave them medallions just in case: BY VALOR AND ARMS, PRIDE RUNS DEEP, they read. Jess Hewitt stuffed hers in her pocket. She knew she'd hang on to it for a long time, though she hadn't really thought about the storm yet. Laura Groves, the ship's bosun, had first heard about the storm the day before, when she and third mate Dan Cleveland had gone to Long Island for a doctor's appointment. She says that she was a little concerned — that it seemed clear they were definitely going to encounter some weather. She thought 20 knots of wind sounded great, but 50 or 60? Not so much. She and the other officers were concerned enough that they met to talk about it. In the end, they decided to defer to Walbridge's expertise. "We each decided that we'd go with what the captain wanted," she says.

Meanwhile, texts started coming in. Jess Hewitt got one from her mom. She was really busy and really tired, so she didn't think much of it. Besides, she says, her mom can be kind of a worrier. That's what moms do. During the tour of the sub, says crew member Josh Scornavacchi, quips about Hurricane Sandy began to increase. The *Bounty* crew joked around a little bit with the navy, saying, *Hey, we gotta beat that storm out.* He says maybe there was some nervousness on people's faces, but they didn't talk about it.

Robin Walbridge ducked back to the *Bounty* before his crew. It was his birthday, and Claudia had been trying to reach him. When she finally did, she said he seemed really excited about the navy visit. He was chattering away, which was always a good sign from her otherwise taciturn husband.

"I have a birthday story for you," he said. She rolled her eyes a little. She was in Rome, and her tour bus was leaving in five minutes. But she and Robin had spoken so little for the past two weeks, and he sounded so excited. She didn't have the heart to say no or hurry up. He began at the very beginning.

"When I was fourteen or so . . ." *Oh, no,* she thought. *This is going to be a long one.*

His story really stuck with her, though. Robin told her about being a young teenager and how, one day, he took a boat out on the water so that he could contemplate life. He already had a deeply philosophical bent to him, and he had big questions he needed to answer — even as an adolescent. On that day, the questions were about as big as you can get, he told Claudia: *What am I going to accomplish in life? How long do I have to do it? How long do I want to live? When will I be ready to go?* The fourteen-year-old Walbridge settled on the age of sixty-two. That seemed far enough away, long enough to live the life he wanted to live. *If I can make it to sixty-two, I'll be happy,* he remembered thinking. His story now had Claudia's full attention.

"Wow," she said.

Her husband kept speaking. "But, you know, this past year, I got scared."

Claudia stopped getting ready for the bus tour. Her heart sank a little. Robin never said things like that. She began to feel worried. He told her about the cough that wouldn't go away, about the chest pain he hadn't mentioned up until now.

She tried to make light of it. "I'm certainly glad you're telling me this now, and not at the time."

"Yeah," he agreed, and then returned to his usual self. "But look. I made it. I'm sixty-three."

She sighed a breath of relief. Later, when

the allegations would mount, when people would speculate that her husband had a death wish or that he had become despondent over the condition of the ship, she would shake her head fiercely. “No,” she would insist. “He was on top of the world that day.” She would remember their conversation — and then repeat the sentence again, drawing out each word into a full stop for emphasis. “On. Top. Of. The. World.”

Claudia says Robin didn’t say much about the weather that day — he knew there was a storm out there, but he told her he was pretty sure he could get around it. *Beside*s, he said, *the forecasters still weren’t certain where it would track. If things got dicey out there, he’d turn north and head to Newfoundland.* “Don’t worry,” he told her. “The storm will just push us along. If anything, I’ll get home a few days early, and we can have a beer on the porch swing.”

He didn’t mention the rot or the condition of the ship or why he thought it was a good idea to go — that just wasn’t his way, and it wasn’t the nature of their relationship to dwell on work stuff like that.

But the work in Boothbay must have been on his mind. As the crew made their way back from the sub and began preparing to depart, says Chris Barksdale, Walbridge was still tinkering with the ballast. He gave a piece of it to Matt Sanders and asked the second mate to go over to the post office to weigh it. That struck the engineer as a little bit odd.

Crew members Anna Sprague and Josh Scornavacchi didn't notice. They were both on the phone with their folks. Sprague had called her dad, Larry, to tell him about the sub trip. He asked her about the storm, and she told her dad she was pretty sure Walbridge already knew. Josh Scornavacchi's mom was considerably more worried. She called her son saying that the media was already calling Sandy a "superstorm" and the "storm of the century." She'd heard that it was going to collide with a nor'easter. Things were serious out there, she said. Besides, last night, she'd had a bad dream. Josh tried to reassure her.

The *Bounty*'s performance in previous storms was the source of a lot of lore on board the ship. Crew members handed down stories from year to year. During Dan Cleveland's first year on board, the ship went head-to-head with Hurricane Paloma. Like Sandy, Paloma was a late-season storm — the seventeenth tropical cyclone of the 2008 hurricane season. And, from the start, Paloma was a serious storm. As it began to develop off the coast of Honduras, weather watchers couldn't help but begin to make comparisons between it and Hurricane Mitch. When the storm reached Category 4 intensity, those comparisons seemed warranted.

The *Bounty* had just left Mexico when Paloma began its march westward. They were on their way to Costa Rica, and the weather was rough from the start. The ship's weather fax told them Paloma was a tropical storm, and Cleveland says he remembers that they immediately reduced their sail to storm configuration. The idea was to slow the vessel down as much as they could so that they wouldn't overtake the storm — they just wanted to stay close enough to make good on the storm's wind. "It's one of those situations where you're in nasty weather for a few days." Still, he says, the *Bounty* sailed well. She sailed fast. Yes, the ship worked hard. And hell, yes, the crew worked hard. You could tell that they were in heavy seas and big winds, he says, by the way the vessel was flexing and moving. But the *Bounty* was a big, slow boat. She liked winds of at least 30 miles per hour to move, says Cleveland. She liked hurricanes.

That kind of easy, breezy confidence wasn't sitting well with the ship's first mate.

John Svendsen had never sailed in a hurricane before — and he didn't see any reason to do so. Two years earlier, he and the *Bounty* had been in enough heavy weather for him to know what it can do to a ship. In November 2010, he, Walbridge, Cleveland, and nine other crew members left Boothbay Harbor on a scheduled voyage to the Caribbean. The ship hadn't gotten far, however, before it encountered its first nor'easter. Waves grew to twenty feet; snow and ice covered the decks. A second nor'easter soon overtook the first, causing the seas and wind to grow further. Then a third storm came in. Things got sketchy. The ship hove to, a nautical term for putting on the brakes. In the case of a square-rigged ship, heaving to means setting the sails at opposite directions, so that the vessel remains stationary and doesn't need constant tending. It's a way of waiting things out, which, at least in theory, doesn't exhaust the crew or destroy the ship. There's a YouTube video of this moment. In it, a crew member straps a small camera to his head and then stands near the ship's main mast. The *Bounty* is listing hard to her port side, as eighteen-foot swells move roughly against and under her hull. The sky is gray; the water is grayer. Wind whips through the rigging, obfuscating most other noise. But a minute or so into the video, you can barely make out a nervous male voice. "Holy shit," it says softly. Then louder, but shakier, "Oh, my god."

The damaged *Bounty* eventually limped into Bermuda. Not every vessel was so lucky.

The first casualty of that tumultuous season occurred in November, when *Emma Goldman,* a two-masted ketch, departed Martha's Vineyard for the Virgin Islands with three on board. Not long after entering open water, the forty-one-foot boat began encountering gale-force winds and waves of at least thirty feet. Conditions continued to deteriorate. At the height of the storm, the boat hit an enormous wave and rolled. All the way over. When it slowly righted itself, the rigging, the masts, and the captain were gone. The remaining crew members, including his daughter, raced on deck. And then they realized that he was worse than gone. He was tangled in all that rigging and being dragged behind the boat: a slow and terrible drowning, and they could do nothing to help him. Eventually, they made the difficult decision to cut him free with a kitchen knife. For three days, the survivors tried their best to bail the boat. Their engine had flooded. They didn't have an EPIRB. They managed to jerry-rig a makeshift sail, but they had no way to steer. They set off flares when they saw passing cargo ships, but no one saw them. A week came and went. Their boat continued to disintegrate. They ran out of water. On the twelfth day, the cargo ship *Triathlon* passed by. The crew member shot off one of their last flares. Miraculously, the ship saw it. However, seas were still so rough it took nearly a full day for the ship to reach them.

A couple of weeks later, the tall ship *Raw Faith* departed from Salem, Massachusetts, also en route to Bermuda. It, too, encountered the gale and began to take on water. The ship had an inexperienced crew of two. One was bleeding from the nose and mouth, apparently the result of an accident on board. The captain's family phoned the coast guard and said they worried he wasn't capable of making good decisions. As the storm raged on, the deck of the *Raw Faith* began to buckle. Her masts swayed. The coast guard sent out the best of its assets: a C-130, two helicopters, and two cutters. There was little they could do in the dark. Meanwhile, the captain of the *Raw Faith* became volatile. He first threatened to launch his lifeboat and jump in. That sent the crew of the first cutter into a controlled frenzy, as they readied their rescue swimmers. Whether or not to deploy them was a question: Seas, the captain of the coast guard cutter *Tybee* reported to sector, were "well beyond safe parameters." He urged *Raw Faith*'s skipper not to do it. The skipper grew increasingly desperate and then began refusing to leave the vessel. He said he'd rather go down with the ship than see it come to some kind of uncertain future. The next call from the *Tybee* had even sector's most seasoned responders at a loss:

"The master wants to put fire to his vessel."

"Negative," came the stupefied response.

"Roger," came back from *Tybee.* "We do not agree with him setting fire to vessel."

The conversation was just so surreal — beyond the edge of anything the coast guard rescue personnel were prepared for. These crews had trained to save people and boats. In their experience, most people were really glad when they arrived.

The *Tybee* tried again. "What would you like us to do?"

Silence. Then this from sector: "Roger. The staff is discussing."

They settled on the strong arm of legislation. "Per D1 Legal it is a federal crime if he intentionally sets fire to his vessel."

"Roger, will relay that."

It didn't work. They tried again, talking about penalties and the significance of federal crime. Something finally clicked inside the skipper's head. He agreed to abandon his ship. A few hours later, *Raw Faith* sank with another coast guard cutter, the *Reliance,* standing by. No lives were lost. The entire ordeal took forty-eight hours and cost more than a million dollars.

A rescue like that takes a lot of resources. And when it happens, it means other ships in distress may well have to wait in the queue. That's one reason AMVER (the Automated Mutual-Assistance Vessel Rescue System) came into existence in 1958. AMVER is a registry of more than twenty-two thousand ships that voluntarily report their positions while at sea and agree to assist in an emergency, and a program a century in the making: It began after ships passing the sinking *Titanic* admitted they did not know the beleaguered vessel was in trouble (they assumed rescue flares were, instead, part of festivities celebrating the ocean liner's maiden voyage). By the early 1960s, computer technology had caught up to mariners' need for cooperation and assistance, and all commercial vessels of more than one thousand tons were asked to register. Remarkably, ship owners and captains agreed — by the thousands. On any given day, about five thousand commercial vessels at sea are actively reporting their positions and signaling their willingness to help if someone is in trouble. The coast guard estimates that, since 2000 alone, more than twenty-eight hundred lives have been saved by the system. They can't say for sure how many lives have been lost.

But these sorts of stories did little to affect the confidence of the *Bounty*'s crew. What mattered to them was their ship — and their captain. *The* Bounty *likes hurricanes,* they all agreed. Yes, they'd be cold and wet and miserable for a few days, but they had always been fine during storms. The officers say no one expressed any concern to them about the storm. The third mate said he felt like there was plenty of risk in staying at dock, too. "Being in a storm at sea as much as I have been and having it go so well so often, I believe you could argue that a ship is safer at sea," Cleveland said. He'd continue to assert that — even months after the ship went down, even after the coast guard investigator in the case, Commander Kevin Carroll, said he couldn't find a single person who agreed with him.

Even Cleveland's supervisor, John Svendsen, disagreed. The 2010 season had been an eye-opener for Svendsen. He remembered the way the *Bounty* encountered first one nor'easter, then a second. The way a third one overtook them, how he and the crew had to heave to. How they watched as the fore royal mast snapped. How Svendsen had to go up and lash it. On that trip, they knew the storms were out there and building. They thought they could get out before the storms. They didn't.

He recalled forty-foot seas in that last gale — and it wasn't even strong enough to be considered a tropical storm. *What,* he wondered, *would a hurricane be like?* He didn't want to find out. He kept checking the marine forecasts. All signs pointed to a significant coastal storm. Winds would hit 25 knots. Seas around Long Island could build to fourteen feet over the weekend. The Bahamas were now under a hurricane warning. NOAA was predicting seas above forty feet there, along with winds building to 65 knots. Northwest of there — near Bermuda — things weren't looking any better. By Sunday, that stretch of ocean between the Carolinas and Bermuda was expecting to see waves of forty-two feet — maybe higher.

Winds would top 50 knots. And, in all likelihood, that's right where the *Bounty* would be. According to the NHC, Sandy would be there, too. And by then the storm would be huge:

> SANDY IS FORECAST TO BE A LARGE CYCLONE AT OR NEAR HURRICANE INTENSITY THROUGH THE END OF THE FORECAST PERIOD.

That's what John Svendsen most remembers about the forecast advisory that day — the size of the system, and the fact that it was only going to get bigger.

Svendsen didn't want to take that chance. And he didn't believe a ship was safer at sea. He'd just received a new 1600-ton master's license. He'd spent the last month on the coast guard's tall ship *Eagle,* working with that vessel's first mate to devise an officers' manual. He'd taken classes in crisis management at Maritime Professional Training, a sprawling forty-five-thousand-foot school in Fort Lauderdale, and courses on weather and risk analysis. The protocols were clear: Obtain all cyclone advisories. Plot the forecasted position of the storm. And, most important, ensure that your vessel will be well clear of any winds over 34 knots. Have at least two escape routes. Make sure there's a haven you can get to in time. Walbridge's plan wasn't going to allow for any of that.

As the crew began to clean up from the navy trip, Svendsen approached Walbridge. Then he did something he'd never done before: He asked Walbridge if they could speak privately. The two walked off the ship and onto a dock on the other side of the pier. Svendsen told Walbridge he was worried about the storm — that it was predicted to be a big system. Really big — "of historic proportion," even. He told the captain they had other options: They could sail to Bermuda, like the last time. They could stay in New London. They could leave now and get to New Bedford, where a forty-five-hundred-foot stone hurricane barrier protects the entire harbor. Failing that, they could find another safe port. He says he was very assertive. But his captain was even more so.

Walbridge said he had sailed through hurricanes. He'd seen the ship do fine in that kind of weather over and over again.

Svendsen pushed again. The weather maps were saying they would encounter winds anywhere from 35 to 60 knots. Those same charts were saying there was nowhere the

Bounty could go to avoid the system. But the captain was resolute. He told his mate that the hurricane was predicted to remain a Category 1 storm and that seas were unlikely to be more than thirty feet. That's not what the forecasts said, but it was what Walbridge believed: winds below 74 miles per hour; seas below thirty feet. Walbridge reminded Svendsen that the ship had weathered those kinds of conditions plenty of times before during his tenure as captain. He felt comfortable. *Besides,* he said, *the* Bounty *was in the best shape he had ever seen.* He told Svendsen he had no reason to deviate from his intended plan.

Okay, replied his first mate. *But I think you should address the crew.*

It was a few minutes after 5:00 P.M. The crew could hear Amtrak's evening train pulling out of the station — they imagined people in suits on their way home to families and two-stall garages. They knew they didn't want that for themselves. They wanted adventure. NOAA had just released its evening storm discussion: Sandy's eye was 125 miles southeast of Nassau. Tropical storm–force winds extended out more than two hundred miles and were growing. But most of the crew didn't know that. They hadn't read the advisory. Hell, most of them hadn't even heard about the storm until Walbridge called them together.

The crew disagrees on what, specifically, was said at this meeting. Several deckhands remember Walbridge telling them that a "ship is safer at sea," though others don't recall that. John Svendsen says Walbridge definitely told them about the conditions they may experience: *Hurricane conditions,* Svendsen remembers Walbridge saying, *60 knots of wind and twenty-five-foot seas.* Some crew members swear Walbridge called Sandy a "Frankenstorm"; others recall that he said they'd be in for a "rough ride." No one remembers Walbridge mentioning the size of the storm. That afternoon, the wind field for Hurricane Sandy stretched out 228 miles in every direction from the eye of the storm. He also didn't mention the fact that the storm was growing — that in a matter of days, it would more than double that size.

The crew also differs in what they recall as Walbridge's plan: Several people, including Tracie Simonin, the onshore manager, maintain that Walbridge said he was going straight east. Others say his plan was always to head southeast as fast as he could; they say he wanted to get far enough south of the storm so that they could cut over and use its fair winds to push them the rest of the way to St. Petersburg.

All the crew members agree that Walbridge made it clear they could leave if they wanted to.

No one even tried.

Laura Groves, the ship's bosun, says she was definitely nervous. "I don't particularly like to sail in hurricanes," she would later explain. She says she wouldn't be surprised if the rest of the crew was nervous, too. But nobody expressed any concerns about the hurricane to her. "I don't think anybody had really strong opinions about it." For her, it's cut-and-dried: The captain said they could leave; he meant it when he said there would be no hard feelings. People would have left if they'd wanted to.

Jess Hewitt says she remembers looking over at the train station with its dark red brick and imposing, sloping roof. This was no backwater station. This was the kind of place from which you could go anywhere if you wanted to. It was just a stone's throw — less, even — from the *Bounty.* It'd be so easy to leave. That's a rare thing in the tall-ship world. Half the time, you're at some industrial dock where it's hard even to get a taxi to come to you. Or you're in some small coastal town that hasn't even heard of public transportation. A person could get where they wanted to go from New London — if you wanted to. If you had the cash.

Jess didn't want to get away, though. She figured that, based on what Walbridge had to say, the storm must not be that bad. She trusted her captain — she's always trusted the experience of her captains. "I was in oblivious innocence," she would say later. Her fellow crew members agree: They say they didn't really realize the magnitude of the storm. Second mate Matt Sanders had taken meteorology and hurricane avoidance at Maine Maritime Academy. He says that, more than anything, what he learned in those classes is that hurricane predictions can have an error margin of 500 percent. (Chris Landsea takes issue with that number: He says the error rate for track predictions is more like 12 percent.) Besides, says Sanders, on that day, the science didn't really matter. What matters was the trust he had in his captain. "The way I made my decision to stay on board," says Sanders, "was I looked at Robin's history and experience and said to myself, 'Well, I'm going to stay on board because he has more experience than I do and maybe I can learn something from this.' "

Experience was something Claudene Christian never turned down. She texted her mom: "They say BOUNTY loves hurricanes! Really we're not too worried about the hurricane. The Capt. loves hurricanes and we're going to make sure to go outside on the East side." Then she posted a Facebook status update: "YES, HEADED STRAIGHT THROUGH THE PATH OF HURRICANE SANDY!!"

Like the weather forecasters, Claudene and her fellow crew members were making predictions of their own: a million little computations, some conscious, some unconscious, but all settling on the likelihood of possible scenarios. It's a process we undergo hundreds of times every day: *What is the chance this boat will sink? How likely is it that I will be sideswiped while walking my dog?* Each of us performs a complex set of calculations that leads us to a best guess. And, at its heart, it's a process that is all about weighing risk, a word that finds its etymology in early Italian *risicare,* meaning "run into danger." It's about gambling. Even the word *hazard* comes from the Arabic word for dice. Daniel Kahneman and the late Amos Tversky, longtime research partners who are still considered the leading theorists on the psychology of judgment and decision-making (Kahneman won a Nobel Prize for his work on risk assessment), say any question about risk comes down to how we choose to gamble. Any kind of gamble demands that we acknowledge what we don't know: "Risky choices, such as whether or not to take an umbrella and whether or not to go to war, are made without advance knowledge of their consequences," they wrote in an American Psychological Association award address. We make these choices all the time, whether we know it or not.

That's particularly true when we confront forces of nature like hurricanes or any other extreme condition. But it's also true in our daily lives. And that, says Dan Moreland, captain of the *Picton Castle,* is something people tend to forget. Yes, sailing is risky. But so is modern life. "Every day, normal people ashore manage enormous, even profound, risks with very little time spent thinking about these risks or about any conscious concept of 'balance' of risk versus benefit," says Moreland. "We routinely get into cars, drive at deadly speeds, passing other such oncoming vehicles with a yard to spare, knowing nothing of the training or skills of the other driver. And we have all heard somewhere some appalling figures of how many people die in car accidents on the road each year. We pretty much just do it. All of us."

How do we make such decisions? According to Dr. Paul Slovic, a professor of psychology and the president of Decision Research, a think tank dedicated to human judgment and risk analysis, we begin with our gut. The first response we have to any situation is an intuitive one: It's based on our feelings. Images and perceptions filter into our brain and immediately trigger feelings. Some of these sensations may be innate — some people are just more adventurous or reluctant than others — while others come from learned experiences. "The neurons in our brains have a mysterious way of calculating risk and benefit without us even knowing," says Slovic. "Those calculations translate into feelings, and we use those feelings as our compass and our guide. It's how we get through each day. We make tradeoffs based on what makes us feel okay." We don't have to calculate this gut response — Slovic says "it just hits you. It comes to you — often in split seconds." And it can be amazingly persuasive. Sometimes, these feelings are so strong that they cut off the possibility for rational thinking and assessment, a much higher-level process that takes more time. Analytical responses are slow and deliberate.

Dan Moreland wonders if Robin Walbridge had enough time to be analytical in the way that Slovic describes. He thinks maybe Walbridge might have been suffering from fatigue, too. "He had been doing a day sail that day, which is a lot of intensely focused work for the skipper, in close quarters. He made his decision and probably figured he would sort things out at sea, as he had done in the past."

The weather forecast that day may have been extreme, says Moreland, but Walbridge's process wasn't. Many captains and organizations have made decisions similar to Walbridge's. "We all have to make decisions that at some point are a form of triage; in repairs, expenditures, equipment, manning or crew selection, even weather/routing decisions. But then is a good time to put hubris, even confidence, aside and use your best judgment."

What about the judgment of the crew? The sailors on the *Bounty* had less than an hour to decide if they would stay or go. Slovic says analytical thinking requires a lot more time than that. Without it, he says, we tend to just apply past experience with the hope that it'll fit. That idea of past experience is key here. Walbridge and some of his crew members had experienced hurricane conditions before and had made it through fine. That, says Slovic, made them a lot more comfortable with the risk involved in this trip. It also made the prospect of disaster feel a lot less likely to them. A successful past experience makes us that much more willing to undertake a risky activity again. It also feeds our belief that we can control the circumstances surrounding that experience. Take driving, says Slovic. We get into our cars every day, and most of us have a successful experience there. So we tend to think driving is safe — that we can control our destiny behind the wheel. Often that leads us to undervalue risk and what we can't manage — like other drivers. A sense of control creates a heavy bias when it comes to letting our brains do the work of rational thinking, and it's in our nature to underestimate the things we can't control.

There are a whole host of other factors that influence how we make decisions. Kahneman and Tversky contend that our perceptions of risk are greatly influenced by how the risk is — or isn't — described to us. If the risk is described in abstract terms, we tend to minimize it. If the person describing the risk appears calm and confident, we'll assume that risk is less of a big deal. Robin Walbridge was confident in his explanation of how the *Bounty* would make it through the storm. His crew followed suit. They trusted that his experience and the experience of the other crew members were enough to see them through.

That doesn't surprise Slovic at all. He says we often look to respected leaders when trying to ascertain risk: If that leader tells us the danger is manageable, we'll see it the same way. The degree to which we feel an emotional attachment to the matter at hand also has significant effects on our decision-making. So, too, do the people around us.

We tend to underestimate the ways in which we are influenced by others. We'd all like to believe that we're autonomous individuals, and to some degree we surely are. But our brains are also a whole lot like lemmings: Once we've established a belief, our mind would rather race off a metaphoric cliff than reconfigure itself. If the people we value and love have articulated their opinion on a subject, it's going to take that much more effort for us to adopt a different belief. If your shipmates tell you that the *Bounty* likes hurricanes — if they regale you with stories of how the ship made its way through big storms before — then you will naturally assume that taking it into another storm is a sound idea. It doesn't matter if the crew was lucky those previous times, or if all the other tall-ship captains weren't about to risk their vessels in this storm, or maybe even if logic dictated that being onshore was a much better idea. The brain is a highly susceptible organ, and it does a clever little sleight of hand in such situations.

This is not a new concept. Francis Bacon, himself no stranger to the risks of seafaring, referred to the concept as *"the idols of the tribe."* In his 1620 treatise, *Novum Organum,* he explains:

> The human understanding when it has once adopted an opinion . . . draws all things else to support and agree with it. And though there be a greater number and weight of instances to be found on the other side, yet these it either neglects and despises or else by some distinction sets aside and rejects; in order that by this great and pernicious predetermination the authority of its former conclusions may remain inviolate.

In other words, says Slovic, we seek to justify what we already believe or have decided, and we'll use new decision-making opportunities as a way to do that. We can't help it: That kind of thing is hardwired into us, and often part of our very existence. We're pack animals. It's how we avoided being eaten by lions on the Serengeti and often how we get through a crisis like an earthquake or other disaster. Peer pressure may not always be a good thing in a high school hallway, but it's gotten us out of plenty of jams in our evolutionary history. For all our machinations, we tend to be a pretty complacent species. We like where we are. We tend to stick where and with whom we've been. It takes a lot of soul-searching and careful thinking to change our minds. And that takes time.

Claudene Christian's parents wonder what would have happened if their daughter had had the night to sleep on her fateful decision. Would she have woken up and got off the boat? Her mom thinks so. Claudene's friends aren't so sure. Michelle Wilton, Claudene's best friend, says she thinks the decision to stay had a lot to do with how much Claudene trusted not just Matt Sanders, but also the rest of the crew — and how much she wanted them to trust her.

But why was Walbridge so resolute?

"That's the million-dollar question, isn't it?" says Walbridge's wife, Claudia. "I certainly don't have the answer. Obviously, he thought they'd make it safely." Tracie Simonin, the ship's onshore manager, agrees: "We've been in seas like that before, even worse, and we didn't think it was insurmountable."

Paul Slovic says that's as good an answer as any. "Experience is such a powerful motivator. That's especially true with natural disasters. We're so primed to be tolerant of our experience with nature. Research shows that our past experiences can be a real prison when it comes to rational decision-making."

Risk is a numbers game, and that's particularly true when it comes to natural disasters. On paper, they can seem pretty unlikely. The probability of a tropical storm hitting Atlantic City in any given year is 4.8 percent; the chance of a hurricane is less than 1 percent. Compare that to Miami, which has a 26.3 percent chance of a storm and an 11.1 percent chance of a major hurricane event. The chance that a hurricane will turn east and fade out to sea increases significantly as the season progresses. Robin Walbridge rolled the dice and put his money on that last eventuality.

It's easy for us to second-guess this decision now. But scholars also have an explanation for that. It's called "hindsight bias," which, says Daniel Gardner, author of *The*

Science of Fear, will "drain the uncertainty out of history. Not only do we know what happened in the past, we feel that what happened was *likely* to happen. What's more, we think it was *predictable.*" Except, of course, that it wasn't really.

We may see the error now, but at the time, Robin Walbridge felt certain he had made the best guess. He made little ceremony as the crew left New London. If anything, he seemed uncharacteristically businesslike.

"Robin said he wanted to make tracks. That was his exact terminology," says Faunt. "We wanted to get as far south and east as we could before Hatteras. We were going really fast."

From inside the nav shack, Walbridge sent an e-mail to a friend: "So we are under way. Sandy looks like she will be bad," he wrote. "We need to get east of it. I would not dare be anywhere close to land."

Walbridge didn't tell the crew he thought the storm was going to be bad. But they knew they would be encountering heavy weather, and that their ship would be working hard because of it. They began to prepare. The first task was to get the royal yard down from the main mast and lash it to the deck. One of the highest pieces of rigging, a royal yard bears the brunt of a storm. If loose, it can cause an inordinate amount of damage — especially if it crashes onto the deck. The *Text-Book of Seamanship,* published in 1891 and long considered the definitive source for sailing square-rigged ships, warns that great "mischief" can occur in that scenario — and can lead to the loss of an entire mast. "Spars are lost too often by the time lost in considering 'what's best to be done.' One of the *essentials* in seamanship is to be *always ready.*"

That's exactly what the crew of the *Bounty* thought they were doing: getting ready. Walbridge tasked Matt Sanders with the job of creating a large map in the galley. He had other members printing out weather faxes and GRIBs files, large computer-generated forecasts that provide both gridded and global forecast models. The idea was that they would all be able to keep track of precisely where both the ship and the storm were at any given time.

Crew members from throughout Walbridge's tenure all agree that his greatest fear as a captain was losing someone overboard. He drilled his crew constantly. He created a makeshift buoy out of a five-gallon drum and a stick with a light attached. It looked crude, he knew, but it'd give an overboard sailor something to cling to — and enough illumination to be found in the dark.

Walbridge didn't call for any man-overboard or abandon-ship drills heading out. John Svendsen says that's because his captain "wanted to focus on making the ship ready for the storm and giving the crew as much rest as possible."

As the crew continued to prepare, Walbridge made two phone calls: one to Jeff Finston, a former first mate aboard the *Bounty,* and one to Ralph McCutcheon. Both men agree that was pretty atypical for Walbridge at the start of a transit, but neither was surprised to hear that Walbridge was under way: McCutcheon had been on the *Bounty* with him in 1996, as Hurricane Edouard battered New England with 80-mile-per-hour winds. It was, McCutcheon remembers, a relentlessly slow and obstinate storm, marked by hours and hours of wind and rain and waves that topped thirty feet. The Hyannis Fire Department lost the roof on its station. At least twelve boats were washed ashore in southern Massachusetts. Walbridge, McCutcheon, and the *Bounty* were in Fall River then, and Walbridge made the decision to lash the ship to the USS *Massachusetts,* but it was no picnic. Later, he'd say he thought that decision was a mistake.

Jeff Finston was thirty-two when Hurricane Andrew formed in the Caribbean. As the storm barreled toward Miami, he was alone on the ship. A couple of days before Andrew's landfall, he received a visit from the coast guard, who arrived with a clear ultimatum: Get this ship off the dock, or we'll sink it. Anything else, they said, was going to cause even more damage to the already threatened harbor. Finston wasn't about to see his ship go down at the dock. So he says that he called five of his "suicidal friends" and decided to head out to sea. They were hauling ass, he says, or hauling as much ass as a hull totally covered with barnacles would let them. They hit the edge of the storm that night. Waves were topping twenty feet and the *Bounty,* never an elegant mover, began to roll. The ship's clinometer, which measures the tilt or heel of a vessel, maxed out at 30 degrees. The ship kept heeling farther. Its rigging, says Finston, was "definitely tickling the water." The ragtag crew stayed on watch throughout the night as conditions deteriorated. Finston swears winds were more than 100 miles per hour, though how much more he just can't imagine. For his part, the first mate spent most of that time seriously certain that this would be his last night on Earth. He says they were all terrified — almost too much to really gauge what was going on around them.

Somehow, though, they survived. As the storm began to clear, they assessed the damage to their ship. A backstay had broken off in the wind. The waves had burst some seams in the bow, which let water into the bilge. But other than that, the ship was — somewhat miraculously — unharmed. The crew's psyche was a little more damaged. Finston says he's spent every subsequent day really conscious of the fact that he's lucky to be alive. He says that he doesn't sweat the little stuff anymore, that all six of the survivors decided to make some definite changes to their lives from that day forward.

Walbridge called Finston as the ship was pulling out of the harbor. The former first mate remembers it vividly. *New London is not a safe place,* Walbridge told him. *We don't want to be in New London.*

He reminded Finston about the 1938 hurricane. When that storm made landfall, winds in New London were recorded as high as 85 knots before the anemometers were destroyed by the storm. A 1,057-ton ship was ripped from its lines and rammed ashore, coming to rest on the tracks just outside the New London train station. Another ship, which chose to lay anchor rather than chance the docks, dragged all eighteen tons of its anchors across the harbor. Storm surge topped ten feet, flooding untold numbers of recreational craft. He felt safer under way. That resonated with Finston: "We've been in storms. We've been on the edge of hurricanes trying to get away from them. This was just going to be another storm," he says.

Walbridge called McCutcheon next. He seemed confident. Ralph asked him if he was going to stow the top yards — keep them out of the wind of the storm. Walbridge assured him they were already on top of it.

The pace on board was hectic when he hung up. Adam Prokosh set to work stringing jacklines around the deck — something they could hold on to or clip into if necessary. He says Christian was excited about the work — that she seemed exuberant, even. He remembers her bouncing around, having a good time. It's tough for her family and friends to believe that. During a break from the storm prep, she called her mom, who was returning from taking Claudene's grandmother to a doctor's office. The ship was already motoring across the Long Island Sound. Soon they'd be in open water — and they'd lose cell reception. Dina didn't know that. She asked if she could call Claudene back in a few minutes. They were in a drive-thru, she explained. Some garbled voice was trying to take their order. Things felt a little hectic. Claudene, though, was emphatic. "No, no, no," she shouted. Dina said she could tell Claudene was upset. Stressed. "I've got to tell you how much I love you and Dad." The hairs on the back of Dina's neck stood up. This sounded like a scared good-bye. She asked why Claudene was talking like that — what was going on? But Claudene didn't elaborate. Instead, she told her mom to hang up — she wanted to leave a message: "I just want you to know — in case something happens — that I love you so much," she said after the beep.

Claudene hung up and went to stand watch. She helped furl sails. She took a turn at the wheel. And then she went up to the bow, to look for ships and other hazards. But she couldn't stand still. She was too frenetic. She needed to keep busy. So she texted a friend and possible benefactor for the ship — told him how serious she was getting with Matt Sanders, how she couldn't wait to spend every second in Florida with him. She complained that the ship was shorthanded, that they were all doing two jobs at once. She told him they were about to head straight into the hurricane. "WOW!" she wrote.

Claudene lost her cell signal. She went back to work.

Just before 8:00 P.M. she picked up a weak bar on her cell phone, so she texted her friend again.

"Relax," he wrote back. "Everything will work out. I talked to Robin. All is good. Just make sure you all get to St. Pete."

Later, after her watch, Claudene hung out with Matt Sanders in the ship's navigation shack. She wanted to know everything he knew — she'd follow him around, asking questions, saying, *Teach me stuff.* That night, she asked him to show her the weather fax of Hurricane Sandy.

It freaked her out.

She went to find Jess Hewitt. It was right around midnight. By then, the *Bounty* was almost due east of New York City, though they were too far away to make out the city's constant glow. Somewhere off their bow, an enormous Norwegian tanker was steaming into the New York harbor. The *River Elegance,* a forty-eight-thousand-ton cargo ship, was barreling straight east, bound — eventually — for China. Other than that, the *Bounty*'s radar screen was empty.

Claudene didn't want to talk about that. She wanted to talk about what the weather fax had said. Hurricane Sandy was not some manageable little storm. It was already a massive hurricane, and it was still growing — growing big enough to affect a huge chunk of the East Coast. The Carolinas were already under a tropical storm watch.

"This thing is huge," Claudene told Hewitt. "Pretend this is Florida," she said, marking a little space in the air. She made a big circle with her arms. "This is the hurricane."

Jess didn't know if she should believe her. "Show me," she said.

So Claudene went and got the weather fax. The storm was a whole lot bigger than Hewitt thought — more than four hundred miles in diameter and growing.

Her stomach turned over. *We're going to have to go to England to avoid this thing,* she remembers thinking. But she didn't say that to Christian. In hindsight, she kind of wishes she had. "Claudene really, really trusted us," she says.

Margot Carpenter/Hartdale Maps

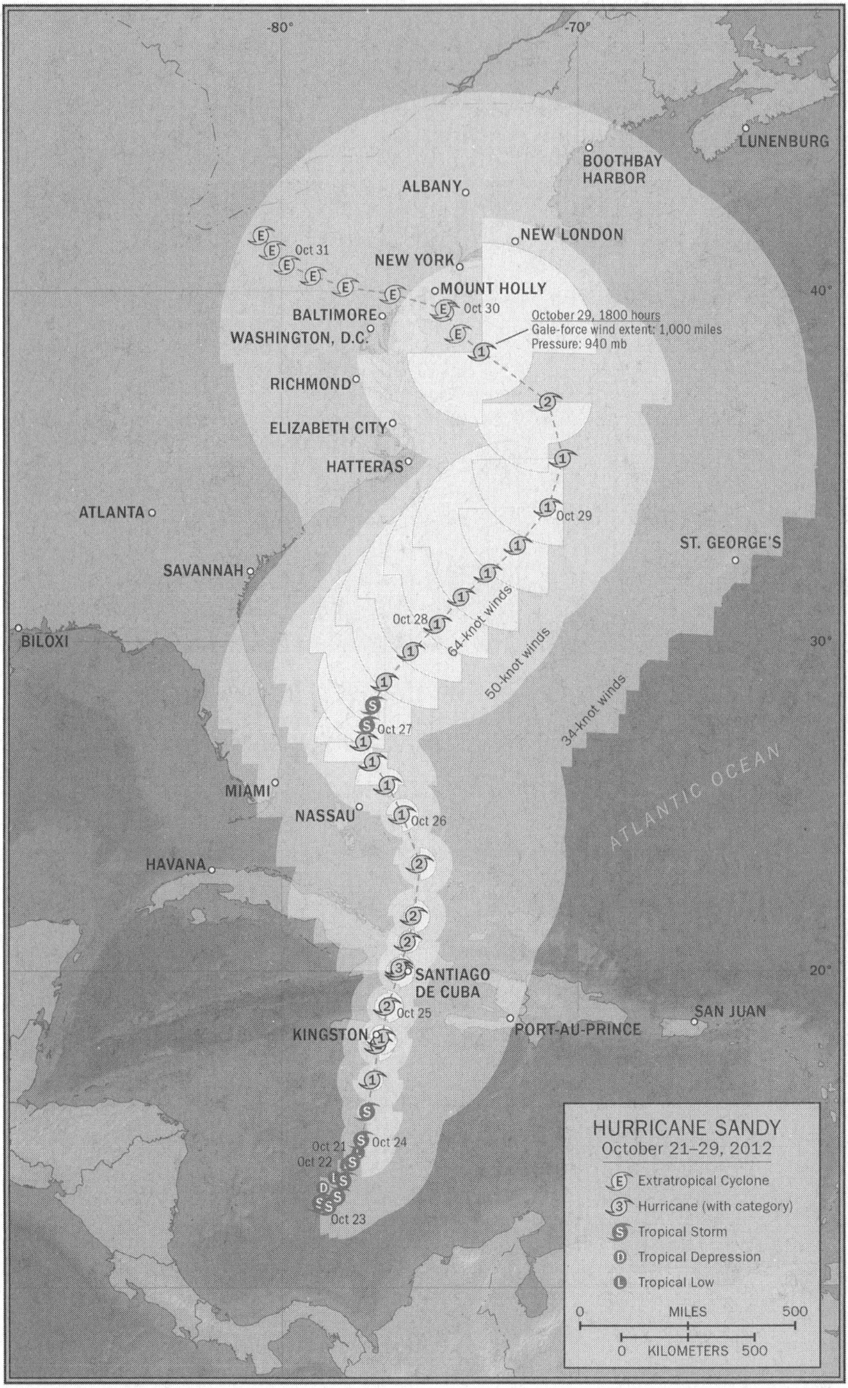

-80°
-70°
40°
30°
20°

LUNENBURG
BOOTHBAY HARBOR
ALBANY
NEW LONDON
NEW YORK
MOUNT HOLLY
BALTIMORE
WASHINGTON, D.C.
RICHMOND
ELIZABETH CITY
HATTERAS
ATLANTA
SAVANNAH
BILOXI
ST. GEORGE'S
MIAMI
NASSAU
HAVANA
SANTIAGO DE CUBA
KINGSTON
PORT-AU-PRINCE
SAN JUAN
ATLANTIC OCEAN

Oct 31
Oct 30
October 29, 1800 hours
Gale-force wind extent: 1,000 miles
Pressure: 940 mb
Oct 29
Oct 28
64-knot winds
50-knot winds
34-knot winds
Oct 27
Oct 26
Oct 25
Oct 24
Oct 21
Oct 22
Oct 23

HURRICANE SANDY
October 21–29, 2012

- Extratropical Cyclone
- Hurricane (with category)
- Tropical Storm
- Tropical Depression
- Tropical Low

0 MILES 500
0 KILOMETERS 500

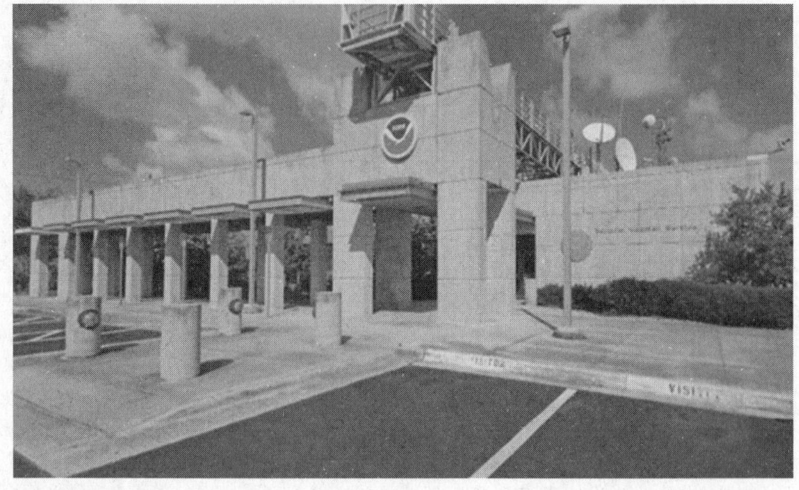

National Hurricane Center (NHC) headquarters, located on the campus of Florida International University in Miami, Florida **NOAA**

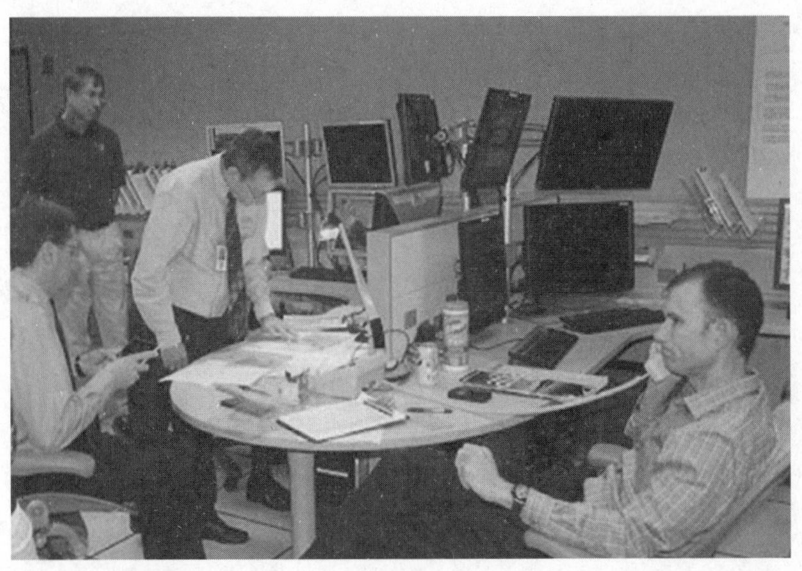

Senior NHC staff participate in a coordination conference call at 10:00 A.M. Sunday, October 28, 2012. From left to right: Director Dr. Rick Knabb, Science and Operations Officer Dr. Chris Landsea, Hurricane Specialist Unit Branch Chief James Franklin, and Storm Surge Team Leader Jamie Rhome. NOAA

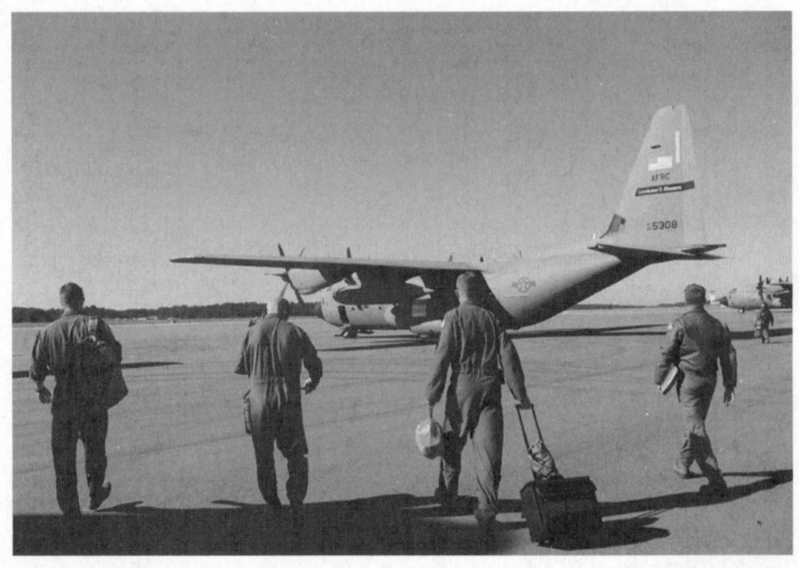

A C-130 Hercules crew from the 53rd Weather Reconnaissance Squadron (WRS) walk to their aircraft for a weather reconnaissance mission into Hurricane Sandy, October 29, 2012, at Hunter Army Airfield, Georgia. The 53rd WRS conducted weather reconnaissance missions in preparation for Hurricane Sandy making landfall along the Eastern coastline of the United States. **U.S. Air Force photo/Staff Sgt. Jason Robertson**

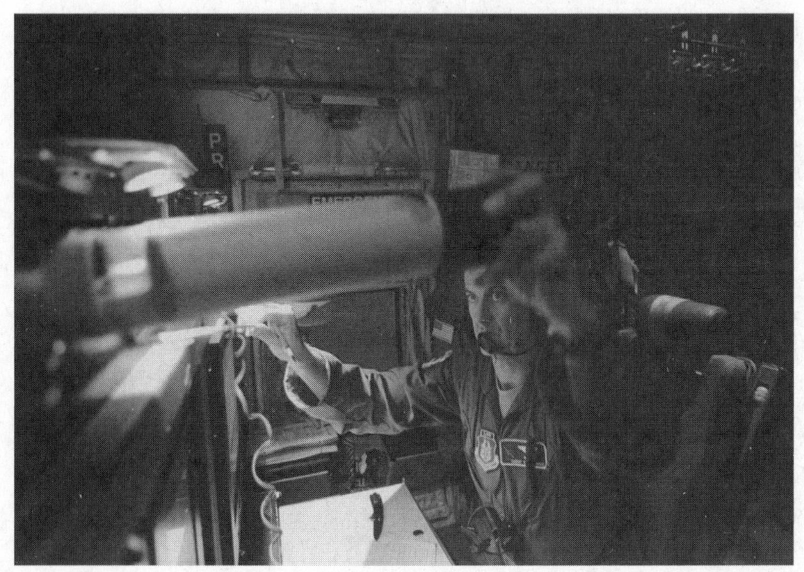

A C-130 Hercules loadmaster, Chief Master Sgt. Rick Cumbo from the 53rd WRS, prepares a dropsonde, which is used to measure and transfer weather data back to the aircraft, while flying on a weather reconnaissance mission into Hurricane Sandy, October 29, 2012, somewhere over the Eastern coastline. U.S. **Air Force photo/Staff Sgt. Jason Robertson**

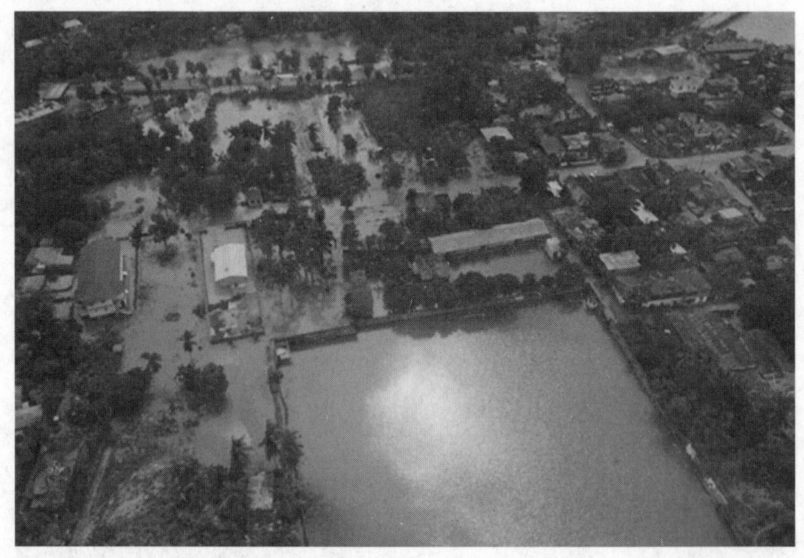

Hurricane Sandy passed to the west of Haiti on October 25, 2012, causing heavy rains and winds, flooding homes, and overflowing rivers. **MINUSTAH/L. Abassi**

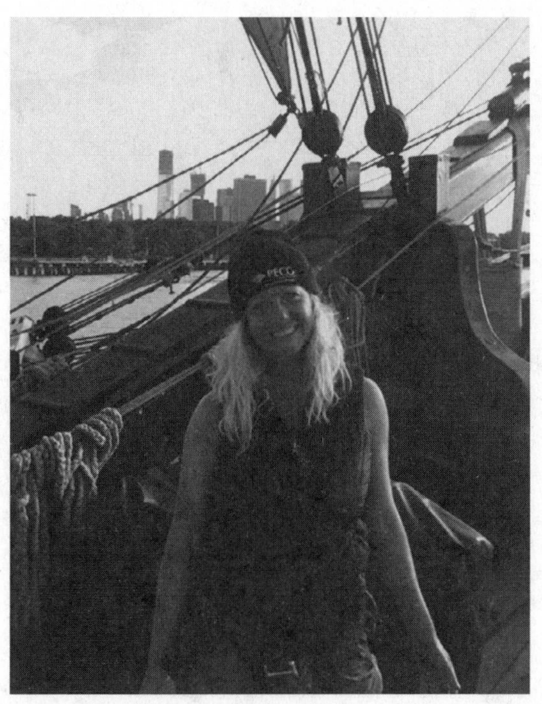

Claudene Christian joined the Bounty *crew as a volunteer in May 2012. She was promoted to a paid deckhand just weeks before the ship departed into the storm.* ***Michelle Wilton***

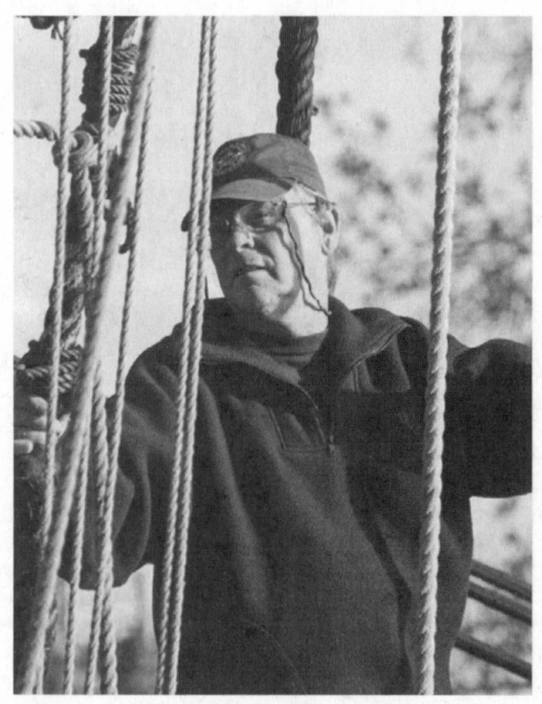

Robin Walbridge took command of the Bounty *in 1995 and spent seventeen seasons as its captain. He was known for fostering a fiercely loyal crew.* **Katie De Prato**

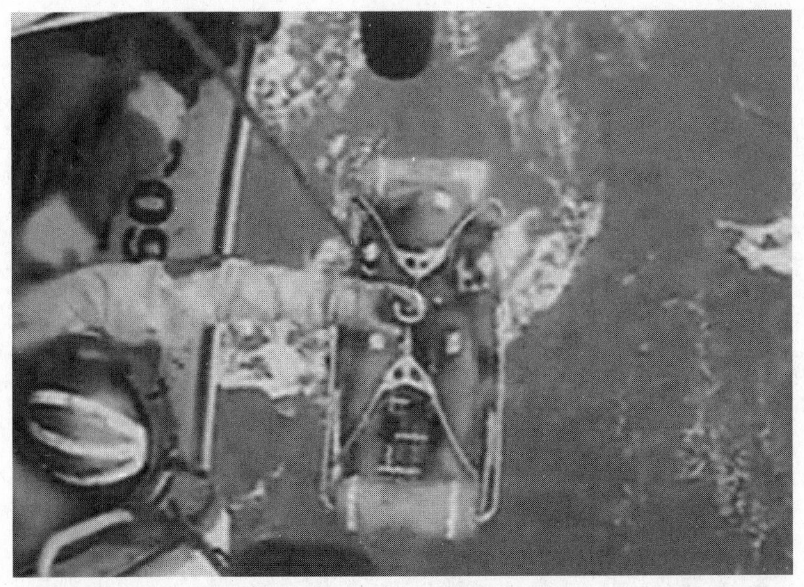

A flight mechanic from US Coast Guard Air Station Elizabeth City pulls a Bounty *survivor into his Jayhawk helicopter on October 29, 2012.* USCG

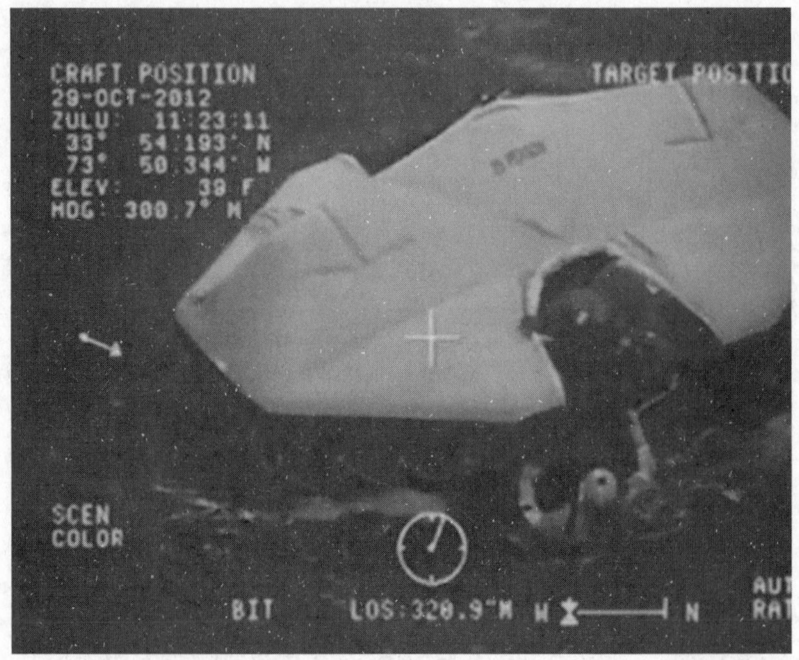

A Coast Guard rescue swimmer assists a Bounty *survivor out of a life raft. This image is a screenshot from a Jayhawk and reveals the helicopter's position and altitude, which is dangerously low, even in ideal conditions.* USCG

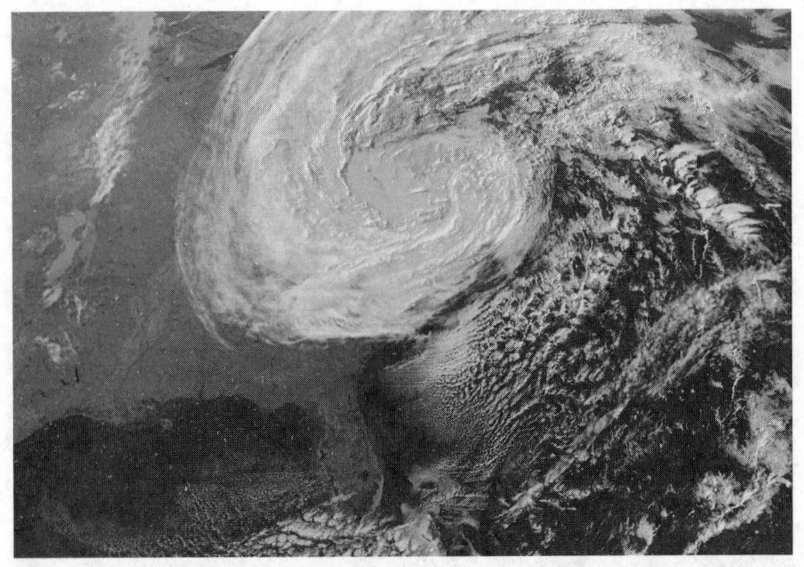

Extratropical storm Sandy, as seen from one of the National Oceanic and Atmospheric Administration's (NOAA's) geostationary satellites, at 6:02 A.M. on October 30, 2012. **NOAA/NASA GOES Project**

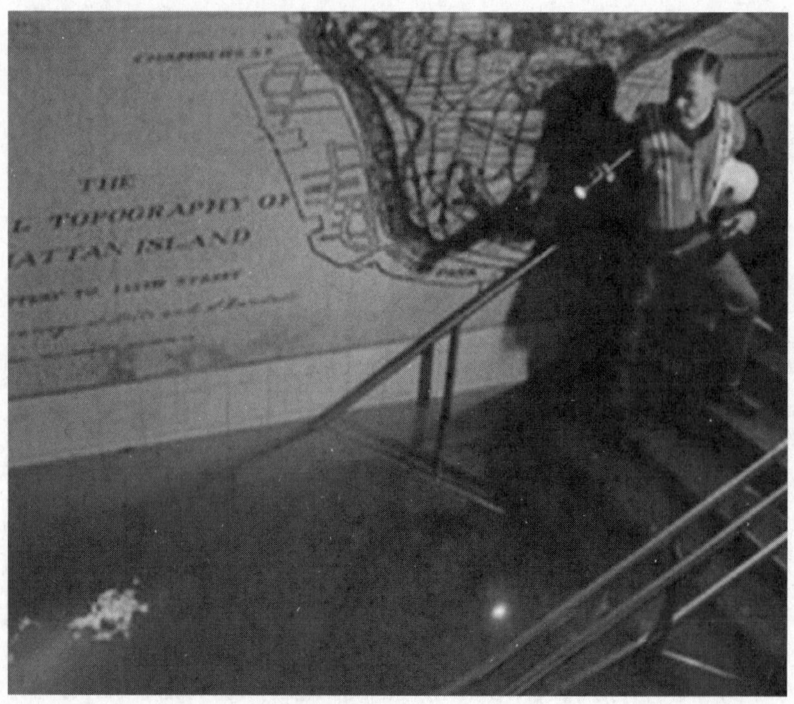

A New York Metropolitan Transportation Authority worker assesses damage to the South Ferry subway station. More than 15 million gallons of saltwater flooded its electrical room, rendering the station nonfunctional. The storm caused the worst damage in history to the city's mass transit systems. MTA

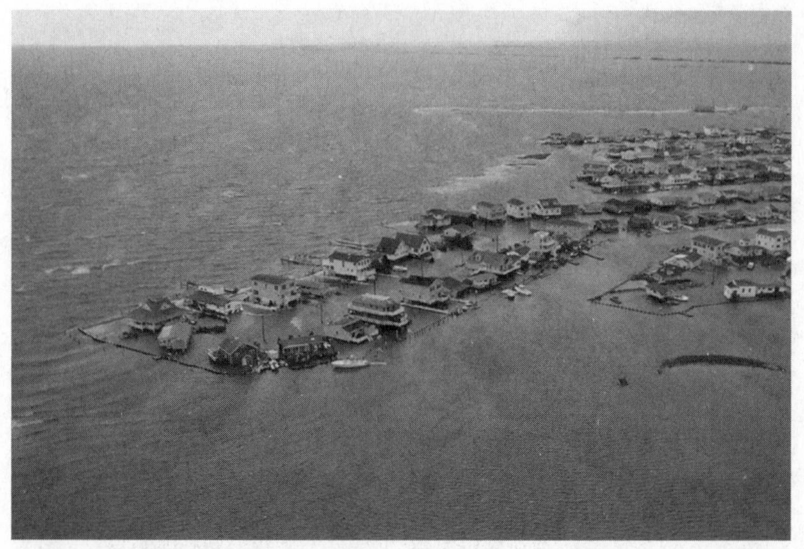

Flooded homes in Tuckerton, New Jersey, a day after Sandy made landfall. An estimated 40,000 Americans were left homeless by the storm. USCG

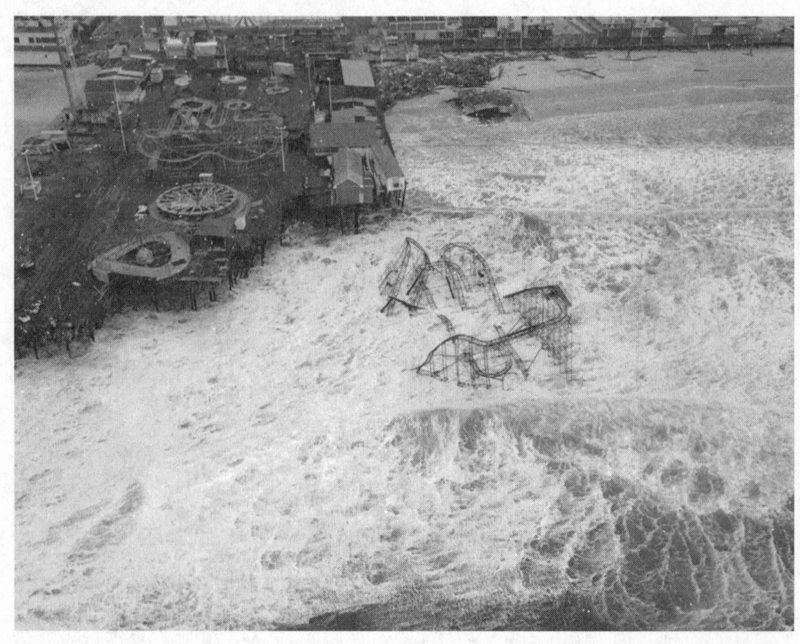

Hurricane Sandy made landfall just south of Atlantic City, New Jersey. Damage to the state was immense and totaled an estimated $36.8 billion, including the destruction of the boardwalks in historic Seaside Heights. **Master Sgt. Mark C. Olsen/U.S. Air Force/New Jersey National Guard**

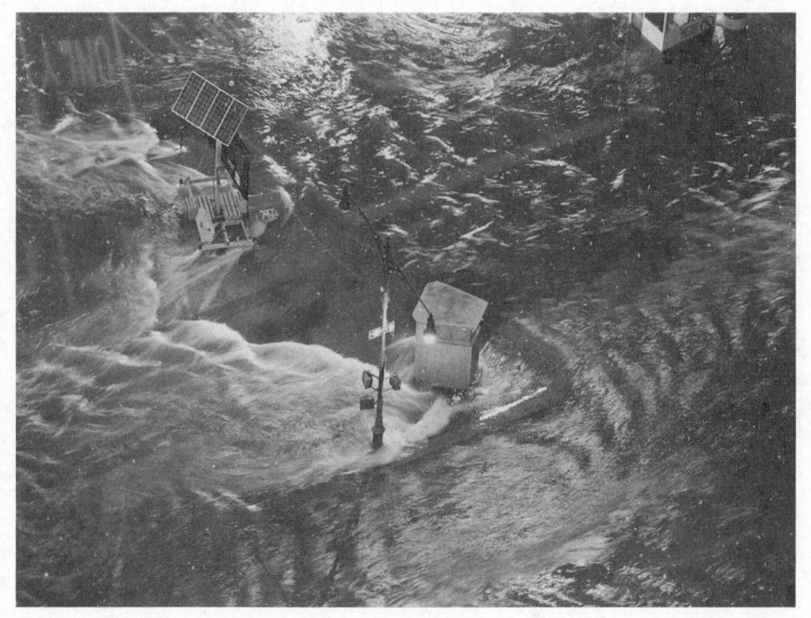

Floodwaters surged into the Manhattan entrance to the Brooklyn-Battery Tunnel during Hurricane Sandy.
MTA/Jay Fine

Friday

1:00 A.M.
Nassau, Bahamas
77°F
Barometer: 29.26 inches (falling)
Winds: 46 mph
Precipitation: Rain
Seas: 8–10 feet

Now a Category 2 hurricane, Sandy began pushing across the Bahamas with winds of 100 miles per hour. They snapped power lines, shrouding the archipelago in darkness. Resorts went on lockdown, sending night owls to their rooms with packaged meals and some drinks. Temperatures dropped to record lows, leaving residents looking for sweaters and socks. They hunkered down in their homes, some pulling their dogs and chickens and goats and horses inside. They tried to make the best of it — they listened to rebroadcasts of Game 2 of the World Series on transistor radios and played cards by candlelight. But soon the winds and rain were joined by walls of water — fierce tidal surge generated miles away and thrown upon the island. It flooded the Grand Bahama International Airport. That same tidal surge ripped docks from their pilings and washed out roads. It contaminated the entire island's water supply and swamped municipal pumps. It submerged cars and poured into houses, where furniture bobbed — headboards and lampshades brushing wet ceilings.

On Grand Bahama Island, Queen's Cove, a sparsely built subdivision of two-story homes that were supposed to be the best in modern convenience, flooded when the nearby canal overtook its banks, submerging empty lots and inundating homes. Residents there clung to rooftops, awaiting rescue. In that same neighborhood, one man refused to leave his home. He was soon trapped by rushing water. His body wouldn't be found until the evacuation order was lifted days later. Hubert Minnis, a member of the Bahamian parliament and leader of the opposition, was one of the first people on the scene. Sandy, he said, was surely not the last storm to rip across his nation. It would take an act of heroic cooperation for them to recover — and to prepare for the next assault. A miracle wouldn't hurt, either. "May God continue to bestow His blessings on our island nation and people," Minnis concluded.

5:04 A.M.
70 miles offshore of Miami
Barometer: 29.56 inches (falling)
Winds: 62 mph (N)
Precipitation: Blowing rain
Seas: 26 feet (building)

Millicent Frick was wide awake. Her cabin aboard the *Norwegian Sky* had become a nightmarish fun house, tilting and swirling. Makeup and glasses crashed around the bathroom. Drawers flew open and slammed shut, sending clothes everywhere. She could hear the wind and waves outside her room. Everything was just so loud — it sounded like the entire ship was being pounded with enormous sledgehammers. There was no way she was going to sleep. Neither was her husband, Ben. Instead, they lay in bed, watching their cabin turn itself inside out.

The day before, Ron Chrastina, the captain of the *Norwegian Sky,* had come over the intercom to announce that they were aborting the day's scheduled trip to Great Stirrup Cay, the 250-acre private island owned by Norwegian Cruise Line. Located just 130 nautical miles east of Fort Lauderdale, the island was in the direct path of the storm. And so, instead, they would spend the day at sea. As they motored out, the rain grew from a light mist to a constant deluge. Winds began to build. It was getting very rough. By the time the group of life coaches assembled in the dining room for a late dinner, Millicent was uneasy. She grew even more so when they were seated near a window, where Frick could see each wave crest just below her. "This was on the sixth deck," says Frick. "Watching those waves, I felt so out of control. We'd sway one way, and then the other way. And the waves were almost up to our window." Her waiter tried to console the group. He told them he'd been in much worse and that the ship was fine. That helped — a little.

But then, just as she was about to try eating, the ship tilted dramatically to one side and didn't right itself. People in the dining room began to scream. "Oh my gosh," Frick gasped. "We're going over." *Get me off this ship,* she added to herself. She was petrified. The ship leveled out. The captain's voice came over the intercom, announcing that he'd run into a snag executing a U-turn. *Everything was fine,* he said. But it was too late for Frick. "The ship kept pounding through those rough waves, slamming down. It was so noisy. I was sick. It was unsettling. More than that, it was terrifying."

Outside the dining room, people were queuing up in long lines for Dramamine. There were signs that plenty of people had been sick, too. Ben was feeling pretty terrible, so they made their way back to the cabin. Every time the ship hit a wave, they'd careen into each other. The whole night, all she could think was, *I want to be off this ship right now.* But that wasn't going to happen anytime soon. The storm had already forced the closing of the Palm Beach port. Port Canaveral, the port of Miami, the port of Everglades, and the port of Fort Pierce were all on restricted access, since conditions there were already too dangerous for many craft. Passengers on the *Norwegian Sky* were wondering if they would be allowed off the ship. Down in the common areas, there were rumors that the port of Miami had closed due to the storm, and overnight, conditions continued to degrade as the storm enveloped them.

The Fricks were glued to their TV, watching as Janice Dean, the meteorologist for Fox News, stood in front of an angry swirl of red and yellow directly atop where the

Norwegian Sky now motored. "You can already see the outer bands spreading out into portions of Florida," said Dean, gesturing to the precise track of the Fricks' ship. "We're going to see the potential for some surf, some big waves, rain, and wind."

The screen cut to a local weather forecaster standing near the water in Miami. It was dark and raining. He struggled to talk over the wind as he reported on damage to homes and flooded parking lots. There were reports of sunk boats in the area, too.

Millicent struggled to fight the feeling of panic that was moving up her neck.

She watched as Janice Dean attempted to explain what was happening within that mess of color. "It's going to become a hybrid," she said. "Sort of a tropical storm–hurricane inside the center of a nor'easter. Something we've really never experienced onshore. It's the 'perfect storm' scenario. And it's going to come onshore and cause a lot of problems. New England and New York, you're really in the crosshairs, which could be really, really devastating." Millions of people could be without power for weeks, she predicted. It could even compromise the election, she concluded.

"Yuck," said one of the hosts. "Let's hope this thing somehow goes away."

Dean didn't look like she thought that was very likely. And neither did Millicent Frick. She and Ben stayed glued to the TV, counting each time Hurricane Sandy was mentioned. Sandy as the dreaded election "November Surprise." Sandy and coastal flooding. Sandy in comparison to Katrina. Each time, the camera cut to the same image of the storm's track: a narrow red line coursing up the coast. The storm was heading directly toward eastern Maryland, where the Fricks' three kids were at home with their grandparents. She hoped to god they were asleep. If they weren't, they'd be watching this very same newscast. That upset her.

The news kept coming. Sandy's damage to Cuba. Sandy's transition into some kind of freakish crossbreed. Sandy's effect on Wall Street. At the end of the hour, the hosts played a word-scramble game with Gretchen Carlson, host of *The Real Story.*

"Can you figure out this long word?" they asked.

Carlson looked at the mess of consonants on the screen and sighed. "I have no idea."

"Think about the weather," urged one of the hosts.

Carlson stammered. "Uh . . . 'monster storm'?"

"Close," they encouraged.

"Oh . . . 'Frankenstorm'?"

"Frankenstorm," they cooed, delighted. "Good job."

Carlson looked exasperated. "Frankenstorm? See now, that's not even a real word now, is it ladies?"

Frick switched off the TV before she could hear their reply.

6:40 A.M.
Savannah, Georgia
66°F
Barometer: 29.94 inches (steady)
Winds: 10 mph (NNE)
Skies: Mostly cloudy

The air had grown heavy at Hunter Army Airfield in Savannah, Georgia. Although it was not yet light out, a large passenger van was already making its way past the front gate and toward one of the large hangars that abutted the two-mile-long runway. Inside, a crew of Hurricane Hunters blinked hard, trying to adjust to the bright lights of the base. Their life had become mechanical: Continuous flights, three crews, all passing one another on tarmacs or in the motel parking lot. Fly. Sleep. Fly. Nothing else. They were entering their fourth day of continuous missions into Sandy. They were tired. They missed their families — the feel of their own beds, a meal that consisted of more than coffee in Styrofoam cups and powdered creamers.

As the van pulled up to the hangar, the crew piled out and began their preflight checklists, happy to have a familiar routine to occupy their tired bodies and minds. Once they were finished, Jon Talbot called them together for a pre-brief. He talked about the flight plan, about what they might encounter between Savannah and the storm. Sandy was beginning to interact with an upper-level trough, and that could mean the extratropical transition was already beginning. Talbot told them what he had gleaned from the NOAA reports. Strong wind shear was causing the storm to weaken, but that weakening was also causing the storm to nearly double in size since it had crossed Cuba. As that growing area met with cooler and drier air, the storm was also beginning to lose some of its tropical characteristics — it was getting sloppy. Unpredictable.

"This is an unusual beast," he heard himself say, not liking the words. "We have to be ready for curveballs because we really haven't dealt with this type of storm before." The crew nodded. Hurricane Hunters don't like the unknown any more than forecasters do. That's especially true when they have to fly through it. Anyone on the crew has the right to suggest they shouldn't go on a mission like this one.

"All eyes on the Eastern Seaboard are looking toward us to get off the ground and go out and get that data. It's a lot of pressure on us," said pilot Major Sean Cross. "But the bottom line is that this mission saves lives, and that's why we're doing it." End of story.

A few minutes later, their C-130 was climbing to twenty-five thousand feet, destined for the Bahamas. As they neared the archipelago, Cross dropped the plane to ten thousand feet. He expected to find pounding rain — the whole crew did. But there was nothing. No sixty-thousand-foot towering monolith of thunderstorm. No eyewalls. No pelting rain.

"That's odd," said Cross.

"Yeah," agreed Talbot. "We ought to be in the thick of it."

The only clue that they were in the vicinity of the storm was the gusting wind.

It bucked the nose of the plane, forcing both pilots to grip the controls. As they did, Talbot looked below. There, the winds had churned the ocean into a white mess, as gusts lopped off the tops of waves and sent spray high into the air.

Oh, man, thought Talbot. *This is going to be stronger than I thought.*

To their south, they could begin to see a shaggy tail of clouds stretching out for hundreds of miles: what had once been the organized bands of Sandy's outer wind fields. The storm had become chaotic, its towers lopped off by wind shear, its bands becoming disorganized by a lack of convection. Without those organizing winds, the tightly coiled storm had begun to ooze out across the horizon, forming a soupy mess that extended nearly two thousand miles. Inside, winds were no longer spiraling down to the surface, but instead were a confused twist of colliding gusts.

This instability made the Hurricane Hunters nervous. Cross took a deep breath and began his flight pattern, cutting toward the southeastern side of the storm. As he did, the lodemaster sent down a series of dropsondes. The crew braced for what should have been the most intense side of the storm. It wasn't. Instead a few clouds drifted on the upper air currents, in sharp contrast to the turbulent weather in the storm's western quadrant. Somehow, the storm had reversed itself. That was the second thing that struck Talbot as odd.

Weirder still was the fact that he couldn't find the storm's eye. It had disappeared from satellite, too. The storm looked disfigured. Lopsided. As if the Cyclops had turned into the Blob.

They kept flying, recording data for the National Hurricane Center, their radio fluttering with the occasional chatter. Then a voice broke in from the US coast guard sector office. A sailboat was adrift somewhere off the Abaco Islands, on the northern tip of the Bahamas. It would take several hours for an Elizabeth City C-130 to get out there. Could the Hurricane Hunters take a look? Cross said he could. Talbot agreed. And so, as the meteorologist continued to take readings, the plane began a search-and-rescue pattern, looking for any sign of the boat. They didn't find any. But what concerned Talbot the most was just how clear a line of sight they had. As the plane punched through the clouds, climbing back up to twenty-five thousand feet for the flight home, Talbot had a nearly unobstructed view of the horizon. They should have been lodged right in the thick of the storm, but instead it spiraled out below them, as if it had been compressed by a heavy hand. Which, says Talbot, was almost exactly what was happening: That high-pressure nor'easter was now spinning down and off the eastern coast of the United States, colliding with Sandy, compressing the tropical storm's uppermost clouds. Down closer to the surface, that same system was merging with Sandy's already powerful winds, creating what Weather Channel senior hurricane specialist Bryan Norcross called "a monstrous hybrid vortex" on his Weather Underground blog that morning.

"This is a beyond-strange situation. It's unprecedented and bizarre," wrote Norcross.

That's precisely what the Hurricane Hunters were witnessing: Sandy was spreading out rapidly as energy from the cold system entered its core, causing it to nearly double in size. The storm's metamorphosis had begun.

"There was definitely some disbelief in that plane," says Talbot. "Not in our entire history had we observed anything like that." And it was about to get much worse.

8:54 A.M.
Atlantic Ocean, 237 miles northeast of Atlantic City
57°F
Winds: 3 mph (ESE)
Waves: .68 feet
Skies: Clear

The *Bounty* crew was up before breakfast, stowing anything that might come loose in heavy seas. A couple of crew members worked on lashing down the gangway. A few more were down below, stashing away gear. They could hear the engines straining, the high-pitched whine that comes only when they are pushed to full throttle. Near the galley, Matt Sanders had hung a giant chart of the Atlantic Ocean that showed the *Bounty* and Sandy. The crew kept coming up with analogies: Rocky vs. the Russian. Godzilla vs. one of those crazy giant insects. The mood was light but electric — kind of like a locker room before a big game.

Up on deck, bosun Laura Groves was pulling together the rest of the crew for a work party: They needed to get down the royal yard — the topmost spar, which would catch the brunt of the wind. It was going to be a lot of work. Not far from them, Robin Walbridge sat in the navigation shack. There, he composed two quick e-mails. The first one was to Tracie Simonin, the ship's onshore manager.

39-45N X 071-18 W

Good Morning Miss Tracie,
You missed an awesome sub tour.

We are headed S X E waiting to see what the storm wants to do. I am guessing it wants to come ashore NJ / NYC.

We are running trying to stay on the east side of it. Bad side of it until we get some sea room, if we guess wrong we can run towards Newfoundland. If it turns and wants to tangle with us that means it is pretty far off shore and we can turn and go down the west side of it. I need to be sure it is well off shore before we can take advantage of the good weather for us. Right now I do not want to get between a hurricane and hard spot. If you can send us updated track info (where it is projected to) that would be great. We know where it is, I have to guess (along with the weather man) where it is going.

Keep you updated,
Robin

Next, he wrote to an old sailing friend.

Looks like I might be able to tell you how far one can drift in a hurricane. Sandy looks like a mean one. Right now we are on a converging course. I am actually headed to the dangerous side of it. Hoping like a deer if I am at it it won't be there when I get there. There is no room to run down the west side of it but if it comes out to play then that will mean there is room on the west side.

At times like this I think about the sailors 200 years ago. There are not signs in the sky, barometer is steady, winds are light. I always watch (knowing there is a storm) for the first tell tale signs. Right now there are none except the electronic weather fax.

Got an awesome tour of SSN Mississippi, US newest nuclear submarine. Quite a boat.

When we heave too [sic] I will keep you posted.

On a square-rigged ship, heaving to is a complicated maneuver and, above all else, a severe-storm tactic. If Robin Walbridge was planning on it, it was because he had a pretty good idea what awaited him out there.

9:33 A.M.
Annapolis, Maryland
63°F
Barometer: 30.21 inches (falling)
Winds: 5 mph (E)
Skies: Overcast

Governor Martin O'Malley signed a hastily crafted executive order declaring a state of emergency. There wasn't time to proofread. "Whereas, the precise path of Hurricane Sandy remains uncertain, the entire state of Maryland must take steps to prepared [sic] for potential destruction and minimize the threat to public safety and the lives of all Marylanders who may find themselves in the path of the storm," began the declaration. It ended with an assertion of O'Malley's powers as governor: to waive regulations for commercial vehicles, to call the national guard into state service, to authorize the distribution of stockpiled supplies, and (if needed) to suspend the statutes and regulations of the state.

10:21 A.M.
Atlanta, Georgia
69°F
Barometer: 30.06 inches (dropping)
Winds: 4 mph (variable)
Skies: Partly cloudy

CNN's Rob Marciano announced that the network would no longer use the word *Frankenstorm* when reporting on the hurricane, following a directive from its management not to trivialize their coverage. "We are refraining due to the severity of the storm," he tweeted to his twenty-seven thousand followers. Inside the studios, severe weather expert Chad Myers sent a text ordering the removal of a banner that used the word. "It's a term that's not appropriate for a storm that's already killed more than twenty people," he told a reporter. "It's too big of an event to make fun of it."

10:28 A.M.
National Weather Service Forecasting Office
Mt. Holly, New Jersey
63°F
Barometer: 30.22 inches (falling)
Winds: 4 mph (NE)
Skies: Overcast

Gary Szatkowski was putting the final touches on his midday weather briefing. "A hurricane or strong tropical storm will affect the mid-Atlantic region late this weekend into early next week," he wrote. There was no longer any reason to play around with probabilities or track potentials. The storm was coming. And it was going to be deadly. "While Sandy could still track a little further to our north, or a little further to our south, we will be feeling her effects one way or the other starting late this weekend (Sunday), continuing into Tuesday of next week."

He wanted to emphasize that point, he says. Max Mayfield, the longtime director of the National Hurricane Center, once joked that the epitaph on his tombstone should read STOP FIXATING ON THE SKINNY BLACK LINE. It's a mantra Mayfield adopted when he realized that residents often made life-threatening decisions based on the predicted track of a hurricane's eye. That's deadly thinking, says Mayfield. Particularly when you're dealing with a storm five hundred miles wide. Sandy was already much bigger than that. As far as Szatkowski was concerned, focusing on where its eye might make landfall was going to "lead to some very bad decisions." The eye could make landfall in Maryland or Massachusetts and still have deadly consequences for people in his region. "People have got to realize that they're not off the hook if they're not in the path of that line," he says. Evidence of that was all around him.

At the five major airports in the region, workers had begun preparing sandbags and testing generators. Contractors at the World Trade Center were battening down cranes and scaffolding. Down in the Chesapeake Bay, the Sultana Project announced that Downrigging Weekend would be terminated two days early: The *Pride of Baltimore II* and the other vessels in attendance needed to get home so that they could prepare for the storm. Nobody aboard wanted to be caught at sea.

Farther south, tropical storm–force winds were now licking the Florida coast. Watches had been issued as far north as North Carolina's Outer Banks. The coast guard set emergency conditions for ports from Baltimore to South Carolina, advising all boaters to stay off the water and seek safe harbor. In Miami, Chris Scraba, captain of the port, set the operating condition to "Zulu," effectively closing the port to all incoming and departing boat traffic. Cruise lines scrambled to reroute passengers and ships. Holland America's *Eurodam* was forced to dock in Jacksonville and wait for conditions to improve. Carnival canceled several of its weekend departures. At Royal Caribbean, Hernán Zini and his team combed charts and satellite images, looking for a safe place to put their ships. The *Enchantment of the Seas* had just left Baltimore carrying twenty-four hundred passengers. She was scheduled to arrive in Bermuda just as Sandy would be passing overhead. Zini called the captain. They both agreed: The ship would head out to sea in search of calmer waters. Another ship, the *Monarch of the Seas,* hadn't managed to make it out of Port Canaveral before the closure. It would have to wait there a day and a half before departing. And once it did, it would remain at sea, rather than make its scheduled ports of call.

At the Elizabeth City Air Station, coast guard base commander Joseph Kelly sent home all nonessential personnel. The crews that remained were busy moving all of their aircraft and emergency vehicles inside. All of them, that is, except for their C-130s. Those were now on their way inland, to the Charlotte airport. Soon, winds on the coast would be too strong even for the coast guard's toughest plane. There was talk of sending the helicopters to Raleigh. But for now their mechanics stayed busy preparing heavy weather bags and discussing who ought to volunteer if they had to go with the aircraft. A couple of them had brand-new babies. They called their wives to tell them what was happening and not to worry. It didn't help much.

And still, the storm kept growing — now reaching out over 800 nautical miles. Sandy had become the largest tropical cyclone on record. News of its transition had exactly the effect Szatkowski predicted: It sounded the warning bell of a five-alarm fire. People were beginning to listen.

11:16 A.M.
Richmond, Virginia
66°F
Barometer: 30.15 inches (falling)
Winds: 10 mph (NNE)
Precipitation: Drizzle

From the executive mansion on Capitol Square, Virginia's Governor Bob McDonnell issued a state of emergency, citing both the track of the storm and its unusual characteristics. Falling temperatures were now predicted throughout the state, along with a chance of snow. "Virginians," he said, "should make sure their family members, friends, and neighbors are prepared for this storm." Across the state, people raised their eyebrows. More than a few even scoffed. No one had heard of snow associated with a hurricane — especially not in Virginia.

12:26 P.M.
Albany, New York
59°F
Barometer: 30.19 inches (falling)
Winds: 9 mph (SSE)
Skies: Overcast

New York State was now under a state of emergency. Its Emergency Operations Center, described by a Homeland Security report as "a cold war relic located in a bunker," was operating around the clock, many of its staff members already clocking in sixteen-hour days. Budget cuts had left the center with just a fraction of its original staff (it had the same number of employees as the center in Iowa, a state with one-sixth the population). Across the state, the floodgates of reservoirs and rivers had been opened. Dams were releasing twenty-five million gallons of water an hour in an effort to accommodate the floodwaters now destined to arrive. "With unpredictable weather conditions, we are taking the greatest precautions — especially after our experience from last year's storms," said Governor Cuomo. "I urge New Yorkers to plan for hurricane conditions and follow news reports to stay updated on the storm's progress."

The response to this declaration from New Yorkers was as fierce as it was varied. "Isn't it too early and too dramatic? I knew liberals are spineless but come on," wrote one reader on the *New York Daily News* Facebook site. "NY Forecasters are always wrong," wrote another. But not everyone was critical. "Preemptive," mused one New Yorker. "I like that. Maybe if they did that in Louisiana prior to Rita, Hurricane Katrina, lots of lives and people's homes and businesses would have been saved. I know one thing if the storm comes and there is lots of damage and lives lost, people would say why didn't Cuomo act. Good job Cuomo." That post got five "likes."

From there, the question rapidly moved into one of comparison. Hurricanes Irene and Katrina were on the minds of many. Just like the *Bounty* crew, these social media followers were making sense of things based on past experience — it's what establishes for all of us the realm of the possible. Even forecasters are quick to say that they learn a lot from previous storms.

The problem, of course, is that no two storms are alike. The average intensity error for the Katrina forecasts was above the ten-year overall average. Irene's were below. Had Hurricane Katrina hit the Northeast instead of the Gulf Coast, the total floodwater driven by the storm surge would have been much greater. High tide on the Gulf is rarely more than a foot; it can be more than ten feet in places like Maine. The switch between high and low tide is more frequent in the north as well, which makes the timing of a hurricane's landfall there that much more important.

After each storm, the Department of Commerce convenes a committee of private and governmental experts to assess the performance of the NHC and NWS. What results is a document called a "service assessment report" that both outlines the successes and failures of the forecasts and recommends future action.

During Katrina, the National Hurricane Center issued what the storm's service assessment report called "unprecedented, explicitly foreboding detail" in their forecasts. The report argues that that language led emergency managers to act swiftly and decisively. That may be one reason why 80 percent of the people in New Orleans's evacuation zones left when ordered. But the report also found that widely varied warning headlines — some of which included language about "catastrophic winds," others about tornadoes or hurricanes — confused the general public. The report argued for more standardized language throughout the course of the storm.

The assessment report published in the wake of Hurricane Irene, on the other hand, criticized the National Weather Service for not adequately conveying the possibility of historic flooding, and it ordered the agency to improve its ability to communicate such threats to media, the general public, and emergency managers. When Irene transitioned to an extratropical system over Maine, the NWS forecasting office in Caribou was forced to cancel its tropical storm warning and replace it with a high-wind warning. Its constituents, it said, were highly confused by the change. The report recommended that the NWS address this problem immediately so that they would have a clear policy should such a transition ever occur again. It also urged the NWS to consider terminology, because during Irene, terms like "tropical storm" had led people to downplay the potential danger.

It also pointed out the need to fully staff NWS offices and ensure that the meteorologists there are well trained, particularly in storm surge and hydrology. The report stated that while the NHC offers weeklong courses on hurricane preparedness and emergency management, cuts to NWS travel budgets meant that forecasters were rarely able to attend. Further budget cuts meant that several key data buoys were out of commission and thus not able to signal ocean conditions for forecasters. Doppler radar at stations like Mt. Holly needed investments of capital if they were going to become more reliable.

The report authors also interviewed emergency managers from New York City and found that the managers "needed a very high level of certainty to justify the evacuation of hundreds of thousands of people and at least three days of lead time to evacuate effectively." The problem, continued the report, was that the maximum lead time for storm-surge guidance was forty-eight hours. That, they said, was sure to be a problem, should another storm strike.

1:30 P.M.
Washington, D.C.
68°F
Barometer: 30.13 (falling)
Winds: 6 mph (E)
Skies: Overcast

At the White House, President Obama ordered a conference call with the heads of FEMA and Homeland Security. The three listened intently as Rick Knabb, director of the NHC, explained what his office was forecasting. Meanwhile, Laura Furgione, acting director of the National Weather Service, and FEMA Deputy Assistant Administrator for Response James Kish were dispatched to Capitol Hill, where they briefed the Senate's Committee on Commerce, Science, and Transportation about the storm. Less than a mile away, emergency operation centers were opening up across Washington. FEMA teams were also on their way as far north as Vermont and as far west as the Ohio River Valley to do the same. States from North Carolina to Pennsylvania were declaring states of emergency, and Maine's Governor Paul LePage authorized a special declaration that would allow power crews from Canada to help residents there prepare for the storm. Meanwhile, down in Norfolk, the US navy was busy sending twenty-four of its largest ships to sea, including its nuclear aircraft carrier, the USS *Harry S. Truman.*

1:42 P.M.
200 miles off the coast of Atlantic City
62°F
Winds: 4 mph (ESE)
Waves: .72 feet
Skies: Clear

The weather was still fair. Perfect, really. The crew of the *Bounty* moved through their watches, then passed through the galley for a quick snack. Jess Hewitt was still talking about the stars from the night before, how clear and bright they were, how Drew Salapatek — another crew member and her sometimes boyfriend — missed a perfect chance to see them by picking sleeping over astronomy. She joined Claudene on deck. Christian had saved a wine bottle from their time in New London. She was making plans to send a message in a bottle. The biggest question on her mind was *to whom.*

The ship passed a couple of sword-fishing boats making slow circles on the ocean as they collected their lines and leaders. Somewhere, just beyond their line of sight, several immense cargo ships were steaming eastward at an ambitious clip. From the ship's navigation shack, Walbridge could just make out their forms on the radar screen. He paused long enough to note their position, then turned to write Claudia an e-mail. She was still in Italy, he knew, but he didn't want her to worry. "Another beautiful day," he began. And it was. Clear and fair, with gently rolling seas. "It's so beautiful out, it's hard to believe there's a storm out there. I'm just waiting to see what Sandy wants to do." He hit send, and an instant later it appeared on Claudia's computer. She was in her hotel room, packing. It was her final day in Italy. She wanted to catch the last of the sights. Robin's e-mail didn't alarm her; she was certain he knew what he was doing.

Back on board the *Bounty,* Walbridge called the crew together for their afternoon muster meeting. He told the crew that the storm hadn't yet picked a direction to go. *We're still not sure if it's going to head out east or for the coast,* he said. They'd try to remain neutral until then. He wouldn't commit until Sandy did first. Walbridge told the crew he'd been checking the weather fax and satellites, but he also wanted them to think beyond that technology.

"Robin was one of those guys who's really old-school," says third mate Dan Cleveland.

He wasn't surprised at all when Walbridge turned the rest of the meeting into a lesson in the history of meteorology.

"Two hundred years ago, when ships like ours regularly sailed the ocean," he began, "would sailors have known a storm was coming?"

The crew looked around at one another. Was this a trick question? Claudene Christian didn't know. But she loved the idea of what history might have known.

He continued. "What signs would they have looked for? How would they have known they were approaching a storm?"

Christopher Columbus was the first Westerner to tackle that issue. In the summer of 1502, he had brought his fleet to Hispaniola when he began to notice eerie changes to the weather there. High, thin clouds raced across the sky, turning an ominous red as the sun began to set. The seas, he said, looked "oily," and were placid for long periods between the growing waves — waves unusually large, he wrote, for such a calm day. And large enough, he surmised, to disrupt the elaborate ecology far below the surface: Turtles and eels, dolphins and enormous squid were all coming to the surface — disturbed, he thought, by the unsettled sea around them. That was a predicament easy for the explorer to understand. The change in weather had also made him tetchy. His joints were aching. His crew was edgy. Columbus had heard talk of these conditions before. And he knew what to do: Seek sanctuary in a southern shelter, where they'd be safe from the worst of the winds. But he had long since overstayed his welcome on the island, and the governor minced few words in denying Columbus safe harbor. Trying to sail through the storm, Columbus concluded, was too risky. So he anchored his fleet in the lee of the island and hoped for the best. It worked. But just barely.

Columbus's ability to survive the storm soon became legendary, and his account of the warning signs was quickly codified. Variations of them were expanded upon by other explorers and sailors in the intervening years, but the basic signs remained very much the same. Henry Piddington's *The Sailor's Horn-book for the Law of Storms,* published in 1848, advises sailors to look for long swell and a fiery red sky marked first by racing clouds and, eventually, a wall of gray or black. Sailors will no doubt notice changes in the behavior of other species, too, adds Piddington: Seabirds, in particular, will either head to land or seek refuge en masse — sometimes on the deck of a ship. Barometers, newly available to the common seaman, were also an excellent tool. Indeed, writes Piddington, crew members, ship owners, and insurance underwriters alike "will all find that *the commander who is watching his barometer is watching his ship,* and that in the most efficient manner."

Father Viñes offered similar suggestions to fin de siècle sailors, advising them to look for bloodred evening skies and growing swell. His book, *Practical Hints in Regard to West Indian Hurricanes,* was somewhat begrudgingly made available to sailors by the US Hydrographic Office, which had it translated and published along with a caveat: "Without accepting these conclusions entirely, the Hydrographic Office hopes that their dissemination among seamen may be the means of calling attention to the various points so clearly set forth by the author, and of proving their value as factors in the great problem of safe navigation." In the book, Viñes warns of the often beguiling first signs of an approaching storm — "dry, bracing, and beautiful weather, clear sky, and exceedingly transparent atmosphere." They are soon joined, however, by vivid sunrises and sunsets aglow with streams of red and purple, along with a slowly thickening cloud cover.

As late as 1940, *Modern Seamanship* — the official textbook of the US Naval Academy — dedicated only two pages to information about hurricane warning signs and avoidance. It wasn't until the Third Fleet encountered a typhoon in the Pacific, resulting in three vessel capsizes, significant damage to another seventeen, and the death of more than 700 sailors, that revised editions included more detailed information. In the meantime, sailors and officers relied upon unofficial apprenticeships in which those who had experienced cyclones could share what they knew. C. Raymond Calhoun was the captain of one of the vessels in the Third Fleet. He remembers being taught such lessons as "Singer's Law," which he describes as, "When the barometer drops .10 inch or more in three hours or less, you're in the path of a typhoon, and you'd better haul ass!" Calhoun was also taught about the "navigable semicircle." It's an idea mariners bank on. Robin Walbridge certainly did.

The official handbook for the International Crew Training program warns that growing swell may extend as far as one thousand miles from the center of an approaching hurricane, and that crews will know they are getting closer when that swell is joined by cirrus clouds: a sign that the storm is about 500 nautical miles away. As the storm rapidly approaches, these high, thin clouds will be followed in quick succession by growing altostratus and nimbostratus formations and, of course, "thick, heavy walls of cumulonimbus clouds," coupled with rain showers. "At this point the center of the system may still be as much as 200–400 NM [nautical miles] from the location of the ship." But by then, the storm's wind and rainbands will already be upon them. What do you do then?

Father Viñes was emphatic: At that point, says Viñes, it's too late for avoidance. The best thing to do is find the least deadly part of the storm. "The track divides the area of the storm into two parts, of which that to the right is called by seamen the dangerous semicircle and that to the left is the manageable semicircle. This classification depends on the greater or less danger usually encountered and on the greater or less effort required to struggle against the storm and to withdraw from its center, according as the vessel is on one side or other of the track. In the dangerous semicircle the gyratory winds tend to force the ship towards the front of the storm, and consequently to throw her in the path of the center." That's the same logic as behind the idea of the navigable semicircle. It's good advice, in the sense that it puts a ship in the lesser of two evils. But they're still really bad options. And recent years have demonstrated that hurricanes don't always bear out this rule. That, says Richard Pasch, came into stark relief in 2007, when Hurricane Noel plotted a deadly course from Cuba to the Canadian Maritimes, taking the lives of at least 163 people along the way. And those unfortunate mariners caught in its path soon learned the hard way that this hurricane had, inexplicably, reversed its semicircles. Anyone looking for safer passage in the left quadrant soon found themselves in the storm's greatest fury.

Robin Walbridge didn't know about that. Nor did he know that Sandy, too, had inverted her dangerous and safe sides. But he did know what the nautical books told him — that mariners often use the back end of a hurricane as a kind of turbo button for their ships, that if you stay a safe distance from the storm itself, you can ride on its tailwinds and increase your speed.

"That was his whole plan," says Claudia. "He'd done it many times before: Just get to where the storm is behind you and it pushes you like a rocket. That's what he wanted to do: to get to the safe side. He knew he could make it there."

3:30 P.M.
New York, New York
64°F
Barometer: 30.14 inches (falling)
Winds: 3 mph (variable)
Skies: Overcast

New York City looked like it was getting ready for war. Throughout Manhattan, volunteers and disaster preparedness teams were stockpiling supplies: 892,000 liters of water; 561,000 meals; 11,900 cots; 165 ambulances. Nearly 62,000 national guard troops were pouring in as well. Officials hoped it would be enough. They knew there was a pretty good chance it wouldn't even be close.

Earlier in the day, Bloomberg's administration had met with Dr. Thomas Farley, the city health commissioner, and Dr. Nirav Shah, the state health commissioner. Later, Farley told the *New York Times* that they both were under the impression that Sandy was weakening — that the impacts to the city would be, at the very worst, on par with those dealt by Irene. It would take days and millions of dollars to evacuate the facilities in the flood zone. The health of patients could be compromised as a result. It didn't seem worth the risk.

Just after 3:30 P.M., Mayor Bloomberg interrupted afternoon programming on five New York TV stations to go live with his afternoon press conference. "Our first obligation is to protect the most vulnerable New Yorkers [in low-lying areas]," he promised. That included six hospitals and forty-one chronic-care facilities in the flood zone. "At this point," Bloomberg told reporters, "we are not — let me repeat that — not recommending evacuations of these facilities." He concluded his remarks with the kind of admission no official likes to make: He just wasn't sure what was in store for his constituency. "You're welcome to go to any of the websites or television or radio and listen to everybody speculate," he told viewers, "but there are probably twenty different forecast tracks for this storm, and any one of them could be right and there's nobody that's going to know anything for a period of time."

That floored Bryan Norcross, the senior hurricane specialist at the Weather Channel. He had been the weatherman for a local TV station when Hurricane Andrew devastated

Miami in 1993. For twenty-four hours straight, Norcross stayed on the air, offering safety tips on the fly, along with updates on the storm. Even after the storm crashed the radar at the National Hurricane Center, Norcross kept at it, using information he was getting from another TV station in West Palm Beach. The event made him a legend in meteorological circles. More important, he says, it taught him a lot about warning the general public. "You've got to get out in front," he says. "It takes days for a warning to really resonate with people. As soon as you tell them to go about their lives and business as usual, people are going to die."

Our ability to convey that threat, he says, is "dysfunctional." Countries like Canada and Japan tie their national weather forecasting to a national news outlet. But in the United States, the National Weather Service has no such relationship. Instead, they issue advisories and warnings and leave their dissemination to the discretion of private media and state or local agencies. For the general public to understand the threat, says Norcross, they need to hear about it for days, and from an authority figure they really trust. Bloomberg, he says, was the perfect leader for that task.

"Bloomberg was the guy everybody turned

to to find out what the story was. He had very strong leadership. And not just for New York City, but for the whole metropolitan area." The mayor was in a perfect place to raise the threat level for this storm. When he didn't, Norcross became concerned. "After that press conference, it was clear to me Bloomberg and the New York City Office of Emergency Management didn't understand the threat," says Norcross. "There should have been warnings. But they weren't being talked about. Somewhere, there was a point of real confusion."

1:51 P.M.
Cape May Courthouse
New Jersey
69°F
Barometer: 30.15 inches (falling)
Winds: 12 mph (E)
Skies: Mostly sunny

Gerald Thornton, the Cape May County director, issued a brief news release announcing the voluntary evacuation of New Jersey's barrier islands, effective immediately. That evacuation order, he explained, would become mandatory on Sunday. It was the first such order of the storm. To emphasize Sandy's impact, Thornton attached to his press release Gary Szatkowski's 10:30

A.M. briefing. "Confidence has increased that the storm will have major impacts on our region," wrote Mt. Holly's meteorologist-in-charge.

3:15 P.M.
NWS Forecasting Office
Mt. Holly, New Jersey
68°F
Barometer: 30.12 inches (steady)
Winds: 5 mph (E)
Skies: Overcast

The pace on the forecasting floor was frenzied. Gary Szatkowski had been there since 7:00 that morning, and he knew he wouldn't be leaving anytime soon. An hour earlier, Governor Christie had echoed Thornton's call for mandatory evacuations of the barrier islands and given communities in the projected path of the storm carte blanche to do what they needed to do to prepare.

"Act first, worry about the DEP later," he told leaders at a press conference. "It's easier to ask for forgiveness than permission. Get done what you need to get done." That earned the governor an enthusiastic round of applause.

No one at the Mt. Holly office bothered to watch the press conference, though. They were already far too busy with the approaching storm. Suddenly, the word *Frankenstorm* didn't seem so alarmist.

"We were dealing with so many things that we hadn't seen before," says Szatkowski. "It was a learning experience. Except that we didn't have any time to learn."

Outside his office, he could hear the phones ringing without pause — people across the region were scared and didn't know what to do. His e-mail box was overflowing, too. No one, it seemed, knew where to go for information. *Could he please add them to an e-mail distribution list? Something?* But the list was frozen — there were just too many people on it as it was. Szatkowski thought about the Twitter feed. His colleagues on Long Island had already switched to social media. So, too, would he. "Please 'like' us on Facebook or 'follow' us on Twitter to receive the notification when we issue a briefing package," he wrote in his public briefing, knowing full well it was a terrible solution: Too many of his constituents still had no idea what to do with social media, let alone how to get there. But it was the best he could do, and the chief meteorologist had other problems to contend with. The models were indicating that wind gusts of 70 miles per hour would soon be arriving, and the higher-ups at the NWS and NHC still hadn't settled on what to call this thing — or who would be issuing the watches and warnings that now seemed inevitable.

Sandy was once again surprising the forecasters. The jet stream was continuing its wonky path, winding up and down the continent. Its twisting, corkscrewing path meant that it could have conceivably sent a hurricane in just about any possible direction, depending upon where the storm met it. Had Sandy been a few hundred miles to the east, it probably would have sent the storm on a dwindling path toward Iceland, which would have caused it to burn out over the sea. But instead, Sandy was meeting the jet stream precisely where it made an orderly turn to the north. A storm inside the jet stream is like a tire slipping into a rut or a bobsled alighting onto its track. Sandy was now locked into a northward trajectory. Only one thing could jar the storm from its course, and that was the massive system cemented over Greenland. That collision would pinball history's biggest storm directly into the mid-Atlantic coast. It no longer really mattered where it made landfall: Sandy was so massive, it was going to affect everyone.

"We were thinking huge coastal storm — the coastal storm of all coastal storms. Our confidence was so high," says Szatkowski.

Tony Gigi was leading the forecast desk that afternoon. The floor was a zoo: Already, a team of reporters had camped out there, and the forecasters were showing signs of stress. Gigi is a conscientious, deliberate guy: When buying a house, he looks first for big trees and streams in the area. "Trees fall over. Streams flood," he says. He's memorized the area around the university where his daughter attends classes and knows the few parking places where her car won't be damaged by crashing limbs or other debris. And he's worked the forecast desk for the NWS for a long time. Even still, he says he'd never before encountered a storm with the kind of destructive power Sandy already had generated.

"It was the most nerve-wracking weather event that I've felt in my life," says Gigi. "It was a lot of stress. A lot of stress."

Gigi remembers being told that there would be many meetings and conference calls going on that day, as the heads of the NWS and NHC determined once and for all how to deal with the storm — what to call it, and who would be responsible for forecasting it. Meanwhile, Gigi was working the short-term desk at the office, which is always the busiest spot in the building. On that day, it felt a little out of control. He had marine forecasts and public products to author, along with a whole host of aviation forecasts, which would determine just how many flights — if any — could get in and out of the busiest airspace on the continent over the next thirty-six hours. The center of Sandy would still be off the coast of Georgia when his short-term forecast expired; tropical storm–force winds associated with the storm would still be more than five hundred miles away. Responsibility for predicting the storm was still the responsibility of the long-term forecasting desk. Gigi's job was to predict what was going to happen for the next twenty-four hours — days before the hurricane made landfall. It was, he said, remarkably easy. The front predicted to merge with Sandy was careering across the continent, dragging cold air behind it. High pressure was infiltrating New England. That dry, cold air was going to collide with the low pressures still draping the region. And whenever two divergent systems like that meet, they create wind. A lot of it. For the next thirty-six hours, Delaware Bay would be seeing gusts that could easily top 40 miles per hour. Gusts of over 40 miles per hour require gale watches and warnings; sustained winds get different titles, like tropical storm watches and warnings. But those kinds of winds weren't going to reach his area until Sunday.

"We're drilled on this," says Gigi. "We have binders. Procedures. When there are gusts of this level, you issue a gale warning."

Szatkowski agrees. "Issuing a gale warning was easy. This was low-hanging fruit."

But just to be sure, Gigi called his colleagues at the Wakefield, Virginia, office to see what they had planned. *Easy,* they said. It's a gale warning. They sent him the text they were planning on using:

> A GALE WARNING MEANS WINDS OF 34 TO 47 KNOTS ARE OCCURRING OR EXPECTED WITHIN THE NEXT 24 HOURS. OPERATING A VESSEL IN GALE CONDITIONS REQUIRES EXPERIENCE AND PROPERLY EQUIPPED VESSELS. IT IS HIGHLY RECOMMENDED THAT MARINERS WITHOUT THE PROPER EXPERIENCE SEEK SAFE HARBOR PRIOR TO THE ONSET OF GALE CONDITIONS.
>
> A STORM WATCH IS ISSUED WHEN THE RISK OF STORM FORCE WINDS

OF 48 TO 63 KNOTS HAS SIGNIFICANTLY INCREASED . . . BUT THE SPECIFIC TIMING AND/OR LOCATION IS STILL UNCERTAIN. IT IS INTENDED TO PROVIDE ADDITIONAL LEAD TIME FOR MARINERS WHO MAY WISH TO CONSIDER ALTERING THEIR PLANS.

Gigi decided to issue a similar warning for his region. This wasn't about Sandy coming ashore; it was about what was happening beforehand. If the storm accelerated, he figured, he could always take down the gale warning and issue a tropical storm warning instead. No big deal.

But that wasn't the reception he and the other NWS forecasters received during their afternoon conference call with the National Hurricane Center. They say Ed Rappaport, the deputy director of the National Hurricane Center, was incensed when he found out about the gale warning. And depending upon which NWS forecaster you ask, you'll hear a different description of his response: Angst. Heartburn. Vitriol.

Rappaport says he doesn't want to comment on that. But he does say he was agitated: He felt like the warning forced his hand and prematurely committed them to issuing nontropical warnings for Sandy.

"We thought we had a game plan," he says. "We really wanted to have another six or twelve hours before a watch went up. The longer we could go without one, the closer we would be to actual landfall and the more likely we would be forecasting the right phase of the storm."

"We all would have been comfortable with that," agrees Franklin.

After the conference call, Mickey Brown phoned Rappaport directly. He wanted to talk about the gale warning.

"We can take it down," said Brown.

Rappaport said it was too late. Besides, he hadn't studied the meteorology of the region enough to make a different forecast for the day. He wasn't about to begin micromanaging forecasters at NWS field offices.

"I'm not following the weather details in your area," he said. "That's your responsibility. If you think the warning is what's best, then I'm not going to interfere with that."

Brown asked him what his preference was.

"Leave it," said Rappaport.

"It's a complicated situation," offered Brown.

"There are times when we have to readjust things on the fly," said Rappaport. "This is definitely not one of those times. We've got a need to be consistent."

As far as he was concerned, the decision had been made: Once Sandy moved north of the Outer Banks, forecasting the storm and informing the public would be the NWS's responsibility, not the National Hurricane Center's.

4:40 P.M.
Miami, Florida
78°F
Barometer: 29.51 inches (rising)
Winds: 21 mph (NW)
Skies: Mostly cloudy

As Senior Hurricane Specialist Eric Blake watched the Hurricane Hunter data stream in, he shook his head once or twice. He ran his fingers through his hair. And then he began to pace.

"Everything about this storm is just weird," he told Landsea, passing by the operations officer's office. "It's a weird, big storm, and you just know it's going to do something really strange."

Landsea looked up from his desk, where he'd been trying unsuccessfully to draw flight tracks for the NOAA reconnaissance jet. The storm was just so big, he couldn't figure out where best to send the plane. This thing really was beginning to look like a monster. Blake offered a welcome diversion. Landsea spun his desk chair around, shaking his head. His lips were pursed. He had a five o'clock shadow. He looked tired. The lecture at the University of Colorado had gone pretty much exactly like he had expected. During the question-and-answer session, someone from the audience asked him what would be so wrong about making a connection between the two if it helped encourage the public to care about global warming.

"What if it's proven to be incorrect?" responded Landsea. "We'll risk losing the trust the public has in us to play things straight."

The questions had then turned back to Sandy: *Didn't the fact that a storm was bearing down on New York prove the climate was changing?*

Landsea tried again. "We know this storm is going to be a real threat for New York. It shouldn't come as a surprise. We've known there's going to be a hit to New York and New Jersey because we've seen it before. It's not global warming. It's the repeat of what we've seen in the past." And on and on it went. He'd been replaying the exchange over and over in his mind ever since.

Landsea looked up at Blake and shook his head.

"Sandy. I've never seen anything like it." He blinked hard. That's how Blake knew he was really thinking — Landsea always closes his eyes. On the other side of the wall, Dennis Feltgen, the public affairs officer, was entertaining questions from reporters, most of whom wanted to know exactly when and where the storm was going to make landfall. They seemed disappointed when he told them he couldn't answer that. "Everybody along the US East Coast needs to be paying attention to this right now," he said. "We're not telling people to rush to the grocery stores. Let's not go overboard with this thing, but you should at least start becoming aware of it."

Nearby, James Franklin was on a conference call with reporters, trying to explain just how large the storm had become. Across the building, Rick Knabb, the director of the National Hurricane Center, was on the phone with President Obama; FEMA administrator Craig Fugate; and John Brennan, assistant to the president for homeland security and counterterrorism. Knabb had been on the job for less than five months. And at forty-three, he was the second-youngest director in NHC history. Landsea was really glad he wasn't in Knabb's shoes that day.

"We were all like, 'What is this thing? What is it going to do? How do you forecast it?' " Landsea couldn't imagine how you explain that to the president of the United States.

"Sometimes it's kind of nice to be at a lower pay grade," he said.

The simple fact of the matter was that no one in the meteorological world had an answer.

"What the hell is going on?" wrote Bryan Norcross on his daily weather discussion on the Weather Underground blog. "The strong evidence we have that a significant, maybe historic, storm is going to hit the east coast is that EVERY reliable computer forecast model now says it's going to happen. . . . The hope we have is that the computer models are not handling this unusual situation well, and are predicting a stronger storm than we get. But we can't bet on it. Even a weaker version will likely mean a nightmare for millions."

A few minutes later he was on the air, talking about the prospect of the storm hitting New York City and what it would mean for America's most populous city.

"Are they going to issue a hurricane warning?" asked his Weather Channel colleague Jim Cantore.

"They've got to do it tomorrow," said Norcross.

5:50 P.M.
Lunenburg, Nova Scotia
58°F
Barometer: 30.12 inches (steady)
Winds: 4 mph (N)
Skies: Mostly clear

The crew of the *Picton Castle* was busy. As dusk settled upon them, they struggled to lash down rigging and add extra chafing gear to their barque. The vessel would remain at the dock, and the crew would remain on her: If the winds shifted, they'd have to motor to an alternate berth. In the meantime, they were under full navigational watch, checking every aspect of the ship each hour. Normally, that level of work is reserved for when a vessel is under way. But Captain Moreland didn't want to take any chances as the storm approached. While the crew worked, Moreland was pacing the dock, trying to arrange alternate housing for the crew: If they got a direct hit, it would become untenable for them to remain on board. But Moreland says he wasn't too worried — their wharf had just been rebuilt, and he felt confident that they'd have decent warning if conditions deteriorated.

His cell phone rang just after he had found the housing. Someone from the main office was on the other end of the line; they'd been on Facebook right when the *Bounty* updated its status: "Rest assured that the Bounty is safe and in very capable hands," the post read. "Bounty's current voyage is a calculated decision . . . NOT AT ALL irresponsible or with a lack of foresight as some have suggested. The fact of the matter is . . . A SHIP IS SAFER AT SEA THAN IN PORT!" Moreland and Walbridge had known each other for more than ten years. The captain of the *Picton Castle* had always considered Walbridge a friend — a true gentleman. But the *Bounty* was an outlier in the tall-ship world, and she needed a lot of work. Moreland was shocked — he would say later that he was "mind-boggled" by Walbridge's decision to set sail: a decision Moreland called "unconscionable on a good day."

Some of those thoughts would take more reflection to develop. With his cell phone still in his hand, Moreland had time only for the most visceral of responses.

"Oh my god," he whispered to no one in

particular. "What in the hell are they doing out there?"

Saturday

2:00 A.M.
Vicksburg, Mississippi
47°F
Barometer: 30.09 inches (steady)
Winds: 10 mph (N)
Skies: Overcast

Brad Leggett knew Claudene Christian was tough. She used to brag that her uncle was a leader of the Hells Angels. In school, she drove a souped-up black pickup truck. She wasn't afraid to jet off to a new city on a whim. But she could also be fragile — especially at night. Claudene would have bouts of fear and say things like she was going to die before her time and that she was afraid she might perish alone. In high school, her best friend Mike had died in a tragic car accident. Claudene had felt haunted ever since: She told her friends and roommates that she sometimes felt surrounded by ghosts; that maybe they were preparing to take her away. She said she just hoped it was so that she and Mike could be reunited.

If that was what Claudene was thinking aboard the *Bounty,* she didn't let on. But she did seem nervous. Worried. She didn't like the noise the ship was making as it pitched against the waves. It sounded like the whole thing might come apart. She told Doug Faunt she didn't like the way some of the other crew members were treating her, either — like she didn't know anything. She wondered if anyone even knew they were out there.

Brad Leggett did. At his house in rural Mississippi, he kept thinking about how frightened Christian had been when they began dating — how she'd flinch every time he sneezed, how she'd curl up so tight when they slept. Sure, Claudene could play the role of someone confident and brave, but she had her fears, and they ran deep. And she wasn't a sailor. Earlier in the season, Claudene had called Brad. They talked about all sorts of things, but what kept replaying in Leggett's mind was what she had said about the ship: that it leaked, that it took on water.

"I was like, 'What? That doesn't sound right,' " Leggett remembers saying.

Christian had shrugged it off at the time. But Brad hadn't forgotten. Nor had he forgotten what her dad had said after dropping her off on the *Bounty* back in May: The ship was worn; it would never pass an inspection.

Brad had sent Claudene a text just before the ship departed, but she didn't respond. Early that morning, he sent another one. *Hey, are you okay?* She didn't write back. That had Leggett worried. The *Bounty* was now off the coast of Virginia. Rain was falling steadily. Wind and swell were growing. And the ocean was all but empty: The nearest vessel was the *Norwegian Jewel,* steaming toward New York, some three hundred miles to their southeast. Sandy, meanwhile, was still thrashing the Bahamas, and the storm had returned to hurricane strength. Twenty-four-hour news shows were showing islands darkened by massive power outages and flooded roads. A supply ship destined for Grand Bahama had been forced to turn back. A governmental administrator patiently answered questions about how that was going to affect the island nation.

"Supplies were low before," he said. "So you can imagine what we are going through now."

The Bahamas were still under a hurricane

warning. Tropical storm warnings were in effect for much of the Carolinas. But no one knew for how long.

The storm, meteorologists were explaining, was growing more peculiar by the moment. Hurricane Hunter data was revealing that the maximum wind field now spread out for more than 100 nautical miles, and the most intense of the winds were still in the western side. Forecasters couldn't say why. Nor were they sure why thunderstorms were confined to that area, too. A warm front was forming a few hundred miles northeast of the center, and another was growing northwest. They were like tumors, and they were making conditions even more perilous. Low-level moisture was making the system unstable as well. The storm had begun its extratropical transition. That, said the broadcasters, required a new kind of playbook for everyone involved.

As Brad Leggett sat in front of the TV, his worry intensified. He grabbed his laptop and sent a quick e-mail to Claudene's dad, asking if he was watching the storm. Rex wrote back right away; he told Brad the ship was planning on going east, all the way around the storm.

"That's the stupidest thing I've ever heard in my life," Leggett responded.

3:00 A.M.
Off the coast of Port Canaveral
71°F
Barometer: 29.49 inches (falling)
Winds: 56 mph
Precipitation: Rain
Seas: 27 feet

Jamie McNamara and other guests aboard the *Fantasy* were wondering why they were at sea. The McNamaras were trying to make the best of it, but that was getting harder every hour. The previous day, Disney spokesperson Rebecca Peddie spoke to reporters about the condition of the vessel: "The Disney *Fantasy* skipped its stop in Castaway Cay today, and instead, guests are enjoying a sunny day at sea a safe distance from the storm," she said. That outraged Jamie McNamara. "She was so far from the truth that I actually laughed, and my husband was offended by her statement. She obviously didn't have a clue as to what the conditions were on the ship, nor should she have commented on it. We were *not* enjoying a 'sunny' day at sea, nor did I feel we were at a 'safe distance' from the storm. We were, in fact, experiencing high winds, closed decks and pool areas, and a complete lack of communication or empathy from anyone on board." Crew members had bungeed the doors to the deck area closed, forbidding anyone to open them after several guests became trapped outside and were unable to open the doors due to the force of the growing winds. All outdoor activities had been canceled, and most of the Disney characters had disappeared from the inside common areas. When Jamie asked about that, a Disney representative told her it was too dangerous for people to walk around in giant mouse and duck costumes. Dinner had been a disaster: The ship was in the thick of the storm now — nearly directly west of Sandy. Passengers had to hold on to their plates so that they didn't roll off the table, and everyone around the McNamaras seemed "really, really frightened." They tried taking their kids to the send-off pageant held in the ship's grand atrium lobby. There, Mickey Mouse was singing his famous good-bye song. People were throwing confetti. *Maybe this wouldn't be so bad, after all,* thought Jamie. But just as that thought flickered across her mind, an enormous wave struck the ship, sending one of the princess characters careening down the large atrium staircase. "We've got to go," said Brian. Jamie agreed and grabbed the kids.

They wobbled their way back to their

stateroom. But that, too, had become a kind of house of horrors, says McNamara — souvenirs and shampoo, wineglasses and shaving cream were all tossing around their cabin like missiles. From the sliding glass door of their cabin, eight decks up, they felt like they could reach and touch the waves. The ship began to roll from side to side, tossing furniture as it did. Bar stools overturned. Bureaus skidded across cabins, sending glassware smashing against walls. Those doors not bungeed began to open and slam as if possessed. Just after midnight, Captain Forberg came over the intercom, urging everyone to remain in their cabins. Later, some passengers would say he sounded nervous — even scared. As he made his announcement, the McNamara family was hunkered down on a single bed, listening to the sound of glass breaking and doors slamming as the ship pitched and pitched and pitched. When one of Jamie's daughters got up to use the bathroom, the bathroom door slammed shut on her hand. She wailed. Brian leapt up to grab her and tried to stuff some towels around the door to keep it from banging. Everett hugged his stuffed animal tighter and looked up at Jamie. "Mommy," he said, "I'm too young to die." That, she says, pretty much broke her heart. "He's not a timid kid."

Those on the sixth-level deck watched as waves slammed against the sliding glass doors of their cabins. Heather McGee was on board with her family. "Everything came off the shelves and countertops. Our son was on the upper bunk, and it had a railing, but every time it would list, it would toss him toward the glass door," McGee said. Worried about the safety of her five-year-old, she and her husband tucked him into their bed, bracing him against the cabin wall.

Made seasick by the swaying of the upper decks, some passengers opted to try their luck in the lower-level atriums, where they sprawled on couches or spooned on the swaying floor. Others took the opportunity to record videos of plates flying across restaurants and entire gift-shop display cases overturning, spewing purses, watches, and tons of Disney memorabilia onto the floor. Windows broke; glasses smashed against walls. Mothers placed their young children in life vests and began plotting how they'd get the kids out of the ship if it capsized.

Just after 3:00 A.M., Forberg returned to the intercom, assuring the passengers they were perfectly safe. *The ship can handle it.*

Please stay in your staterooms. Later, Captain Forberg admitted to some of the passengers that the conditions they encountered were far more harrowing than had been predicted — and more than he expected. Still, that did little to placate them, some of whom were already in the process of creating a Facebook page for passengers with complaints. Within hours, it would have more than one hundred members. "It was quite possibly the worst night of our lives," says Keri Suess, who surveyed the damage done to gift shops and the ship's opulent restaurants, now a chaos of broken glass and downed chairs. Her young son stood by. She looked at him. "What was the captain thinking when he sailed a ship full of small children into such a powerful storm?"

5:46 A.M.
New York, New York
61°F
Barometer: 30.03 inches (steady)
Winds: 7 mph (ENE)
Skies: Overcast
Waves: .75 feet (building)

The city was still dark. Outside, available taxicabs cruised up and down largely empty streets, patrolling for early risers looking to get to a train station or airport. A few intrepid joggers worked their way down the esplanade on the banks of the Hudson. Down on the piers, someone turned on a weather radio just in time to hear an urgent broadcast from the Upton National Weather Service forecasting office. The computerized voice warned of an increasing threat "of moderate to significant coastal flooding" beginning Sunday night and into Monday. Tides could be two to three feet above astronomical norms. Battery Park could see more than eight feet of floodwater. Historically high surf could, of course, make these flood levels many feet higher. "A coastal flood watch means that conditions favorable for flooding are expected to develop," the voice continued. "Coastal residents should be alert for later statements or warnings . . . and take action to protect property." The joggers kept going, oblivious to the warning.

8:30 A.M.
Chesapeake Bay
63°F
Barometer: 29.99 inches (falling)
Winds: 8 mph (NE)
Skies: Mostly sunny

It was a perfect morning for a leisurely sail off of the Pasadena peninsula, and that's precisely what Jan Miles and his wife were doing. Leslie had packed a picnic, and the two were out on their fiberglass sloop, enjoying an easy morning. A couple hundred miles to their south, Lieutenant Mike Myers was enjoying a similarly leisurely start to his day, dawdling over pancakes with his three daughters. As a copilot on one of the Elizabeth City C-130s, Myers doesn't get a lot of downtime, so he says he knows how to make it count. Somewhere nearby, his pilot, Wes McIntosh, was out for a nine-mile run: *Crazy,* Myers thought, *but that's an alpha pilot for you.* Their phones rang simultaneously: Sandy was getting close now, and winds were increasing. Before too long, the crosswinds would be too high for the C-130 to take off from the airfield. McIntosh's crew was moving to Raleigh.

Those staying behind would begin storm prep immediately. The coast guard's Wilmington sector office was hard at work preparing for the storm as well. Any mission launched in the area is overseen by the command center there, where they do everything from handling initial calls of distress to coordinating search-and-rescues, all from a hermetically sealed command center that looks a whole lot like the forecasting floor of the National Hurricane Center. Like the NHC, sector North Carolina has to be able to withstand a major storm with both its electronics and people intact. They may evacuate their family members, but the staff of the sector are going to weather a storm so that they can do everything they can to keep people safe. During Hurricane Floyd, as water lapped at their building, the sector staff coordinated heroic rescues off of buildings throughout the state. During Irene, they oversaw oil cleanups and statewide damage assessment. There was plenty of both, and the hurricane still weighed heavily on the mind of Sector Commander Anthony Popiel.

"Mother Nature can be very cruel," he says. "She plays to win every time."

That becomes Popiel's mantra during a storm event. As sector commander, he has the power to close down North Carolina's ports and to decide if and how a rescue can initiate. That means he needs to know everything he can about the conditions outside his command center, too. On that particular morning, he was on the phone with the National Weather Service, listening in on the day's briefing. The storm was getting closer, bringing with it low-slung skies and monstrous swells. Despite the warnings, surfers were beginning to congregate at beaches. Pleasure boaters were out securing their boats. The nearest coast guard cutter, *Elm,* was on standby in Atlantic Beach, having been repositioned to better weather the storm. Just to be sure, Popiel gave a quick call to confirm the ship's readiness. Someone was going to need rescuing, Popiel knew. Whether or not they could be saved would come down to just how well the coast guard could perform in adverse conditions.

8:57 A.M.
Atlantic Ocean, 425 nm northeast of Norfolk, Virginia
62°F
Barometer: 29.67 inches (dropping)
Winds: 18 mph (NNE)
Waves: 5 feet (building)
Skies: Overcast

Clouds now blocked out the sun. Aboard the *Bounty,* those standing morning watch couldn't say for certain when the sun rose — they just noticed that the sky got a little lighter gray. Chris Barksdale, the ship's engineer, awoke to an unfamiliar sensation: seasickness. The rocking of the boat made him feel unsteady. He was glad for the jack-lines.

After breakfast, Robin Walbridge made his way to the nav shack to find an e-mail from Tracie Simonin waiting for him. She was sending the 6:00 A.M. storm advisory from the National Hurricane Center. It said that Sandy had been downgraded to a tropical storm. The headline read, SANDY WEAKENS BUT IS EXPECTED TO REMAIN A LARGE STORM WITH WIDESPREAD IMPACTS INTO EARLY NEXT WEEK.

That weakening was temporary. By 8:00 A.M., Sandy was again hurricane strength and growing. The advisory for that hour read:

> HURRICANE FORCE WINDS EXTEND OUTWARD UP TO 35 MILES . . . 55 KM . . . FROM THE CENTER . . . AND TROPICAL STORM FORCE WINDS EXTEND OUTWARD UP TO 275 MILES . . . 445 KM. THE WIND FIELD OF SANDY IS EXPECTED TO GROW IN SIZE DURING THE NEXT COUPLE OF DAYS.

Simonin didn't send that second advisory to Walbridge, so he thought it was still a tropical storm. Just before 9:00 A.M., he sent her a return message.

> Hi
> Thanks for the update, because of it I feel okay about trying to sneak to the west of Sandy. New course 225 T.
>
> It looks like it will stay off shore enough to us to squeak by.
>
> Thx.

Then he tacked his ship and set a collision course for the eye of the storm.

9:05 A.M.
Port Canaveral, Florida
70°F
Barometer: 29.49 inches (rising)
Winds: 37 mph (NW)
Skies: Overcast

The Disney *Fantasy* had been hovering about a mile southeast of the port for hours, waiting for conditions to improve. The ship was supposed to have docked at 7:00 A.M. Passengers were lining up at the customer service desk and in the atrium, waiting for a free phone that would allow them to reschedule missed flights. Few of them saw the small pilot boat as it battled its way out to the cruise ship, its bow slamming hard against the sea. Waves splashed up and into the pilot house on board. Around it, the skies were low and gray.

It took several tries for the boat to pull up alongside the enormous cruise ship. And even there, on the ship's leeward side, the wind was raging. A pilot, dressed in bright blue and red foul-weather gear, emerged from the protection of the pilot house, struggling to hold on to a support bar as he picked his way across the bow of his boat. The 45-mile-per-hour gusts of wind whipped at his jacket, wrapping the hood around his neck. His step was timid, as if he was unsure of his footing. Aboard the cruise ship, two officers stood in their dress whites, each wearing a thick red harness and clipped to a heavy bay door. They were holding a rope ladder — standard procedure for the mandatory boarding of a pilot before entering the harbor. The pilot boat, no match for the heavy waves, beat hard against the cruise ship, pulling the ladder this way and that. Every second or third wave was enough to catapult the boat high above the bay door, forcing the officers to step back, straining against the anchored lines that held them in place. Spray drenched them. Drenched the pilot. Drenched the skipper, who had driven the boat out beyond the safety of the harbor. He reversed the boat, trying again to line up with the bay door. The pilot reached out for the ladder, just making contact. He lost his grip. He tried again. And again. On the fourth try, he made a tiny leap toward the ladder, grasping it with both hands. The officers pulled him up as the boat turned into the waves, its onboard camera now blurred by salt and foam. An hour later, the eleven-hundred-foot ship, flanked by three tugboats, struggled into the port.

Amid the crowd of tired, tousled passengers in the atrium, the McNamaras sat clustered together atop their luggage.

Around them, the chaos of the previous night was still apparent. Furniture was overturned. Gift shops were in shambles. They could smell alcohol from the duty-free store, where dozens of bottles of expensive liquor had broken. Jamie passed the time by composing a letter of complaint in her head. "Disney has failed miserably in this situation," it would begin.

10:58 A.M.
National Hurricane Center
Miami, Florida
79°F
Barometer: 29.31 inches (steady)
Winds: 18 mph (W)

The FEMA hurricane liaison room isn't much bigger than a walk-in closet. Painted a dark gray and overflowing with state-of-the-art communications technology, it operates like a souped-up television studio, capable of broadcasting teleconference calls with meteorologists and lawmakers around the country. It was getting a lot of use. The next FEMA coordination call was scheduled for 11:00 A.M., and Chris Landsea struggled to make his way through the growing scrum of reporters now overflowing the glassed-in seminar room where they were supposed to be sequestered. But their number had grown too big over the past twenty-four hours, and even Dennis Feltgen, the National Hurricane Center's bulldog of a public affairs officer, was having a difficult time corralling them. Landsea let out an audible sigh of relief as he slipped into the FEMA studio, where he joined NHC director Rick Knabb just a few minutes before the call. The cameras in the studio had been running nonstop as various members of the NHC did their best to explain just how serious Sandy had become. Landsea could hear the staff making a similar statement to reporters out on the forecast-desk floor. Earlier in the day, Feltgen had issued the official press release stating that the National Hurricane Center would no longer be issuing advisories as soon as Sandy became post-tropical. Once that transition occurred, the NHC web page would no longer include forecasts or advisories for the storm, either. Instead, explained the release, National Weather Service forecasting offices like Mt. Holly would continue to provide detailed information on local impacts. The Hydrometeorological Prediction Center would assume responsibilities for issuing public advisories about the strength, location, and track of the storm. The Ocean Prediction Center would continue marine advisories so long as the storm remained over water.

Reporters in the fishbowl seemed confused. What was the Hydrometeorological Prediction Center? Where did its advisories appear? James Franklin took a deep breath and explained it again. Chris Landsea watched, glad again to be at his pay grade. This was serious.

"We were all trying to communicate that this is not Irene," Landsea says. "It's much, much worse. Irene traveled south to north, so New York City really just got a glancing blow. Sandy was on a direct westward march, which means she was going to bring her full force to bear on New York and New Jersey."

The FEMA studio's soundproofing did little to dull the din outside on the forecast floor. Landsea could tell the situation was heating up out there, and he was glad to be sitting in the relative still of the studio. This scheduled call was supposed to be with FEMA reps in the area and in Washington — a chance to emphasize to them just how dire the situation had become. But 11:00 A.M. came and went, and the television monitors remained blank. Five minutes passed. Then ten. Landsea was getting antsy; he had so much work to do out on the floor. He felt Knabb shift a few times. He was no doubt feeling anxious, too.

Landsea turned to the FEMA coordinator setting up the call. "What do you think the delay is?"

"Hard to say. But usually it's because they're trying to get someone important on the line."

Landsea nodded and then stood up a little straighter. And then he continued to wait. Minutes later, the ninety-inch screen blinked on. The face of President Obama, phoning in from Air Force One, appeared. The plane was on its way to New Hampshire, one of the last stops on the campaign trail.

"Hi, Mr. President," Knabb said a little sheepishly.

"How long is the worst of the storm going to last?" Obama asked. "How soon can we get going with recovery efforts?"

That impressed Landsea.

"We're not sure," said Knabb. "It's a slow-moving storm. There's going to be a lot of damage."

Knabb went on to explain that the Hurricane Center was about to issue its first public advisory with specific storm-surge forecasting. They were predicting four to eight feet of inundation for New York City;

if the storm hit during high tide, that would be more than enough to swamp the subway system and cause perilous conditions for hundreds of thousands. Regardless of when the storm arrived, flash flooding was expected to affect others throughout the region. Cruise lines were in the process of emptying their terminals, and fleet commanders, including Hernán Zini, were working around the clock to find new berths for their ships. The Port Authority was closing everything from the Newark Container Terminal to the South Brooklyn Marine Terminal.

President Obama wondered aloud if that was enough.

"I want to bring all available resources to bear to support state and local responders," he told them.

Craig Fugate, FEMA administrator, was also on the call. He told Obama that the agency was already on the case. The New York transportation authority would activate their incident command center first thing the next morning. Despite the fact that the storm surge from Irene got within one foot of flooding subway tunnels and rendered entire sections of the commuter rail system impassable, people were still furious over the city's decision to close mass transit during Irene. Klaus H. Jacob of Columbia University's Earth Institute thinks that view is pretty shortsighted. If Irene did anything, he says, it demonstrated just how vulnerable New York is to the effects of major storms: Everything, from the city's electrical grid to much of its public transportation to housing for some of its most vulnerable residents, exists below ground level within the surge zone.

Storm surge has always been a problem for New York. Key structures, including the Holland and PATH tunnels, are at risk of flooding every time a nor'easter strikes. In 2004, the remnants of Hurricane Frances flooded the city's subway system. Three years later, a massive thunderstorm system brought with it enough rain to shut down the city's subways again, stranding hundreds of thousands of commuters. In both cases, neither the subway's drainage system nor its pumps could keep up with the deluge. Elliot G. Sander, chief executive of the Metropolitan Transportation Authority at the time of the 2007 stoppage, blamed the National Weather Service for not predicting the storm. The state homeland security chief agreed, telling reporters that "the National Weather Service blew it." A spokesperson for the NWS countered, saying that they issued both a flood advisory and a flash-flood warning.

Ross Dickman, the meteorologist-in-charge at the Upton, New York, NWS forecasting office, says that part of the problem, too, is that different city and state organizations use different services to get their weather. The Department of Sanitation, for instance, uses AccuWeather. The MTA uses the NWS. Their forecasts can be significantly different, particularly when it comes to things like precipitation amounts and the timing of storms. Dickman says that the Office of Emergency Management has asked the different weather services to coordinate, but the meteorologist says that's beyond the scope of the NWS. "We can't coordinate with private-sector people," he says.

He and Klaus Jacob both agree that the debate over who should predict what is moot so long as the city maintains an antiquated subway system in a flood zone without adequate pumping and water retardation equipment.

Currently, more than 11 percent of New York City exists within the flood-risk zone; that includes nearly four hundred thousand people. That number is expected to more than double in the next fifty years, as both sea levels and population figures continue to rise, putting the city's infrastructure in even more jeopardy than it already is. Sea levels in New York City have risen more than one foot since 1900. By 2050, more than 50 percent of power generation for the New York City metropolitan area will be located within the one-hundred-year floodplain. If these trends continue, the chance of surge inundating Manhattan will drop from one in every hundred years (what it was last century) to one in four years. With every sea-level increase comes a new forecasting challenge. "You're starting from a new zero," the National Hurricane Center's storm-surge expert, Jamie Rhome, says. "The exact same storm is going to produce an even worse storm surge in a future time."

We've tried different methods to combat this kind of problem. In 1953, a severe winter storm brought a storm tide of nearly twenty feet to parts of Europe. More than eighteen hundred people died in the Netherlands. Three hundred were killed in England. Both nations responded by building surge barriers, including the iconic Thames Barrier in London. After the 1938 hurricane, several New England towns built their own versions of surge barriers, ranging from seawalls and dikes to more elaborate structures. A 2005 study suggested that a series of barriers erected at key points around Manhattan could prevent catastrophic flooding; engineers involved estimated that the project could be constructed for approximately $10 billion. That same year, Hurricane Katrina breached at least one levee in New Orleans and overtopped many more, prompting inquiries into a flood-containment system many saw as grossly underfunded and mismanaged.

The city of New York never formally pursued the idea of a barrier system. But after the flooding incidents in 2004 and 2007, the transit authority made some improvements, like elevating ventilation grates and reconfiguring entrances into subways so as to arrest the flow of floodwaters, but in the event of a major storm surge such measures would be far from sufficient.

"We're playing Russian roulette," Jacob had warned in a *New York Times* article just months before Sandy's arrival.

City officials agreed, but they didn't have the funds to begin a new and less deadly game. What they could do, they said, was to be sure to include "customer advocates" in an effort to ensure that decisions were made with the general public in mind.

11:34 A.M.
Hartford, Connecticut
60°F
Barometer: 30.05 inches (falling)
Winds: 5 mph (N)
Skies: Overcast

The state of Connecticut was preparing to do battle with Sandy. And just to drive home that point, Governor Dannel Malloy decided to hold his storm-briefing press conference at the State Armory. There, inside a drafty gymnasium, he stood on the stage from which he usually welcomed soldiers returning from Iraq and Afghanistan. There was no such message of gratitude and hospitality on this day, however. Instead, the governor told his constituents to prepare themselves for disaster. The Upton, New York, NWS forecasting office was indicating increasing confidence that there would be major impacts to the region, he explained. That included the possibility of significant and widespread flooding, along with strong surf. Major beach erosion and local washovers were expected. "Folks, this could be bad," said Malloy. "Really bad." Flooding could be on par with the hurricane of 1938. People could be without power for weeks. To make matters worse, he said, Sandy was predicted to be an exceptionally slow-moving storm, which meant that surge and winds would have a cumulative effect on the region. Portions of coastal towns, including Bridgeport, Fairfield, and Westport, were already under voluntary evacuation orders. Those orders would become mandatory by noon on Sunday. All state parks and beaches would be closing that day as well.

"We have to prepare for the worst and hope for the best," said Malloy.

1:09 P.M.
Cape May, New Jersey
64°F
Barometer: 29.94 inches (falling)
Winds: 18 mph (NE)
Skies: Partly cloudy
Seas: 6–9 feet

At the coast guard training center (TRACEN), three hundred new recruits had just received word that they would soon have to evacuate. Nearby, at Coast Guard Station Cape May, enlisted personnel were working hard to relocate the station's response boats to safe havens. Work at both sites paused momentarily as four state police helicopters passed overhead. They flew in formation and low enough to make out the words *Homeland Security.* Aboard one of them, Chris Christie and several of his staff were preparing for the governor's second press conference of the day. They had begun their morning at the state's Regional Operations Intelligence Center in West Trenton before staging an event in East Keansburg, just across the lower New York Harbor from Coney Island. Now, some two hundred miles and several hours later, they were late for the briefing. At the Anglesea Fire Company, a crowd of reporters huddled in the driveway, awaiting the governor's arrival. He appeared nearly fifty minutes late and wearing a blue fleece embroidered with his name and title. Sandy, he said grimly, was a severe and potentially devastating storm. Conditions were going to get much worse than they had with Irene. Christie announced that he was calling for the mandatory evacuation of the Jersey shore, including the Atlantic City casinos. Tolls had been waived on the Garden State Parkway and Atlantic City Expressway so that people could get out faster. He chided cynical New Jersey residents who were considering staying behind.

"Everyone is saying, 'Crap, this isn't going to happen. The weatherman is always wrong.' " *Not this time,* Christie promised. "Let me be clear about this," he said. "We should not underestimate the impact of this storm and we should not assume the predictions will be wrong."

2:17 P.M.
New York, New York
64°F
Barometer: 29.96 inches (steady)
Winds: 11 mph (ENE)
Skies: Mostly cloudy

Governor Cuomo had moved to his New York City office. There, he hosted yet another press conference, which included updates from the state health commissioner and Port Authority representatives. But what most people really came to hear was what the governor would say about mass transportation in the city. They didn't have long to wait. Standing with Joseph Lhota, chairperson of the MTA, Cuomo announced that the transportation authority had begun preparing for a suspension of bus, subway, and commuter rail lines. It was part of the MTA's hurricane plan, which calls for action whenever winds top 39 miles per hour and storm-surge forecasts reach four to eight feet. The Upton National Weather Service was predicting that winds on Monday would reach 40 to 50 miles per hour, with potential gusts of 70 to 80 miles per hour. New York, Connecticut, and New Jersey were under a flood watch; Upton was predicting total water levels to top eight feet at Battery Park, with major flooding in places like the south shore of Long Island. Neither Cuomo nor Lhota could commit to a definitive shutdown, they said, but given the process of first relocating and then storing cars and buses, they felt it prudent to begin now. Lhota told his customers — all 8.5 million of them — that they should plan to complete their travels by Sunday.

That included commuters in places as far away as Staten Island, where the railroad runs the length of the island, from St. George down to the neighborhood of Tottenville. About six miles northeast of Tottenville is the neighborhood of Great Kills — the last stop before departing Staten Island's south shore. Great Kills has a protected harbor, a national recreation area, and a main drag with some pizzerias, liquor stores, and a bike shop that promises easy layaway. Parts of the town can feel a little rough — some of the gas stations and storefronts on Hylan Boulevard have bars on their windows. But down by the water, a marina stays flush with powerboats. Up on the hill, tree-lined streets separate well-manicured lawns. Neighbors there tend to keep an eye on one another. Older residents look after younger families, sometimes unawares.

Several neighbors quietly kept track of the Moore family. They liked them a lot. Damien, thirty-nine, had immigrated to the United States from Donegal almost twenty years earlier. He still had his Irish accent, and that tended to endear him to people in a community with plenty of pubs with names like Flanagan's and McGinn's, along with a swim club that hosted a special "Irish night" every year. He was employed by the city as a sanitation worker. Moore's wife, Glenda, was a nurse. She was also thirty-nine. The two were married in 2009. Their son Connor was four. Brendan was two. They both had curly hair. Brendan's was dark, like his mom's. Connor's was bright red: classic Irish hair, some people said. Connor loved to swim; Damien had set up a pool for him, though he couldn't persuade Brendan to join in. Neighbors assumed it was because he didn't like water. Besides, it had long since become too cold for a dip.

That afternoon, an elderly neighbor watched Damien as he hung Halloween decorations outside the house. The boys had their costumes; they were already planning a trick-or-treat route. The Moores didn't know how long they'd be staying in Great Kills. They both worked in Brooklyn, and the commute was wearing on them. Brenda's sister lived there, too. It'd be nice to have family nearby. Damien's parents still lived in Ireland. He went back when he could, but it was too much to take the boys.

The Moores told neighbors they were thinking about moving. In passing conversation, people agreed they'd really miss them: The kids were always so happy, and their parents clearly adored them. They were kind of an ideal family, really.

3:43 P.M.
Miami, Florida
85°F
Barometer: 29.58 inches (rising)
Winds: 23 mph (NW)
Skies: Scattered clouds

Whenever a storm begins to form in the Atlantic Ocean, the Caribbean Sea, or the Gulf of Mexico, an automated system operated by the National Weather Service begins using a sophisticated ensemble computer model known as Sea, Lake, and Overland Surges from Hurricanes, or SLOSH. The SLOSH model can take into account the unique characteristics of an area and plug that data into thousands of possible hurricane scenarios, ultimately creating what is called the Maximum Envelope of Water (MEOW), a kind of worst-case scenario for surge in a particular area, and the Maximum of the MEOWs (MOM), which details a worst-case scenario for a perfect storm of a particular category. The data from MEOW and MOM is used by emergency managers to make key decisions about evacuation zones and policies. Once a storm is under way, these programs use a complex series of physics equations, past storm information, and current data to produce storm surge estimates. And 224 storm-tide sensors, maintained by the US Geological Survey, provide information about water level and wave heights, which gets rolled into the modeling as a storm nears.

There are two types of SLOSH models: One creates forecasts for tropical storms, the other for extratropical storms like nor'easters. Initially, Sandy fit cleanly into the capabilities of the tropical SLOSH model. However, as the storm began to change over the Bahamas, it began to fall in between the capabilities of the two models. It takes a human forecaster to see that shift and to adjust the surge forecasts accordingly. Normally, when a storm becomes extratropical, the National Hurricane Center's involvement ends. And that means that Jamie Rhome's does, too. The mission of the NHC is clear: "To save lives, mitigate property loss, and improve economic efficiency by issuing the best watches, warnings, forecasts and analyses of hazardous tropical weather, and by increasing understanding of these hazards." If a storm isn't tropical, it isn't part of their purview.

Sandy, though, was clearly serious enough to allow for a little mission creep. And because of the storm's severity, Rhome and his supervisors decided he should remain involved, even though doing so was uncharted territory. "I was doing laps outside my normal swim lane," he says.

Rhome's subcontractors can provide him with data and help him interpret what the models are saying, but they aren't allowed to speak for the federal government. When it comes to issuing a forecast or helping an emergency manager make an evacuation decision, the entire United States must rely on one guy. Luckily, he's really good at his job. Rhome grew up in a small town in the North Carolina Piedmont, and the accent has stayed with him, though he can drop it at an important meeting with the World Meteorological Organization or at a White House briefing. He reads a lot about how stress affects the body, which is good — his body manages a lot of it every hurricane season. It's not uncommon for him to go three or four days without sleep during a storm.

"I walk the precipice of burnout nonstop," he says. He'd love to have a bigger staff — James Franklin says everyone at the National Hurricane Center would love for him to have a bigger staff — but funding and a hiring backlog have prohibited that so far. Besides, says Rhome, there aren't a lot of candidates for the job out there.

"So few people can do this. Dozens of academics claim they do it better, but it's not the scientific prowess, it's the ability to focus one's self under such intense pressure and public visibility."

Rhome was feeling a great deal of both that Saturday afternoon. Sandy was now 250 miles north of the Bahamas. Emergency managers from eleven different states (Rhome can't begin to estimate how many counties or towns) were calling, asking for information about the surge and its effects on their communities. Mostly, though, he was on the phone with Ross Dickman at the Upton National Weather Service office. Both meteorologists agree that surge forecasting is a collaborative effort: Rhome has the model data, Dickman or a forecaster in another area has the local knowledge.

"In the Gulf of Mexico, surge goes almost universally inland. But the varying topography in places like New York causes very localized flooding." That, Rhome says, can be very hard to communicate to people.

Sandy's surge was predicted to be higher than Irene's, though it was still too early to say just how much. Four to eight feet for New York City was Rhome's official prediction. Weather Underground's director of meteorology, Jeff Masters, gave the prospect of a flooded subway system a 30 percent chance. In meteorological circles, that is a very high percentage.

Rhome had been calling Dickman every few hours. When he called just before three o'clock, the two double-checked their figures. Rhome asked if the forecast still fit what Dickman was looking at. The meteorologist said that it did. Rhome felt good. Out on the forecasting floor, Rick Knabb, the director of the National Hurricane Center, was hosting yet another press briefing. "There's no avoiding a significant storm-surge event over a large area. We just can't pinpoint who's going to get the worst of it," he told reporters.

"What time do you want to get back on

the horn?" Rhome asked Dickman.

"As soon as you're able," said Dickman.

He'd been getting calls all day from the New York City Office of Emergency Management (NYCOEM). The calls were becoming increasingly urgent.

"They wanted a graphic, something that would show where the surge was going to go." Dickman says you can't do that — at least, not with the software available to the National Weather Service at that time. "Tides, timing — there are so many little variables," he says. "It's virtually impossible to ask a human to try to identify a specific number in a spreadsheet of data points."

Instead, Dickman told them what he felt certain about: Surge levels were forecasted to be four to eight feet above the astronomical high tide. Waves up to eight feet were expected in New York Harbor. The total water level could be as high as twenty-one feet. Their 5:30 advisory would now include a coastal flood warning and surf advisory for Sunday night into Tuesday morning. The voice at the other end of the line seemed frustrated. Their office had trained to make decisions based on data received from the National Hurricane Office. Upton wasn't signaling information in the same way. Dickman told him he was working in concert with Jamie Rhome — that the two had arrived at the surge predictions together. That wasn't enough. The NYCOEM needed the information in a way its team of geographic information systems (GIS) specialists could deal with. They said they weren't feeling very confident about what Upton was sending them. Dickman told them it was the best he could do.

5:09 P.M.
Wilmington, Delaware
65°F
Barometer: 29.92 inches (falling)
Winds: 12 mph (ENE)
Skies: Partly cloudy

A state of emergency was now in effect for the state of Delaware. It included, among other things, the mandatory evacuation of the state's coastal communities. Sandy's track kept shifting, said Governor Jack Markell, but it had nevertheless become clear that the state was going to be affected by high winds and rain. Shelters in all three of the state's counties would open at noon on Sunday. They would provide what Markell called "some basic food," along with cots for the elderly and people with special needs. Everyone else, he said, should bring sleeping bags and pillows, along with books and games and anything else that might keep a family occupied. Within days, he said, the towns located on the coast would inevitably be cut off from the rest of the state. When that happened, first responders would not be able to help anyone who stayed behind. Markell trusted that residents would obey his order.

"This is not a police state. People need to take personal responsibility here," he said. "This is serious stuff."

6:23 P.M.
New York, New York
63°F
Barometer: 29.96 inches (steady)
Winds: 7 mph (variable)
Skies: Partly cloudy

Mike Bloomberg was late for his 6:00 P.M. press conference at the city's Office of Emergency Management. His press secretary, Marc LaVorgna, sent out a tweet to the media:

> Sit tight for a few min if ur waiting for @MikeBloomberg's storm update. Just wrapping up final briefing with all City agency heads.

Back behind the briefing room, Bloomberg

was listening intently to the reports from his Office of Emergency Management, along with the Department of Health and Mental Hygiene. They were looking at the forecasts, trying to account for the possible impacts — particularly from storm surge. The mayor wanted to reach consensus.

"You're looking at a lot of information," says Cas Holloway, the deputy mayor for operations. Holloway was Bloomberg's right-hand man. He was in charge of oversight, for ensuring the coordination of the city's coastal storm plan. "You're trying to figure out what you think these impacts are going to be: Are you going to order tens of thousands — or even hundreds of thousands — of people to evacuate? And if you do that, what is the basis of your decision?"

He says the city had been criticized for its decision to evacuate during Irene, but that the mayor and his staff stood by that decision. In the year since the storm, the decision had been vetted and evaluated, and it stood up to inquiry.

"We had no hesitation about evacuating," says Holloway. "We'd done it before."

Joe Bruno, commissioner of the New York City Office of Emergency Management, was thinking about Irene, too, though for different reasons. He says he talked to the NWS meteorologist who was embedded in the NYCOEM. That forecaster told him that surge levels were predicted to be four to eight feet. The 5:00 P.M. advisory issued by the NHC said the same thing.

"Everything we saw looked a lot like Irene. With Irene, we didn't see the impacts; we handled it quite nicely. So we felt confident we could ride out Sandy at four to eight feet."

That's what he remembers telling Bloomberg: "What we have now, Mr. Mayor, is very similar to Irene."

Good, said Mayor Bloomberg, *let me know if anything changes.*

They had arrived at consensus.

A few minutes later, Mayor Bloomberg made his way into the briefing room. As his phalanx of staff members and emergency managers filed in behind him, he chatted with the sign language interpreter standing next to him, telling her about connections he had to a high school for signing — the principal there, he said, was also the sister of the city's commissioner for immigrant affairs. The interpreter smiled politely. "Excellent," she said. "Seems such a small world."

"Yeah," agreed Bloomberg. "Yeah, it is." Cas Holloway stood behind him. He fidgeted with his blue blazer, then crossed his arms and joked with a few city commissioners and representatives from Con Edison, the electrical company for New York, as they clustered on the small stage, vying for room with state and POW/MIA flags. Bloomberg wore a light blue cashmere sweater with the sleeves rolled up. He looked calm — like he was at a fund-raiser or a cocktail party.

"Are we ready?" Bloomberg asked no one in particular.

"We're getting there," he affirmed, again to no one in particular.

And then he began. He explained that he was there to bring everyone up to date on the emergency situation. He said that President Obama had asked Craig Fugate, director of FEMA, to call earlier in the day and offer FEMA's services.

"I assured him that we had, we think, everything under control," said Bloomberg. FEMA, he said, would be better deployed helping other parts of the country that didn't have the infrastructure New York did.

"This is a dangerous storm, and I think we're going to be okay," said Bloomberg. "If things are the way it's planned and if everybody does what they're supposed to do, we will get through this very nicely and look back on it and say, 'Maybe we can offer some help to other parts of the area.' "

Sandy, he predicted, would be less dangerous than Irene.

Bloomberg said he wouldn't be ordering evacuations for any part of New York City. "We are making that decision," he explained, "based on the nature of the storm. Although we are expecting a large surge of water, it is not expected to be a tropical storm– or hurricane-type surge. With this storm, we're likely to see a slow pile-up of water rather than a sudden surge, which is what you'd expect with a hurricane. Which is what we saw with Irene."

All city workers, he continued, were expected to report to work on Monday. City services would continue as scheduled, though he advised people to weigh down their trash-can lids so that they wouldn't blow away. Commuters should expect some delays on the Staten Island Ferry, he said. And then he wrapped up his remarks.

"Let me reiterate: As of now, we are not ordering any evacuations."

The storm was going to bring a lot of wind. And there'd surely be damage. But, Bloomberg said by way of conclusion, Sandy was "nothing that we don't think we can handle."

More than one person disagreed.

6:37 P.M.
Miami, Florida
75°F
Barometer: 29.73 inches (rising)
Winds: 11 mph (WNW)
Skies: Partly cloudy

Jamie Rhome was watching Bloomberg's press conference from the FEMA liaison room. It'd been days since he had slept for more than a couple of hours at a time. He'd been trying to plow through the fatigue. The mayor's statement sent a jolt of adrenaline through him. Suddenly, he felt very awake. "The threat of storm surge was already quite high," he says. "I was obviously really concerned."

The NHC surge expert isn't supposed to give briefings at the city level. Nor is that person supposed to micromanage evacuation decisions. Rhome is a rule-abiding kind of guy. But this was far from a normal situation. "Time had elapsed for New York City," he says. "So I made the difficult decision. I broke ranks and stepped in."

He called the first person he could think of: Donald Cresitello, project planner and hurricane specialist for the US Army Corps of Engineers. The two scientists had worked together to develop evacuation zones for the New York region. They were Facebook friends. They were peers — Cresitello was thirty-three, Rhome was thirty-five — and they could level with each other. Rhome says he remembers thinking it was really important that he impress upon Cresitello just how concerned he was about what was about to happen to New York City.

Cresitello says his heart sank when he saw Jamie's name come up on his cell phone. "There's a joke in this industry that when the National Hurricane Center has time to call you, it's a sure sign you're screwed," he says. Cresitello had just gotten off the phone with one of his bosses, who had called to ask why New York City wasn't evacuating. He remembers feeling flabbergasted — and even more so when he picked up the phone to talk to Jamie.

"It's an unprecedented event, Don," said Rhome. "I need to speak to NYCOEM."

Cresitello told him he'd set it up.

It was Kelly McKinney, the deputy commissioner of NYCOEM, who picked up the phone when Cresitello called a few minutes later. Cresitello said NYCOEM should expect a phone call from the National Hurricane Center momentarily. McKinney says it was that moment when the magnitude of the situation really hit him.

"What does the NHC want to talk about?"

"Your evacuation decision. I think there's been some miscommunication here," replied Cresitello. "There's going to be an issue."

All McKinney could think was, *There's got to be information we don't have.* This was serious.

6:55 P.M.
NWS Forecasting Office
Mt. Holly, New Jersey
61°F
Barometer: 29.94 inches (falling)
Winds: 4 mph (ENE)
Skies: Clear

Gary Szatkowski was dumbfounded. Floored. He stood akimbo, looking at the television screen above the Mt. Holly forecasting desk, where Bloomberg was now taking questions from reporters. Did he really just hear the mayor of New York say that this storm was no big deal? He looked at his forecasters. They were tired. They had been working nonstop to get word out about the storm. Bloomberg had all but sabotaged their plans.

Criticism was going to come hot and heavy, he predicted.

Szatkowski sighed. That criticism, he knew, was going to land firmly in his lap.

The phones at the public affairs desk had been ringing steadily throughout the day, but within moments of Bloomberg's press conference, they were on fire. Residents in his area were confused: Governor Christie had said go; Bloomberg said stay. What should they do? Media representatives from newspaper editors to on-air meteorologists were calling as well. Information was coming from too many places, the partners complained. No one knew where to look. No one knew what "extratropical" meant. A gale warning didn't carry nearly the impact of a hurricane warning, they explained. Neither did a coastal flood warning. They needed language that would make sense to their viewers and readers: People heard those kinds of warnings, and they worried about the cost of a flooded basement, not that they might be swept to their deaths in a raging torrent. A high-wind warning didn't do much more. Worst of all, people were confused. They didn't even know if they were affected by any of the warnings. Why couldn't the National Hurricane Center post the warnings issued by the forecasting offices? What were the emergency managers supposed to do? Neither New York nor New Jersey used emergency alert systems for coastal-flood and high-wind warnings, so they weren't even certain how people would get the news.

"You're getting so caught up in the technicalities, you've lost sight of the big picture, which is getting the word out and warning people," one on-air meteorologist told him. "It makes my job much harder when I have to keep explaining what a post-tropical storm is when I could be telling people how to prepare." Officials at the Port Authority of New York and New Jersey agreed.

Szatkowski asked them what they wanted him to do.

"Break the rules," said one New Jersey official. Another agreed.

Szatkowski raised his eyebrows. "Break the rules? *That's* an interesting comment."

They persisted. He became frustrated.

"Look," he heard himself saying. "Pretend I'm your doctor. I shouldn't have to lie to you about your condition to get you to take your medicine."

James Franklin was experiencing the same phenomenon down at the National Hurricane Center. Again and again, he heard the same request — a plea, really. *Just break the rules. Call it a hurricane. It'll save lives.*

That rankled Franklin. "I know we got a lot of criticism for our decision," he says. "But media people didn't necessarily appreciate just how complicated a situation it was to begin a new procedure on the fly."

7:10 P.M.
Atlanta, Georgia
60°F
Barometer: 29.81 inches (rising)
Winds: 11 mph (WNW)
Skies: Clear

Franklin's answer didn't sit well with Bryan Norcross. He was back at the Weather Channel headquarters in Atlanta, and he, too, had been watching the press conference. He had been certain that Bloomberg would call for massive evacuations. "I was shocked," he says. "It was clear to me that New York was confused. They ended up with a threat analysis that was just plain incorrect." The day was ticking by. New York City and much of the mid-Atlantic region would be feeling the effects of Sandy in less than twenty-four hours. But the National Hurricane Center remained true to its decision, and posted no tropical warnings. Now Bloomberg was telling people they didn't need to evacuate.

"We all looked at ourselves and were like, 'You've got to be kidding,' " says Norcross.

What to do? It's a challenge, says Norcross, because he knows that it's not a meteorologist's role to make policy decisions. But this was different.

"When you feel like governmental folks are misinformed or not thinking right, when something has gone wrong, people are being led astray. You just feel like when you are absolutely certain that a misunderstanding is in the works that will affect people significantly, you feel the need to take action to mitigate it."

This, he says, was clearly one of those times.

"We had confidence in our analysis of the threat and how New York should react to it. We were ready to support the mayor in his decision to evacuate. Now, instead, we had to find ways to express our concern."

He took to his blog, criticizing both Bloomberg and the National Hurricane Center. He called Bloomberg's statements "incomprehensibly inexplicable." He accused Bloomberg of playing down the storm and behaving "bizarrely out of character." The same could be said for the National Hurricane Center:

> The normally well-oiled machine that is the Bloomberg administration seems to have slipped a communications cog. And in a possibly related cog-slipping develop-

> ment, the National Weather Service decided NOT to issue a Hurricane Watch for the Northeast coastline . . . are you ready for this . . . because it would be confusing to switch from that to a Coastal Flood Watch and a High Wind Watch after the storm — which will come ashore with hurricane-force winds — morphs into another kind of storm according to the meteorology dictionary. Whether the missing Hurricane Watch sent the Mayor off-kilter, we'll see. But the criticism came hot and heavy . . . enough that the Weather Service wrote up a big media release to explain why the clearest possible communications is a bad thing. I grant that a technical reading of the "rules" says that you can't put up a Hurricane Watch and a Coastal Flood Watch and a High Wind Watch at the same time. But I'm betting the rules didn't envision a super-mega-combo freak of a storm slamming into the most populated part of the country. When all hell is breaking loose, sometimes you've got to break a few rules to do the right thing.

He was trying, he says, to do what is always the right thing for any forecaster to do: Save people's lives. He explained that even if forecasters had their predictions only partly right, there would still be more surge than during Irene:

> The forecast calls for a massive, destructive storm to affect tens of millions of people. If the forecast is wrong, hooray. But so far it's been right, and the odds are this is going to be really bad for a lot of people. Everybody's goal should be to be sure that as many people as possible are as ready and aware as they can be.

He reread his post and thought about what he really wanted to see happen. "Let's all get on the same page," he added.

But it was too late for that.

James Franklin says that he and his hurricane specialists think of Bryan Norcross as a really good friend to the NHC. "But not on that day," he says.

7:20 P.M.
Miami, Florida
73°F
Barometer: 29.75 inches (rising)
Winds: 7 mph (W)
Skies: Scattered clouds

Sandy was now just over three hundred miles southeast of Charleston, South Carolina, trudging forward at 13 miles per hour. Wind and rain were lashing the barrier islands there, and buoys were reporting waves nearly thirty feet high. Surf was moving entire dunes, beginning to clip houses on the shore side of North Carolina's Outer Banks. The winds had begun groaning the night before and had increased in the hours since: a constant, raging noise that seemed to seep inside your body. People there were complaining of headaches and fatigue — effects, longtime residents said, of the rapidly dropping barometric pressure. The waves kept building, removing entire chunks of Highway 12, the only road onto Hatteras Island. Residents there were still recovering from Hurricane Irene, which had washed away homes and left the island without a bridge for months. The state had suspended ferry service to the nearby Ocracoke Island as well; any resident still there would have to ride out the storm.

That's precisely what Jack Markell, governor of Delaware, wanted to avoid in his state. By 5:00 P.M. he had ordered the evacuation of fifty thousand residents living on the coast. Already, twelve-foot seas were being reported across a swath of ocean more than one thousand miles in diameter. Buoys off the coast of Florida and Georgia were reporting wind speeds of 69 miles per hour. NOAA's hurricane research division rated the winds a 2.3 out of 6 in terms of destructiveness. The resulting surge, on the other hand, they deemed a 5.2: about as dangerous as you can get. Both the ECMWF and GFS models were predicting that the storm would make landfall sometime late Monday or early Tuesday.

In Washington, D.C., Amtrak announced the cancellation of routes ranging as far as Chicago, New York, and Miami. The Department of Defense appointed dual-status commanders for the mid-Atlantic: special high-ranking officials authorized to command both federal and state national guard forces so that they could make available troops and supplies at the request of governors in the region. At the US Northern Command headquarters, located at Peterson Air Force Base in Colorado Springs, helicopters and rescue teams were elevated to twenty-four-hour prepare-to-deploy status.

All of these decisions were based on interpretations of exceedingly complex sets of data. There are a lot of these sets, and they mean different things to different people. That, says Jamie Rhome, is particularly true when it comes to storm-surge models. "It's very confusing and very technical — even for meteorologists, it's very, very hard to understand."

Rhome had a problem. From where he was sitting, he was pretty sure that New York had made a mistake — that they had gotten something wrong with the numbers. It's not part of his job description to reach out to emergency managers, nor is he supposed to play a part in their decisions to evacuate or not. But he felt confident this was a good time to "break ranks and step in."

"Once I saw that they weren't evacuating, I knew they weren't understanding the forecast. So I reached out and offered my services."

Rhome called McKinney. The two worked through the data again and again. "We were talking about the threat of a national disaster. Confusion is normal. But I wanted him to be confident," says Rhome. "Confident enough to make the decision to evacuate."

He told McKinney the amount of surge forecast for New York was plenty for the city to feel it. He told him there was a high probability the city would soon be flooded.

By the end of the conversation, Rhome had a feeling NYCOEM still didn't get it. So he hung up and went in search of bigger guns. He didn't stop until he found Rick Knabb.

8:00 P.M.
Atlantic Ocean
325 miles east of Elizabeth City, North Carolina
64°F
Barometer: 29.62 inches (dropping)
Winds: 27 mph (NNE)
Waves: 8.41 feet (building)
Precipitation: Rain

John Svendsen had been below deck trying to get some rest when Robin Walbridge decided to change course. The first mate was still hoping they might make a run for Bermuda — it'd be tight, he knew, but they could get there in time. The barometer was dropping rapidly, so Svendsen knew the storm must be close. And there were signs all around him. The seas were really turbulent now — there was no debate about that anymore. The wind shrieked through the rigging, and the ship lurched and bucked at unexpected intervals. People were starting to fall and get hurt. Their ship was injured, too, though just how badly was anyone's guess. Each time it hit a wave at an awkward angle, they could hear the loud hiss of water coming inside. Down in the engine room, Walbridge and Matt Sanders were losing their fight to keep up with the incoming water. It gurgled up over the floorboards of the room. It wouldn't be long before those sole boards came loose and began to float. One of the generators was spitting and sputtering, emitting a weird smoke no one had ever seen before.

They were in Sandy now, surrounded by tropical storm–force winds. The crew attempted to take wind readings with a handheld anemometer. They got one reading as high as 90 miles per hour before it broke. One of their mainsails ripped. Someone needed to run the pumps at all times, so the watch schedule lost its structure — crew members stayed on watch later and later, or rose from naps ahead of schedule to try to help. But it wasn't working. The starboard bilge pump kept losing its prime, despite everything they did to try to fix it. Exhausted crew members stumbled off watch to try to get some sleep, only to discover that their bunks were flooding. They began congregating in the great cabin at the ship's stern, where at least it was dry. No one got much sleep. Their captain remained in the engine room, attempting to repair corroded fittings on one of their auxiliary pumps. Things were not going as planned. The ship was in distress, and everyone on board knew it. That night, Adam Prokosh was on watch in the ship's navigation shack. Since leaving New London, he'd been watching the ship's AIS. Throughout the voyage, he'd been monitoring the traffic around them as the *Bounty* steamed southward. But now the screen was empty. That alarmed him.

We must be all alone out here, he thought to himself. He kept the thought to himself.

"At that point," he says, "it wasn't worth reporting."

9:00 P.M.
Chesapeake Bay
64°F
Barometer: 29.87 inches (steady)
Winds: 12 mph (ENE)
Skies: Partly cloudy
Waves: .5 feet

Back at his house, Jan Miles was watching the AIS feed as well. He could feel the winds building out of the northeast, and he was worried about his ship and crew.

"There's always this zone we occupy at times like this," he says. "You wonder to yourself, 'Should we have gone sooner? Should we have not gone at all?' " He kept his eye on the tiny icon indicating the *Pride*'s position as it made its way out around Eastern Neck and into the western portion of Chesapeake Bay. From there, they'd have just 15 nautical miles until they reached Baltimore. Still, Miles wasn't taking any chances. He began making notes of places where the *Pride* could duck in, should the weather deteriorate. He wanted his vessel on a dock. He wanted his crew safe. But for now, watching the slow progress of his beloved clipper was more fun than anything else — a wonder of technology that he could relish at his kitchen table. He picked up his phone and sent his co-captain Jamie Trost a jaunty little text: *Hey, I can see you!*

Trost and his first mate pulled up the AIS as well. They moved the range in and out, marking their progress in the empty waters of Chesapeake Bay. It was really empty. They enlarged the scope, looking for other ships. They found few. They enlarged the field even farther, so that it encompassed most of the Eastern Seaboard. There was one small dot on the otherwise empty screen — a tiny little fleck, two hundred miles off the coast of North Carolina. They clicked on its icon and recognized the call sign at once. They both groaned. Trost picked up the phone and called Miles.

"It's the *Bounty,*" he said. "They're out there."

Jan had but one thought: *Oh, Jesus.*

Sunday

1:33 A.M.
Miami and New York

Sandy's eye was now 275 miles southeast of Cape Hatteras, North Carolina. Hurricane Hunter data recorded sustained winds of 75 miles per hour. Hurricane-force winds spread out for more than one hundred miles; tropical storm winds extended for another five hundred. The Weather Channel reported twenty-nine-foot waves off the coast of North Carolina. Water levels were rising from South Carolina to Virginia. The storm was getting closer.

Don Cresitello of the US Army Corps of Engineers was on a conference call with so many people he couldn't keep count. He knew Jamie Rhome and Rick Knabb were on there. Cas Holloway, New York's deputy mayor, was, too. So was Joe Bruno, the commissioner of NYCOEM.

Rhome and Knabb were explaining that

the surge forecast had increased again: It was now five to ten feet. Flooding seemed imminent. But New York officials still seemed uncertain about what to do.

Cresitello was getting agitated. They'd be feeling the first effects of the storm within hours. He hadn't been home to prepare his own house for the flooding. But still the conversation went around and around.

"There were still all these questions," he says. "There shouldn't have been questions anymore."

He and Rhome kept bringing up the decision to evacuate during Irene. "There's going to be more water than Irene," Cresitello remembers saying.

"How much more water?" asked one of the voices on the line.

"I'm not able to tell you that," said Cresitello. "But it doesn't really matter."

The city needed to evacuate, he told them, and they were running out of time. It's Cresitello's job to analyze worst-case scenarios. He's worked with social scientists to determine how people behave during disasters. It takes us a while to realize that we're actually in danger, he says. It takes us even longer to decide to act. Of the people willing to evacuate during a storm, only about 10 percent actually go to shelters. The rest, he says, decide to hightail it out of town. That's a transportation nightmare in places like New York City. So Cresitello and his team spend a lot of time determining just how many people the streets and mass transit systems can handle at one time (they call this "load analysis"). He says the city needs about twenty-four hours to achieve what he calls a "safe clearance time," and that doesn't take into account health-care facilities or other places with special needs. Ideally, they'd get seventy-two hours to prepare before storm-force winds arrive. No one in New York had that kind of time anymore.

He felt himself getting more heated.

"Look," he snapped. "You've got to realize that you're about to have water in your streets. You guys called an evac for Irene. It didn't seem to be an issue then. What's the problem here?"

Someone at the NYCOEM — he can't remember who — said they'd rerun the numbers.

Cresitello hung up and tried to get a few hours of sleep. Jamie Rhome went home to try to do the same.

As soon as the conference call ended, Commissioner Joe Bruno phoned Cas Holloway.

"Cas," he began, "it looks like the game seems to be changing."

Holloway asked him to explain. Bruno told the deputy mayor that they were no longer looking at Irene. "This could get a lot worse," he said. New York Harbor was going to flood. Predictions were going up.

Holloway said he'd be right over. They spent the next three hours poring over data.

5:00 A.M.
Miami and New York

Two cell phones rang simultaneously. Two very tired hurricane specialists answered them. One of them was Jamie Rhome. The voice on the other end told him Rick Knabb needed him back at NHC headquarters.

"New York wants to hear from you again," they told him.

He sighed and grabbed his car keys.

Don Cresitello received the other call. He was out on Long Island, struggling to help his dad haul out his boat. Dawn was still hours away.

"You've got to be kidding me," he said, pulling out his phone. "Really?"

As far as he's concerned, though, the call was more than worth it. By the end of the conversation, Cas Holloway and Joe Bruno felt confident. Holloway told Bruno he wanted to be the one to inform the mayor. Bruno said great. "Bloomberg's a smart guy. I knew he was going to get it."

Holloway says that's exactly what happened. He told the mayor that surge values had changed overnight. "The values are looking higher than we anticipated," he said. The city's health commissioner was recommending evacuation.

Bloomberg agreed. Holloway turned his attention back to Bruno and his staff at NYCOEM.

"At that point," says Bruno, "It was like, 'Let's go. Let's get our talking points in order.' "

8:30 A.M.
Bermuda
70°F
Barometer: 29.76 inches
Winds: 65 mph
Precipitation: Rain
Seas: 21 feet

Just before dawn, the *Norwegian Gem* made its way along the western coast of Bermuda, looking for a safe haven from the storm. Residents in Somerset Village, a small town on Mangrove Bay, could make out the ship's characteristic hull, painted with a rainbow of precious stones, as it slipped past. For most of the residents, the ship's passage was hardly worth noting. Boat people have lived in Somerset Village for centuries, and pirates once used it as a favorite hideout. The current iteration of Somerset Village is much quieter: The one-street town has a boat club and a bank, along with a handful of hotels, pubs, and shops. Between the early hours on a Sunday morning and the slow-moving hurricane overhead, most of these were closed. The town was barely waking up, in fact — a few couples were walking along the south shore; a couple of cars trundled past the quiet restaurants. At 8:30 A.M., Bermuda Weather Service radar picked up evidence of particularly heavy thunderstorm activity in one of Sandy's disorganized bands.

Minutes later, a telltale tornado snaked from the clouds, siphoning water off the bay in a large white flume. It overturned boats and a diving raft before making its way toward land. People on the beach ran for cover. A car swerved to miss part of a roof that was torn off by the wind. Another was crushed by falling debris. The tornado soon dissipated. The storm that spurred it did not. If anything, it was growing more unstable. And ever larger. Inside, the organized core had returned, creating a perfect conduit for heat and energy as Sandy surged across the unusually warm waters of the northern Atlantic, picking up speed as she did. Out over the Midwest, an enormous cold front was making its way across the country. The two were on a collision course now. Three different cruise liners had already canceled their planned stops at the island. The *Bermuda Islander,* the container ship responsible for making a weekly run of goods and supplies from New York to Hamilton, was stranded in New Jersey until both ports could be cleared of weather advisories.

"Don't know if I have ever seen #Bermuda and parts of the US coast with TS Warnings for the same storm. #Sandy," the Weather Channel's Jim Cantore tweeted.

11:00 A.M.
200 miles east of Hatteras
62°F
Barometer: 29.32 inches
Winds: 54 mph
Waves: 33 feet
Precipitation: Rain

Chris Barksdale's hand was throbbing. He was pretty sure he'd broken it after careering across the deck of the ship. He slunk down to his bunk and tried to get some sleep, but the screech of the struggling hull kept him up. Even the earphones he grabbed from the engine room weren't enough to muffle the noise. Eventually he managed to nap a little. He awoke to the sound of water streaming into the ship. It sounded to him like a waterfall. He got up to let John Svendsen know, and then he joined Robin Walbridge in the great cabin. The *Bounty* was still off the coast of Elizabeth City, trudging in a diagonal line toward shore. The eye of the storm was three hundred miles to their southeast. They were in the thick of it now. Walbridge had just finished writing Claudia an e-mail. She had arrived back from Italy and was trying to get adjusted to East Coast time. "I am thinking we will have the worst of the storm in the next 24 hours," he typed. "And then we should start to come out of it. Can't wait to see you."

Now the two middle-aged men were alone. They didn't talk much — they were comfortable with big silences. There was no warning before the monstrous wave struck the side of the ship. The force of it threw Walbridge across the cabin. He spiraled backward, unable to regain his balance, and crashed into a heavy, bolted-down table. The table didn't give. Walbridge crumpled to the floor. Barksdale was sure he had broken his back. "I'm going to be okay," Walbridge said. "I'm hurting, but I'm okay."

The engineer wasn't sure he believed him.

11:23 A.M.
New York City Office of Emergency Management
57°F
Barometer: 29.84 inches (falling)
Winds: 16 mph (ENE)
Skies: Overcast

Another press conference. Mayor Bloomberg looked uncharacteristically casual in a gray fleece pullover and purple turtleneck. "Last night we said this was a serious and dangerous storm," he began. "Nothing has changed there." What had changed, he said, was the magnitude of the storm surge. Overnight, the National Hurricane Center had increased its prediction by several feet. "We've got to take some preparations today," he said. All the city's public schools would be closed on Monday. And then the big news. "In light of these conditions, I'm going to sign an executive order mandating evacuations." People in low-lying areas would need to vacate by 7:00 P.M. "Let me stress that we are ordering this evacuation for the safety of the approximately 375,000 people who live in these areas. If you live in these areas, you should leave them this afternoon."

That was particularly true, he said, for residents of the twenty-six public housing projects within the flood zone. Elevators there, he said, would be shut off that evening. "It really is important that you leave," he said. "If you don't evacuate you're not just putting your own life in danger, you are also endangering the lives of our first responders who may have to come in and rescue you."

As for the hospitals and chronic-care facilities in the surge zone, Bloomberg explained that they were not part of the evacuation order. "The reason for all of this is that the shelters have facilities, they have backup generators, and it's dangerous to move people when they're elderly," he said. "So on balance, we think they'll be fine. Every one of the shelters has been contacted more than once, and we're satisfied that it's an intelligent decision to leave them in place."

Cas Holloway says that Bloomberg's decision was an attempt to balance the risk of the storm against the risk of moving the infirm. "Our ultimate decision was not to evacuate, based on what we thought the impacts would be. The threat was not going to be at a level where evacuation was the right move. Moving people has its own risks, and they didn't appear to be outweighed by the storm."

11:45 A.M.
NWS Forecasting Office
Mt. Holly, New Jersey
57°F
Barometer: 29.78 inches (falling)
Winds: 16 mph (NE)
Skies: Overcast

The National Hurricane Center's surge forecast that morning raised Sandy's landfall inundation prediction: It was now six to eleven feet, and the report targeted New York Harbor as the place most likely to be hit. They also revised the headline for that forecast: It now read LIFE THREATENING STORM SURGE. At the National Weather Service offices in Upton and Mt. Holly, forecasters were struggling to find ways to get this information to their clients. The National Weather Service does not mandate formal training for predicting surge and coastal inundation. They recently created a data-conversion tool to help with surge guidance, but most of the meteorologists who have access to it haven't been trained on its use. The SLOSH model is available to emergency managers and private meteorologists as well, but they weren't sure how to use it — and some were under the impression that you couldn't use the model for a storm of Sandy's track: None of them had ever before tried to run data for an extratropical storm about to crash headlong into New York City.

Joe Miketta was sympathetic. He's an expert on National Weather Service products, but he, too, finds them difficult to navigate. That's one reason why, when given a choice about where to get his own weather, he uses an iPhone app created by one of his local TV stations. Technology, he says, is changing. The National Weather Service doesn't always keep up.

That's what the Committee on the Assessment of the National Weather Service's Modernization Program found during its recent examination of the NWS. The committee was convened to evaluate improvements made as part of the $4.5 billion restructuring of the agency — a decade-long attempt to make good on the Weather Service Modernization Act of 1992, which sought to better integrate science and weather and to improve public outreach. The subsequent report concluded that the NWS was still very much structured based on the meteorology of the 1990s and had failed to accommodate dramatic advancements in science and technology. According to the report, that is particularly true in matters of hydrology and technology: Private-sector weather services, said the report, "are exceeding the capacity of the NWS to optimally acquire, integrate, and communicate critical forecast and warning information based on these technological achievements." As a result,

> critical components within the NWS are lagging behind the state of the science. Furthermore, enormous amounts of data generated by new surface networks, radars, satellites, and numerical models need to be rapidly distilled into actionable information in order to create and communicate effective public forecasts and warnings. The skills required to comprehend, manage, and optimize this decision-making process go beyond traditional meteorological and hydrological curricula. Hence, the NWS workforce skill set will need to evolve appropriately.

That evolution wasn't going to happen in time to assist with the forecasting of Sandy. And Miketta was doing the best he could with the tools available to him. That morning, he was on the phone with officials in Delaware — he and Gary Szatkowski had decided it made sense to divide the region so that they could be consistent in their delivery of information: Szatkowski drew the Garden State; Miketta focused on Delaware.

The officials in Delaware were getting a little frustrated, he thought. Emergency managers wanted to provide graphs to help officials decide about whether or not to evacuate the state. Miketta tried to explain that they didn't have those available. He told them to think in terms of records. They asked for examples. The 1962 nor'easter was the best antecedent he could come up with. A lot of people still thought of it as the storm of the century — or at least the storm of that century. It was enormous and incredibly slow moving: a deadly combination that brought gale winds and surge for five tide cycles on the coast and blizzard conditions across North Carolina and Virginia. Bryan Norcross lived in New Jersey at the time and had since helped to make the storm famous: He still tells stories about finding bits of his aunt and uncle's house scattered throughout their coastal town, about how refrigerators and books and pieces of cars washed up on the shore for months after the storm dissipated. *That was all interesting,* said the Delaware emergency managers, *but how does it help us?* Miketta told them about the twenty-foot waves that hit coastal towns like Dewey Beach, about the way the surge overtook canals and rivers. He told them to go back and look at the data — it'd give them a pretty good indication about what they were up against.

A few cubicles down, forecaster Dean Iovino was on the phone with emergency managers and state police in New Jersey. Like the rest of Szatkowski's crew, he was working sixteen-hour days at this point. He was tired and stumbled over his words a little as he tried to explain to them just what the predictions meant: namely, that walls of water were going to push up the rivers of New Jersey, flooding towns far removed from the coastline. The threat was more than serious, he said. He wanted them to understand just how serious, but he felt like he didn't have the words.

We've got to do a better job, he remembers thinking. "Meteorologists — we lose ourselves in the science." And when it comes to surge science, even the best don't know a great deal.

Governmental officials and emergency managers asked Iovino how far the water would move inland. He admitted that he didn't know for sure. Surge models don't extend inland. River flooding models don't go down far enough to include tidal zones. There isn't a third model to fill the gap. He told them they were estimating as best they could.

Iovino called his parents, who still live in his childhood home in one of those communities. He tried to stay calm, to explain that they may be in danger. They reminded him they'd lived there all his life and had always been fine. "Look," he tried again. "Water is going to go places you've never seen it go before." They told him they planned on staying anyway.

They weren't alone. Tony Gigi was having a hard time persuading his daughter to leave Rutgers — she was worried that classes had not yet been canceled. His mother-in-law refused to leave her home in Yonkers, despite his best attempts to get her to stay with her son for a few days. Few of the 350,000 people under mandatory evacuation orders from Mayor Bloomberg were taking action, according to police officers who were patrolling the neighborhoods and knocking on doors. They were met with everything from contempt for weather forecasting to heart-breaking stories about people who lacked the bus fare needed to get to a shelter. One wheelchair-bound couple couldn't figure out how to leave their house. One woman told them she and her kids were going to hole up and watch movies. "It's going to be great," she said. "I'm just too lazy," another resident told a *New York Times* reporter.

The message that people were in danger had gotten garbled, says Bryan Norcross. People didn't understand the threat. Barry Myers, the CEO of AccuWeather, was now also urging the National Hurricane Center to change its mind about issuing a hurricane warning.

"What we have is a hurricane becoming embedded in a winter storm. It's clearly unprecedented. But to refuse to issue hurricane warnings can cause confusion." The Hurricane Center, he said, was too focused on labels and not focused enough on how the general public was responding. Marshall Moss, his vice president for forecasting, agreed. He told reporters he thought meteorologists were being blinded by technical considerations.

"The discussion is getting too weather weenie," he said.

The force of this criticism surprised James Franklin. "We usually play for the same team, but we clearly weren't this time." That, he thought, didn't seem entirely fair.

"Media people don't necessarily appreciate just how complicated a situation it is to get up a new procedure on the fly. You don't always know what the consequences are going to be."

Press conferences were proliferating. President Obama held his own. "My first message," he said, "it that you need to take this very seriously and follow the instructions of your state and local officials." Still, people remained — more than 70 percent of all residents who had received mandatory evacuation notices.

Once a governor or other elected official declares a state of emergency, a very specific — and often rigorous — legal protocol goes into place that grants powers not otherwise available. It allows officials to, among other things, "direct and compel" an evacuation, and legal precedent supports taking forceful action in such an instance. A report issued by a bipartisan congressional committee mandates that it is also the government's responsibility to take care of people they have evacuated. That's an important point, given that as many as 30 percent of all

Americans surveyed said they wouldn't be able to leave their homes without assistance. A disproportionately high number of people who stay are sick and elderly, and many of them are at great risk whenever they are transported. Nevertheless, a mandatory evacuation is just that — mandatory. In most states, disobeying is a misdemeanor punishable by jail or a stiff fine. In New York, you can serve up to ninety days for disregarding an evacuation order. North Carolina holds evacuation holdouts financially responsible for the cost of their rescue.

Neither penalty does much to dissuade people who have already decided to disregard an order, nor does a common police tactic of going door to door and asking for next-of-kin information in an effort to emphasize just how dangerous a storm is going to be.

"The big bad wolf can huff and puff all he wants, you know?" one Cape May, New Jersey, resident told reporters. "This house is going to be fine."

On Staten Island, residents who disregarded the evacuation order gave a variety of reasons. Some said they had lived there all their lives — more than sixty years, in some cases — and had never seen their homes flood. They told their family members that all their neighbors were staying, so they would stay, too. Others said they wouldn't go without their pets. Some didn't have cars or couldn't drive. John Paterno, a sixty-four-year-old originally from a small town near Poughkeepsie, had moved to Staten Island to be closer to the city. He was legally blind, and his cerebral palsy meant he used a wheelchair most days. Every time a family member suggested he consider an assisted-care facility, he shot down the idea in an instant. His cousins kept an eye on him as much as they could, stopping by a few times a week to run errands or help him with meals. As the storm approached, he told his sister he didn't want to evacuate — that he would feel too vulnerable in a shelter. Instead, he, his dog — a pit bull named Bear — and a cockatoo hunkered down in the living room of his single-story bungalow.

At the southern tip of Staten Island, some residents in the neighborhood of Tottenville were making similar decisions. Theirs was a friendly, middle-class neighborhood. The kind of place where old meets new: on one street, sprawling contemporary homes with backyard pools; on another, older, narrow houses and power lines slung with old sneakers. The Dresches lived somewhere in between, in the last house on a dead-end street. George Dresch, a plumber, bought the house in 1983 and spent years renovating it before moving in. In the years that followed, he and his wife, Patricia, built an addition on the back of the house. They filled rooms with family pictures and Elvis memorabilia. Their eldest daughter, Jo Ann, got married and moved to Nashville, where she worked as a chef. Their youngest daughter, Angela, was in middle school. She was obsessed with music and dance and Facebook and all the other things thirteen-year-old girls tend to love.

The Dresches saw hardly any traffic at their end of the street. Just beyond their side yard, a narrow dirt path led through trees and brush to the beach and Raritan Bay. A fence and some trees separated their backyard from the Coral Bay Café, a bright yellow seafood and Italian place with an outdoor patio and purple table umbrellas. When the café was closed, it could seem like you lived in the middle of nowhere.

A year earlier, when New York called for evacuations ahead of Hurricane Irene, the Dresches obeyed. They locked up their house and went inland. So did most people on their street. Their house weathered the storm just fine. But while the Dresches were gone, looters broke into their house and took everything they could carry. No one saw a thing: It was a perfect time and place for burglary.

George Dresch didn't want that to happen again. They would have been fine if they had weathered Irene at home. He assumed they'd be fine this time, too. Friends told the *New York Daily News* it was "a hesitant but collective decision."

Gary Szatkowski didn't know the Dresches personally. But he knew people were choosing to stay, and that was bad enough. Mayor Bloomberg's press conference from the previous day was playing on a continuous loop in his mind. He'd barely slept Saturday night — he kept thinking about the people in the flood zones, about how their lives were in his hands. The forecasts for this storm were good, he knew — good enough that no one in the region should lose their lives.

"We're not perfect, but we can tell you that something really bad is coming at you. That ought to be enough."

In Washington, D.C., the buses and Metro were about to stop running. Amtrak services were about to cease, too. New Jersey had already begun shutting down its transit system; commuter services had been suspended as far away as Boston as well. Even the New York City subway and bus services were about to be put on lockdown. Consolidated Edison was shutting off steam to large buildings. Still, there were hard decisions to make. New York City had mandated the evacuation of several hospitals, but not Bellevue, the oldest public hospital in the country and home to more than 750 patients, including some of the most notorious convicts from Rikers Island, diagnosed with a whole host of psychotic conditions. The forensic psychiatry unit is located on the nineteenth floor of the hospital. Patients are carefully organized and sequestered to prevent major incidents. The unit's director, Elizabeth Ford, didn't know how long she could ensure their safety. At nearly two hundred feet above sea level, the winds would be much worse on their floor. Without power, the elevators wouldn't work, and there would be no water or heat. Ford told *New York Magazine* that she didn't know of any evacuation plan. And she had no idea where she would send the sixty-one criminals under her care, should it come to that. Sixteen of them spoke only Chinese. Others were beyond dangerous.

"These are not patients that other city hospitals want. That's just the fact."

They would have to ride out the storm. Ford asked her staff to stay close to the hospital. She told them to pack for several days, to bring all the bottled water and flashlights they could find. The city and state health commissioners, she told them, had ordered the hospital not to evacuate. Neither would Langone or Coney Island Hospital. They had ordered massive evacuations during Hurricane Irene. Doing it again, they said, was just too risky. The hospitals had made dramatic improvements since Hurricane Irene. Their executives insisted they were ready for Sandy. Besides, said Alan Aviles, president of the corporation that runs Bellevue, the chance of an actual emergency seemed unlikely. "The National Hurricane Center was saying that there was only a 5 percent probability of a storm surge over eleven feet in the area that would impact Coney Island, and they weren't even showing a 5 percent probability on the East River," he told *The New York Times.*

People are not getting it, thought Szatkowski. He was receiving reports of tourists milling around Times Square. Of gawkers loitering on the Atlantic City boardwalk. They weren't concerned.

It's a problem the National Weather Service has been confronting for years.

In a 2011 white paper, Chris Landsea and Eric Blake estimated that approximately 90 percent of residents on the Eastern Seaboard have never experienced a hurricane. That number is rising as millions of people move to the coast. However, if anything, say Landsea and Blake, advances in storm prediction have made people more blasé than ever about preparation.

Szatkowski was in complete agreement. Counting Sandy, the region had experienced mandatory evacuations precisely three times in forty years (the other two were Irene the year before and Gloria in 1985. Luckily, the latter hit at low tide).

"That's infrequent enough that people should have known we were serious. Still, I got that people weren't getting it. They were hearing conflicting reports, and the raging subtext of that conflict was 'Don't go anywhere.' "

Szatkowski says he was pretty emotional. "The best technical aid was not going to sway them. I didn't need a vivid graphic, a bigger font, or to bold more of the text. I needed to go outside the box."

"In poker parlance," he says, "it was time to move some more chips across the table."

And so he did what no meteorologist had

ever done in the forty-two-year history of the National Weather Service: He wrote a personal plea and published it along with his noon advisory:

> If you are being asked to evacuate a coastal location by state and local officials, please do so.
>
> If you are reluctant to evacuate, and you know someone who rode out the '62 storm on the barrier islands, ask them if they could do it again.
>
> If you are still reluctant, think about your loved ones, think about the emergency responders who will be unable to reach you when you make the panicked phone call to be rescued, think about the rescue/recovery teams who will rescue you if you are injured or recover your remains if you do not survive.
>
> Sandy is an extremely dangerous storm. There will be major property damage, injuries are probably unavoidable, but the goal is **zero fatalities.**
>
> If you think the storm is over-hyped and exaggerated, please err on the side of caution. You can call me up on friday (contact information is at the end of this briefing) and yell at me all you want.
>
> I will listen to your concerns and com-

ments, but i will tell you in advance, i will be very happy that you are alive & well, no matter how much you yell at me.

Thanks for listening.

He signed his name and included both his office telephone and personal cell phone numbers. And then he walked out to the forecasting floor. He didn't show anyone the plea — he says he didn't want any fingerprints on it other than his. There could be big consequences for something like this. He could tell that the staff was concerned — caught off guard. Maybe a little in shock, he concedes. No one told him not to do it, though he doubts he would have listened if they had. Instead, he walked back to his office and hit send. This time, he didn't hesitate — not even for a second.

12:33 P.M.
Atlanta, Georgia
51°F
Barometer: 29.83 inches (steady)
Winds: 18 mph
Skies: Overcast

At Weather Channel headquarters, Senior Meteorologist Stu Ostro was having a reaction very much like Szatkowski's. Coastal waters from Virginia to Cape Cod were now under hurricane-force wind warnings. He took to his blog and urged compliance: "Regardless of what the official designation is now or at/after landfall — hurricane (including if "only" a Category 1), tropical storm, post-tropical, extra-tropical, whatever — or what type of warnings are issued by the national weather service and national hurricane center — people in the path of this storm need to heed the threat it poses with utmost urgency."

The station's Twitter feed posted his statement again and again. "Please retweet," it read. Within an hour, the statement had gone viral.

At 2:00 P.M., President Obama hosted another national press conference from FEMA headquarters in Washington. "Obviously, all of us across the country are concerned about the potential impact of Hurricane Sandy," he said. "This is a serious and big storm. And my first message is to all the people across the Eastern Seaboard, mid-Atlantic, going north, that you need to take this very seriously and follow the instructions of your state and local officials, because they are going to be providing you with the best advice in terms of how to deal with this storm over the coming days."

He urged people to check on their neighbors and friends to make sure they were prepared. It still wasn't clear where the storm was going to land, said Obama, so he and the FEMA team were going to be relying heavily on state and local governments. "My message to the governors, as well as to the mayors, is anything they need, we will be there. And we're going to cut through red tape. We're not going to get bogged down with a lot of rules. We want to make sure that we are anticipating and leaning forward into making sure that we've got the best possible response to what is going to be a big and messy system."

Ostro liked the sound of that.

4:12 P.M.
Savannah, Georgia
75°F
Barometer: 29.60 inches (steady)
Winds: 24 mph (WNW)
Waves: 2.7 feet
Skies: Scattered clouds

Sandy's tropical storm–force winds now spread out for nine hundred miles. "That's the driving distance between New York City and Atlanta," tweeted the Weather Channel.

The coast guard had closed New York Harbor. Blizzard warnings were now in effect for the mountains of West Virginia. And still Sandy continued to grow, fed by both the warm waters of the Gulf Stream (a tremendous current originating near Hatteras that conducts heat out of the Caribbean and into the North Atlantic) and the second, larger air trough now sweeping down from the Great Lakes. No longer was there a vertical wind shear to tamp down the storm. Instead, it again grew high, high, high into the troposphere. Off the coast of Hatteras, buoy 41001 was registering waves of more than twenty feet and gusts of 74 miles per hour. Sean Cross and his crew of Hurricane Hunters were on their way back inside the storm.

"I've kinda got this feeling that Sandy is going to be just one nasty little girl," he told a Weather Channel cameraman before boarding the plane.

The pilot didn't have to wait long to see the nastiness. Minutes after departing from Savannah, the plane entered the outer wind fields of Sandy. Cross didn't attempt to hide his surprise.

"This thing is so wide and so large it's everywhere. It's just encompassing an entire region of the Atlantic Ocean. I mean, it's massive."

In a typical hurricane, storm-force winds extend about twenty-five miles from the eye. But in Sandy, winds more than 50 miles per hour now extended 150 miles outside of the storm center. He told everyone to strap in, then braced himself against the window of the plane. An instant later, they were in a sea of dramatic turbulence. The non-meteorologists, of course, loved it.

"Wooooo-eeeeee," whistled one of the crew members.

"Rockin' and rollin'," cheered another.

Val Hendry, the meteorologist aboard the flight, was silent. The storm was stretching out for nine hundred miles, and it had lost much of its orderly definition. She couldn't tell where the eye was located — assuming there still was one — and she had no idea where to begin looking. Without that information, it would be impossible to measure the true intensity of the storm.

Cross turned on his microphone to speak with the Weather Channel cameraman on their flight. "I said she's a nasty little girl? She's a nasty *big* girl."

Val Hendry and pilot Sean Cross couldn't be more different. She has a soft voice and an even softer presence. She is bookish. Understated. A clear contrast to Cross's bravado. And at that moment, all of her attention was focused on just where the center of the storm was located. What she determined would have multimillion-dollar implications for an Eastern Seaboard still uncertain about where this storm was going to land. They knew that the worst of the surge would be just north of the storm's center. A few miles in either direction could mean the salvation — or destruction — of New York City. Inside the Hurricane Hunter liaison office at the National Hurricane Center, Chris Landsea was peering over the shoulder of a computer specialist who was busy feeding Hendry coordinates, watching as her data streamed in on several of the computer screens. Every few minutes, another dropsonde reading would appear. It seemed as if the storm was shifting — as if it might make landfall far enough to the north that the New York region would be spared. But it would be an hour before they knew.

Landsea tried to pretend that he wasn't crazy impatient to know for sure. He started to pace a little, wandering between the relative quiet of the liaison office and the chaos of the forecast room, which had now become a full-fledged media circus. On his third or fourth circuit, Hendry's final word came in: The storm was still headed directly toward the city. A reprieve was all but impossible now.

Neither Hendry nor anyone else on board the C-130 had time to consider the implications of what they had found. Their plane was now engulfed in the storm. No one bothered to hide their disbelief.

"It's freaking snowing," said Cross to no one in particular. "This is so bizarre."

Even the normally taciturn Hendry agreed. "Oh, yeah," she said with real enthusiasm. "This is bizarre."

Cross turned on the plane's deicers.

Jon Talbot was following their movement from their temporary base in Savannah, and this was one of the last things he wanted to hear. Portions of Virginia and North Carolina were reporting snow accumulations of more than an inch. He knew it had to be much worse inside the storm.

"This is worrisome to me because this thing is combining with the cold air, and this is going to add a lot of energy to the storm."

Cross agreed. "It's going to be really bad. We know that now."

They turned back toward Savannah and had just crossed the Hatteras buoy when they got a look at the ocean below. The sea surface looked as if a giant pane of glass has been horribly, violently shattered.

"Man," one of the crew members whispered. "I would not want to be in a boat in that."

8:30 P.M.
Staten Island, New York
59°F
Barometer: 29.70 inches (falling)
Winds: 26 mph (NE)
Skies: Overcast

The Dresch family had finished dinner hours ago. Angela was somewhere upstairs, probably on Facebook or Instagram. Her mom, Patricia, was on the phone with Angela's older sister, Jo Ann. She and her husband, Brad, were in Nashville, where they had been glued to the TV, watching news of the growing storm. Jo Ann wanted her family to evacuate. Brad remembers that the conversation seemed like a debate. Patricia told her that they had made the decision to ride out the storm.

11:00 P.M.
140 miles off the coast of Hatteras
62°F
Barometer: 29.23 inches (falling)
Winds: 64 mph (N)
Waves: 40 feet
Precipitation: Heavy rain

Scholars estimate that nearly a million people died in tropical cyclones during the last half of the twentieth century. They have no way of extrapolating how many people died before that. They have even less of an idea how many people experienced a hurricane and lived to tell about it. The eyewitness accounts gathered over the years are intermittent and uneven at best, but they share the hyperbole needed to attempt a description of what it is like to be trapped inside a storm. One mariner wrote in 1831 that the "distant roar of the elements" was enough to make him mad. The sound, he said, was like "winds rushing through a hollow vault." Washington Irving called it "a terrific noise" capable of convincing many that "the end of the world was at hand."

That's how it felt aboard the *Bounty.* The vessel was in trouble. More than that, it was in crisis. Adam Prokosh had taken a fall at least as serious as Walbridge's. Claudene Christian was tending to him as best she could. There'd been an electrical fire in the galley, where the force of the waves had also pulled tables from the hinges. Waves had crashed through the windows of the great cabin. The engine room was so inundated with water that equipment was arcing and sparking. The crew had had to abandon it, lest they be electrocuted. Twice, John Svendsen had asked Walbridge to call the coast guard. Twice he had refused. The captain was in obvious pain. A few crew members wondered if he was able to think straight with that much discomfort. They doubted they'd be able to. Claudene Christian was frustrated — she still felt like she had been trying to help, but people weren't listening to her.

Laura Groves passed around motion-sickness medication, but not everybody could keep it down. It was just so rough out there. Conditions continued to deteriorate. The engines failed, leaving the ship helpless against the waves and winds. The generators stopped as well. The ship went dark. A few crew members donned headlamps, but there weren't enough to go around. "I need a light over here," people kept yelling.

It was time to prepare to abandon ship. John Svendsen went above deck to try Tracie Simonin on the satellite phone, but the wind was blowing so fiercely he couldn't tell if she answered or not. He ended up talking to her voice mail. Eventually he sent an e-mail to her instead, and it found its way to coast guard Chief Petty Officer Jeremy Johnson, the command duty officer at Sector Wilmington. The *Bounty* needed help, but Johnson didn't know how to get it to them. He checked the position of all navy and coast guard vessels, but they had long since cleared out of the area. He dialed up the AIS and found a lone cargo ship in the vicinity. It was too dangerous for them to turn back. Johnson contacted his supervisor, Billy Mitchell, who was at home helping his kids prepare their Halloween costumes. His daughter was going as a geisha girl. His son was dressed up as the Flash. Rain was falling outside. There was a little wind.

"It was like watching a horror movie where the audience knows the hero is in trouble, but he doesn't yet realize it," says Mitchell.

Just how bad things had gotten on the *Bounty* was anyone's guess: Billy Mitchell's team at sector was already engaged in a convoluted game of telephone between the *Bounty*, its home office, and the coast guard communications center. He needed to talk to them directly, but the only way to do that was to get a plane in the air.

He called Captain Joseph P. Kelly, commander of the Elizabeth City Air Station. It was almost midnight.

"I need a big metal antenna in the air," said Mitchell.

"You're asking me to send my folks into a hurricane," Kelly shot back.

Mitchell asked if he had concerns. That struck Kelly as almost absurd.

"Of course I have concerns," said Kelly. "You're asking me to put my assets and my crews in danger. Ultimately, I'm responsible for their lives."

Kelly is a funny, warm, jovial guy. He likes to laugh and quote country music lyrics. Mitchell is hilarious, too, though more in a hipster kind of way. They're both as easy to get along with as anyone you might meet. But things had taken a serious turn. Every coast guard mission is rated on what's called a GAR score, based on its predicted dangers. A green rating means the crew can pretty much just notify the operations boss on their way out. An amber score and they need to get clearance from that boss. Only Kelly can authorize a more dangerous mission.

"If it's in the red, nobody goes anywhere

until I get briefed and I feel good about it," he insists.

But, he adds, it can be a challenge to persuade his crew as much: "They're go-getters. They want to go out. That's just who they are." Sometimes, he says, it's up to him to hold them back.

It was a decision bigger than either he or Mitchell was capable of making, and they knew it. Within minutes, a conference call had been convened, including a representative from the 5th District admiral. They were trying to weigh the cost-benefit of sending personnel into the storm. What, specifically, was to be gained? What could be lost? *A great deal,* thought both Mitchell and Kelly.

"Look," said Kelly. "We're in a storm the size and power of Katrina. It's ugly out there."

Mitchell was resolute. If asked, he is quick to say that he doesn't wear his heart on his sleeve, but he was certain that someone or something wanted the coast guard out there. He wanted Kelly and the others on the phone to understand that he didn't need a plane on top of the *Bounty* — he just needed them to get close enough to communicate. He had to know what was happening on the ship. "Just let them try," he said. "They can always turn back."

As soon as Captain Kelly got off the conference call, he picked up his personal cell phone and called C-130 pilot Wes McIntosh in Raleigh. He and his crew were already prepping for their departure. The *Bounty* crew, Kelly explained to McIntosh, had indicated they could make it until morning. Kelly didn't want anyone risking their lives if the ship was going to be okay.

"Listen, I'm very concerned about this," he said to McIntosh.

The pilot told him they had been looking at the radar.

"Good," said his commander. "Then you know that bands of heavy weather are stretching from the shoreline to ninety miles out."

McIntosh said he did. They wanted to go.

Kelly sighed. It was, he thought, a lot easier to be a pilot than to be a commander sitting at home worrying about one.

"Okay," he conceded. "Get your crew. But you are to go no farther than you need to establish comms. If you can talk to them from the shore, then that's where you stay."

He repeated himself. "Just establish comms. That's all you need to do now."

"Roger," replied McIntosh. "Got it."

The pilot took a deep breath. It was either going to be an exhaustingly long night or a tragically short one. And it all depended upon the *Bounty.*

Monday

2:28 A.M.
Elizabeth City, North Carolina
62°F
Barometer: 29.31 inches (dropping)
Winds: 27 mph (NW)
Precipitation: Rain

Joseph Kelly was pacing around his house, stopping every few minutes to check the weather. Storm surge in Maryland was more than four feet. Waves tore through the pier in Ocean City. Twenty-foot waves were being recorded as far north as Islip, on Long Island, New York. Sandy's predicted change in direction was happening. "The turn toward the coast has begun," tweeted the Weather Channel. Kelly's phone rang just after he read that. It was the coast guard base, saying that McIntosh's C-130 crew hadn't been able to drop dewatering pumps for the *Bounty.*

Kelly was incredulous. And more than a

little mad. "What do you mean they tried to drop pumps? I said establish comms. That's it."

The operations chief on the other end didn't know what to say to that. He stammered a little. Kelly hung up and got dressed. There was no way he was going to sleep now. He'd always told his pilots that he would support them even if he disagreed with their decision, so long as they could demonstrate a logical thought process. He was really hoping that McIntosh had one now.

3:40 A.M.
130 miles off Cape Hatteras
62°F
Barometer: 29.21 inches (falling)
Winds: 57 mph (N)
Waves: 38 feet
Precipitation: Rain

They were the only two planes in the sky for hundreds of miles. That struck both crews as eerie. Wes McIntosh and his coast guard crew continued to circle over the *Bounty,* ducking down to make radio contact with Svendsen, then returning to a safer cruising pattern. His crew was sick and getting pretty banged up. That worried him. Not far from him, the Hurricane Hunters had their own concerns. Jon Talbot didn't like what the data was telling them. Dropsondes on board found a small surface area where winds were registering above 90 miles per hour. Thunderstorms were continuing to build around the storm's center. They flew through a perfectly round eye twenty-eight miles across and made note of that, too. "#Sandy is still a fully tropical cyclone at this time," tweeted the Weather Channel. "No doubt about it."

One hundred and fifty miles off of Hatteras, the *Bounty* crew was huddled in the great cabin. Some of the headlamps had started to flicker out. They were waiting, but for what they didn't know. Walbridge had thought they could make it until morning. Now he wasn't so sure. Josh Scornavacchi had snagged a guitar out of the lazarette. He was hoping there'd be time for Claudene Christian to sing one last song. But they didn't get a chance. Their captain told them it was time to go. They struggled to climb into their survival suits. Claudene Christian had never practiced getting into one. Jess Hewitt showed her how and cracked a few jokes. "Remember the number of your suit," she told Christian. "That way you'll know where to put it back." That made her friend smile.

Walbridge always warned his crew never to take anything with them in an emergency. "You can't go back for anything," he would say. "Anything." But he did, somehow. Even injured, he managed to make his way down to his cluttered little cabin. He took Claudia's picture off the wall and stuffed it into his suit. Doug Faunt grabbed his teddy bear. Jess Hewitt took the medallion given to her by the crew of the *Mississippi:* BY VALOR AND ARMS, PRIDE RUNS DEEP. She also grabbed a hair tie and a cigarette lighter: She planned on having a smoke as soon as they made it back to shore. She went back down for a couple of other things, too: Prokosh's captain's license — it was a bitch to get a replacement one, she'd always heard — and his pea coat. He had to be freezing. Claudene asked her to go back again. She really wanted her journal, she said.

An hour later, and they were all up on deck. The ship was listing. The skies were clearing. Every once in a while, they could pick out the lights of the C-130 directly overhead. McIntosh and his crew had done exactly what their commander had told them not to do: They flew in and tried to help. When conditions there got too bad, they'd fly back to their safe holding space on the side of the storm.

"It was important. We were holding their hands," says Mike Myers. "We were trying to say, 'You're not alone. Keep fighting.' "

Somewhere off in the distance, the Hurricane Hunters' C-130 was struggling through its own flight pattern.

4:28 A.M.
130 miles off Cape Hatteras

On board the *Bounty,* the crew congregated into two groups, braced against whatever they could find to keep from tumbling down the steeply pitched deck. Jess Hewitt thought about capsizing and tried to reassure herself: *I just need to keep breathing. If I can keep breathing, I'll be okay.* She and Drew Salapatek clipped their climbing harnesses together. *You better not leave me,* she told him. Meanwhile, Claudene looked around: Matt wasn't nearby. She caught sight of him up near the mast. She smiled and darted to him. Even in the storm, Anna Sprague remembered thinking it was "a cool move."

Claudene never wanted to be alone. Especially in the dark. She nestled in with Sanders. "It's going to be okay, baby girl," he said. That was his nickname for her: *baby girl.* He kept saying it over and over again:

"It's going to be okay. It's going to be okay."

Above them, the C-130 kept circling, ducking down just long enough to check on the status of the ship. Every time they did, the turbulence became unbearable. The crew in the back were vomiting. The cargo bay door was covered in it.

Everything appeared to be in stasis. Until suddenly, it wasn't. A wave — bigger than the rest — struck the side of the ship. The vessel screamed and rolled from a 45-degree angle to a 90-degree one. They were dangling over the water now. Debris rained down around them. A few crew members jumped. Some tried to hold on. Matt Sanders caught his foot — it was pinched and he was stuck. Claudene panicked. "What do I do?" she screamed. "What do I do?"

"Claudene, you just have to go for it," Sanders replied. "You have to make your way aft and get clear of the boat."

So she did. Or tried to, anyway. The last he saw of her, she had worked her way back to the mizzen — back to where her original group had been crouching. She was standing on a rail, looking as if she was trying to decide whether or not she should jump. There was no more singing. He never saw her again.

■ ■ ■ ■

The human body will do anything to avoid drowning. It begins with an involuntary desire to gasp. *Go ahead,* your cells plead, *take a breath.* The pulse accelerates. Carbon dioxide levels in the blood rise, creating first heightened alertness, and then anxiety. Once that carbon dioxide reaches a pressure of 55 mm in your arteries, there is no longer any reasoning with your nonthinking self. It will force you to take a breath. If you are still underwater when this decision is made, that is what you will inhale. And if you do, your larynx will spasm — violently — again and again as it attempts to divert the water to your stomach instead of your lungs. In the process, this spasm will also force you to exhale any last remaining air that you didn't even know you had. Your body will do anything — everything — to keep your lungs safe. And this commitment will work, up until the very last second. No matter what, your nonthinking brain will preserve your lungs, the place where air converts into life. Autopsies of drowning victims reveal gallons of water in their stomachs, bellies distended in a last-ditch effort to preserve their lungs. So long as it is conscious, the brain will drink until it can breathe.

In the storm-churned sea, the *Bounty* crew were gulping down gallons of oily seawater as they tried to thrash away from the ship. No matter how hard they tried, they could not find enough air. They flailed against debris, trying to grab anything that might save instead of kill them. Most of them were quickly separated. Not Jess Hewitt and Drew Salapatek. They were still tethered together and now trapped underwater. Jess struggled and writhed and bit at her harness, all too aware of what was happening. But still she was pulled down, down, down. She felt like she had become a giant weight. *I can't fight this,* she thought. She prepared to give up. And just then, she popped to the surface. Somehow, Drew had wriggled out of his harness and saved them both.

For now.

Jess faced the *Bounty,* now lying on its side. Each time a wave rolled by, it would possess the ship, raising its enormous masts and spars high into the air before slamming them down again. One of her crew mates got caught on the mizzen mast and was lifted twenty feet in the air. He thought he heard a voice say *Jump, Jump!* So he did, into the recirculating suction caused by the vessel. John Svendsen was there, too. Jess watched in horror as the rigging slammed down again, one of the spars smashing against the first mate's head. She turned away and tried to swim; she didn't want to see any more.

6:10 A.M.
Staten Island, New York
57°F
Barometer: 29.36 inches (dropping)
Winds: 29 mph (NNE)
Precipitation: Light rain

Sandy picked up speed, moving northward. The strange blocking pattern over Greenland was preventing the storm from moving out to sea, and the trough over the United States was only deepening the storm's nor'easter characteristics. Inside, winds were gusting at nearly 100 miles per hour, and an eyewall had reemerged. Inexplicably, Sandy was again becoming a hurricane.

"A meteorologically mind-boggling combination of ingredients is coming together," wrote Stu Ostro of the Weather Channel.

Sandy's new eye was now just 220 miles southeast of Atlantic City. Tropical storm gusts of 40 miles per hour had arrived on parts of Long Island and as far north as Boston. High-wind warnings were in effect in seventeen states, including Georgia, Maine, and Ohio. On the Weather Channel, Con Edison spokesperson Chris Olert was explaining that the company had already disconnected steam customers. Thousands of people were without power in Connecticut and on Long Island. Blackouts continued as far south as Georgia.

On Staten Island, traffic was light. The train stations were dark. Wind rocked signs, scattered leaves and trash. It had been raining for most of the night. Damien Moore finished getting ready for work and began his drive into Brooklyn. His neighborhood in Great Kills wasn't in the evacuation zone. It seemed like everything would be fine.

6:41 A.M.
Hatteras Island, North Carolina
53°F
Barometer: 29.24 inches (rising)
Winds: 38 mph (W)
Waves: 23 feet

Water streamed across Highway 12, the single route onto the island, tearing off a section of asphalt as it did. It ripped homes off their foundations, crumpling some as if they were made of gingerbread. Even as the storm began to pass, seas remained above twenty feet and winds were as high as 60 miles per hour. Even above the thundering sound of both, residents could hear the telltale *whompa-whompa* of a Jayhawk helicopter. Someone was in trouble. They didn't know that one of the most dangerous rescues in coast guard history was unfolding — that five crews were risking their lives in conditions too dangerous for their superiors to require them to attempt a mission. The crews had chosen to go.

Aaron Cmiel was piloting the C-130 that replaced McIntosh's. The storm cracked his windshield, but he kept flying. The first helicopter launched as soon as its crew got the call. The Jayhawk pitched against the wind as pilots Steve Cerveny and Jane Pena strained to keep it at an altitude of two thousand feet for the flight out. They'd never been in conditions that nasty. None of the crew had. Inside the wall of clouds, everything was pitch-black, and it was easy to get disoriented. Their flight mechanic, Mike Lufkin, scanned the horizon for air traffic like he had been trained to do. And then he laughed a little, thinking there was no way anyone would be stupid enough to be out in this.

As the helicopter neared the *Bounty,* the clouds began to break a little. Lufkin remembers thinking the sea looked more gloomy than anything else — a dark gray-blue marked by a widening debris field. He'd never seen anything like it.

Neither had Pena. She scanned the horizon, trying to make out human forms, a life raft, anything. She pulled her night-vision goggles back on and was blinded by a beacon of light. Attached to it was what looked like a five-gallon tub. And attached to that was one very battered John Svendsen. Cerveny lowered the helicopter so that swimmer Randy Haba could execute a rescue. Pena tried to keep her voice calm as she called out approaching waves. She fought to be heard over the instruments, over the warnings going off in the cockpit — the recorded female voice urging "ALTITUDE! ALTITUDE! ALTITUDE!" every time a wave broke under them. They were coming from everywhere — there was no rhythm to them. Just chaos.

Lufkin lowered Haba for a direct deployment: no basket, just a strap that he could wedge under Svendsen's armpits to raise him up. Haba felt confident he could handle the conditions — until he got down there and encountered his first wave.

"It was pretty much like an airplane hangar barreling down on you," he says. The wave crashed over him. He dove down as far as he could.

Haba says he lost track of time after that. He kicked against waves, felt himself raised and lowered by Lufkin. He lost his mask and snorkel. He checked a raft: empty. He checked another one and saw seven very scared faces staring back at him. The *Bounty* crew members had found one another, had made a daisy chain and fought like hell for what seemed like hours to get into the raft, their survival suits so filled with water they couldn't lift themselves. They had been tumbled and tossed. But they were floating now. And they were together. Nobody wanted to leave. Haba clambered into the raft. The crew was wide-eyed and very, very quiet.

"Just relax," he told them. It didn't help. How could it? He looked around the raft, trying to make quick assessments about everyone's condition. Doug Faunt was hunched over, clutching his belly. He had swallowed so much seawater he was really sick. He was also clearly the oldest in the bunch. Haba picked him to raise first. Lufkin struggled to lower the basket, but the winds were so strong they kept stripping it away from him. He tried weighing it down, but that just made it sink. He tried and tried and tried, eventually getting it close enough for Haba to get Faunt inside.

One by one, they packed the *Bounty* crew members into the very small cargo hold of the Jayhawk. They tried not to notice the smell of shit and vomit, the rising heat from bodies that had worked too hard for too long.

A second Jayhawk arrived on the scene and found another raft. Another rescue swimmer was lowered.

"Hey, guys," he said. "I heard you need a ride." He became a national hero for that.

Back on base and at sector, coordination was hovering just above controlled chaos. Rescue swimmers were beginning to collect *Bounty* survivors. But how many? And which ones? The phones were ringing non-stop. One of the calls was from the British consulate: They'd heard news that the HMS *Bounty* was in trouble and wanted to know if it was one of their ships. Sector officials divided the list of crew members and began making phone calls. Commander Anthony Popiel says most of the people didn't believe him when he called.

Within minutes, though, the story was all over the news. Jamie Trost had been up all night, keeping an eye on the *Pride of Baltimore.* He was one of the first people to see the headline. He texted Jan Miles: *They went over.*

The sound of the text awoke the captain. He grabbed his phone. It woke up his wife, too.

"What's going on?" she asked.

He shook his head. "They went over." There wasn't anything else to say.

In times of natural disasters, it's not uncommon for people to tell stories of visitations from loved ones the moment they died. The night the *Fantome* went down during Hurricane Mitch, relatives of every crew member who died experienced a kind of vision: Some say they were visited by the overwhelming smell of decay; others say their loved ones came to them in a dream and told them everything would be okay. That proved particularly comforting. But the survivors of the missing on the *Bounty* received no such comfort. And certainty was a long time coming.

Dina Christian called Brad Leggett to tell him that the first coast guard helicopter was on its way back from the ship.

"They've picked up six survivors," she said. "But I don't know which ones."

"It's always women and children first, isn't it?" Leggett asked. "She's got to be one of them."

Ralph McCutcheon, Walbridge's friend and former shipmate, was just waking up then, too. It had been decades since he had turned on the morning news; he says he's always been more of a coffee-and-newspaper kind of guy. But that morning, something told him to make a beeline for the television set. He couldn't say why — he still can't say why. Not that it really matters. Because once he turned it on, he learned that all but two of the crew had been recovered. McCutcheon knew one of them had to be the captain.

"Robin is a traditionalist. And, traditionally, the captain always goes down with his ship."

Claudia McCann had no idea the ship had even gone over until a reporter contacted her, saying that two people were missing.

"I knew immediately that it was him," she says. "If the boat was going to go down, he was going to be the last one off." But she also knew that he would have his survival suit on. "He's one tough cookie. I was optimistic they would find him."

Her phone was ringing off the hook now: Everyone from the *Today* show to CNN to international magazines was calling. She didn't want to talk to any of them. Seventeen years of wondering if her husband was okay had hardened her a little bit, but she still had feelings. She wanted to be alone, in the bungalow Robin had made perfect. She still believed he would be coming home.

Rex Christian held no such belief. When the coast guard called him to explain that Claudene was missing, he threatened to go get his gun.

"Apparent suicide threat," the sector communications officer noted in the case file.

8:11 A.M.
Atlanta, New York, Philadelphia, and Virginia

"And so it begins," wrote Bryan Norcross on his blog that morning. "Mega Monster Sandy" was about to smash into the Northeast. "There's no good news from the Hurricane Hunters or the computer forecast models. If anything, the storm is providing more drama in its first act than was expected. Water is coming over seawalls. Flooding and whipping winds have already started. Just from the fringe of Sandy."

He was still fuming over the National Hurricane Center's decision. But it was too late now, he thought. People's lives were in danger. He urged them to stay indoors — away from rooms where trees could fall and crush them. He told them to cover their windows, especially in high-rises, where wind would stress the glass, causing it to explode. “Even Wednesday and Thursday we’ll know that a giant storm is nearby,” he concluded. “That’s it. Hunker down, be smart, and stay safe.”

By the time his column appeared on the Weather Underground website, the day’s first high tide approached, and surge began to overtake the New Jersey coast. LaGuardia Airport was recording gusts of 60 miles per hour. The wind and the tide ripped away eighty feet of boardwalk in Atlantic City, where it careened down what had once been streets. Officials in North Wildwood reported major flooding as the tide continued “roaring in.” In Ocean City, flooding had brought together the ocean and bay in one uninterrupted froth of surf. All roads leading to the town were now submerged. Anyone still there was trapped. Officials told Kathy Orr, meteorologist for the Philadelphia CBS affiliate, that they’d never seen anything like it.

Inside the Upton NWS office, water was streaming inside the ceiling. Mickey Brown had stopped by to check on his staff. He’d never seen anything like this, either. Four thousand feet above him, winds were nearing 100 miles per hour.

At 10:31 A.M., Governor Cuomo sat flanked by a US Army Corps of Engineers colonel and a general from the national guard, both wearing battle fatigues. They were broadcasting live from the New York State Office of Emergency Management. Cuomo announced that the storm surge in New York City was already rivaling Irene levels. Later that afternoon, he would be closing both the Holland and Brooklyn-Battery tunnels. He assured residents that the state was prepared. "We think we've done everything we need to do."

To his south, NWS offices were issuing blizzard warnings for the Shenandoah region. Even veteran meteorologists were surprised. "History is being written as an extreme weather event continues to unfold, one which will occupy a place in the annals of weather history as one of the most extraordinary to have affected the United States," wrote Stu Ostro. "This is an extraordinary situation, and I am not prone to hyperbole."

WHOA, read the top headline for *Business Insider,* THE WEATHER CHANNEL METEOROLOGIST JUST COMPLETELY FREAKED OUT ABOUT HURRICANE SANDY.

Ostro was beating the drum of storm preparation and evacuation, urging people to get out, regardless of what Sandy was called. But residents across the mid-Atlantic weren't sure. Social scientists from the Wharton School of the University of Pennsylvania had been engaged in telephone polls all morning: Most residents thought they were under a hurricane watch. They told surveyors that they were expecting maybe some hurricane-force winds, "but then displayed limited degree of concern over this prospect," noted the report. Even residents living next to the coast continued to believe that the surge effects would be minimal — despite having seen the destruction brought by the morning tide. Of them, only half had flood insurance policies. But they said they weren't concerned about that, either. That they took the time to answer a phone survey with about seventy questions on it is pretty telling, too.

Still, at least people were now paying attention. The National Hurricane Center web page passed a billion hits. The Weather Channel set a new record for viewing, with an estimated 39 million households tuning in that day. Their website and mobile apps got an additional 450 million visits. Sandy had become the biggest news in the history of the channel.

Nevertheless, residents in the flood zone remained — and only 17 percent of them said they thought they were in any real danger. It didn't matter that this storm had already washed away Highway 12 and stranded residents on Cape Hatteras, or that Route 1 had been swamped in Delaware. A mere 150 people had checked into the three shelters open in Philadelphia. They brought with them "dogs, cats, turtles, and a spider," Mayor Michael Nutter told the *New York Times.* The tone of the article was light.

On Staten Island, Angela Dresch was home from school and feeling kind of bored. She scrolled through Twitter and Facebook, looked at some posts by her favorite boy band. Regina George, the fictional character from the film *Mean Girls,* posted a snarky tweet: "Is it raining?" Angela thought that was pretty funny. She retweeted it. Outside, waves had swallowed the beach and were snaking their way through the trees and brush. Her dad was pretty sure they wouldn't get much farther than the first floor of the house.

Across the New York Bay, in the Rockaways, a father of four was being interviewed by his local radio station. "I don't think my safety's at risk," he told the DJ. "We're going to tough it out and play Wii all day until the power goes out."

He wouldn't have long to wait. By 10:00 A.M., the neighborhoods around JFK Airport in Queens were reporting flooded streets and houses. Water was breaching the dunes in Maryland and Delaware. It stranded a police car. A woman in Delaware returned home to find a notice on her door: IF YOU DECIDE TO STAY, DON'T CALL EMERGENCY SERVICES, BECAUSE WE WON'T BE ABLE TO HELP YOU. She turned around and left.

New York Department of Health officials told reporters they remained confident that the impact to hospitals in the flood zone would be minimal. State Health Commissioner Shah speculated that, at most, one might lose power.

"Conditions are deteriorating very rapidly," said Bloomberg at a morning press conference. His voice was uncharacteristically clipped and hurried. He barely paused between sentences. "You're sort of caught between a rock and a hard place," he told residents in the flood zone. "You should have left, but it's also getting too dangerous to do so."

By 3:00 P.M. two feet of water had pooled in sections of Atlantic City. It was as high as eight feet in places. Officials there estimated that 80 percent of the city was flooded, and the storm had not yet made landfall. Those residents who had ignored the evacuation order were now calling for help. The city's 911 system failed after a gasoline tank spilled inside City Hall. They managed to get the system back online, but by then it was too late. Special national guard flood vehicles attempted to reach the city, but high winds turned them back. The city was on lockdown. One official said it was like being "under siege."

In Far Rockaway, waves were biting at the boardwalk. Gusts of wind pulled apart the roof at the NWS Eastern Region Headquarters. When Mickey Brown went out to investigate, he found entire sections of the roof waving. Drainage pipes were pulled loose. Water began to pour inside.

"It was one of those times that you think twice about Mother Nature," he says.

He knew it was going to get worse as the next high tide appeared. Surge was expected to reach eleven feet. Too many people weren't prepared. "There will be people who die," promised Martin O'Malley, Maryland's governor. Dannel Malloy, the governor of Connecticut, agreed.

"The mother is yet to come," he told reporters.

4:00 P.M.
Elizabeth City, North Carolina
50°F
Barometer: 29.14 inches (steady)
Winds: 24 mph (W)
Precipitation: Rain

Time wasn't doing much to clear up the flurry of misinformation about the *Bounty.* The crew hunkered down in a cheap motel wearing clothes purchased at Walmart by the Red Cross. Calls to the ship's owner were going unanswered. The crew needed help, and the last thing they wanted to do was talk to the media. Facebook posts were mounting by the minute, some saying that Claudene had been found alive, others that she was still missing. As the day progressed and no official word was given, Brad Leggett became increasingly concerned.

Something ain't right, he thought to himself.

Out in California, Claudene's longtime friend, Wendy Sellens, was having similar thoughts. The two had been friends since grade school, and Sellens had always admired her friend's audacity. She hoped it would be enough to get her through. "Claudene is really good in a crisis," thought Sellens. "I know she can keep a clear head." But that didn't keep the adrenaline from flowing, or Sellens's mind from settling on the idea that Claudene may very well be experiencing her greatest fear. "I was freaking out," she says. "And we were all so confused."

Rex and Dina Christian didn't want to wait any longer for official news, so they hopped the next plane for North Carolina.

The cutter *Elm* was on the scene now, rolling on thirty-foot seas. The *Gallatin* was on its way from Charleston. At Elizabeth City, Jayhawk copilot Kristen Jaekel had been working desk duty all night and was itching to get on one of the recovery flights. Her aircraft commander tapped her that afternoon.

I'm in, she thought. *I get to play!*

That's a remarkably common response from these flyers. Rescue swimmer Randy Haba had thought the same thing earlier, when he had gone out to pull survivors from the churning seas. *I get to be in the game.*

"We're competitive by nature," says Jaekel. "We all want to be the one to participate. Everybody wants to be the one to help somebody."

Jaekel was just twenty-nine. This was her first SAR case.

They set out to explore the drift pattern established by sector. Below them, they began to see signs of debris: a few disused life rafts, a cooler, some spars, a couple of survival suits. That alarmed Jaekel at first, but her pilot explained to her the way you can tell that they're empty — how they look unnatural, with a leg flipped over backward or a tangle in the arms.

Theirs was the last flight of the day. The sun would be setting soon. The *Bounty* had righted itself, regulated by the additional water it had taken on, and Jaekel felt a chill every time they flew over it. There was a survival suit tangled in the rigging. They were sure it was empty, but still.

Fuel levels were getting critical. They decided to leave their search area, just in case. The next survival suit they came upon looked a lot different than the others. The helicopter circled around again. There was nothing distorted about this suit, said Jaekel, and there was something graceful about the way it crested each wave. She looked down again and saw a halo of blond hair.

"It was a dead giveaway," says Jaekel. "I didn't know who it was. I didn't even know her name. But I knew this was the person we were looking for."

Jaekel still gets teary when she recounts the rest of the story: about how they had just twenty minutes to complete the mission, how they expedited their safety checklist to make sure there would be enough time, how the helicopter mechanic lowered the swimmer faster than he'd ever lowered anyone, how he struggled to place his rescue swimmer as close to Christian as possible, how her suit was so filled with water that the flight mechanic had to really struggle to get her inside. Brian Bailey, her senior pilot, says he was doing constant calculations in his head: They'd have very limited places to land.

"We get paid to worry," he explains. "There was no Plan B in this case."

He says the best way to get the helicopter back safely is to compartmentalize between what is happening in the front and the back of the helicopter, and that's what he told Jaekel to do. She tried not to look as the swimmer and mechanic cut away Christian's suit and began CPR. The rescue swimmer didn't even take off his helmet before beginning to do compressions. Jaekel could tell the woman lying on the floor of the helicopter wasn't responsive. Her jaw was so stiff that they could barely intubate her. Her face was covered in bruises and contusions. Still, the crew worked on her for the two full hours it took to return to

Elizabeth City. As they flew, sector made the call to the Christians, about to board yet another plane on their way to their daughter. When the helicopter finally landed, the swimmer hopped out, too. He didn't want Claudene to be alone at the hospital.

Jaekel was visibly shaken. Bailey tried to comfort her. "If we can't bring them home alive, at least we can bring them home." That helped a little. But she made a point not to turn on the television set when she got home: She didn't want to see photos of Christian alive and thriving. It just didn't square with what she had witnessed in the back of her helicopter.

When Claudia McCann heard word of Christian's death, she says she deflated a little. *Why can't they find Robin?* She began to wonder if he had gone down with his ship. She thought about Claudene's family and the survivors — about what they all must be feeling. That was the hardest thing of all, she says.

Wendy Sellens tried to avoid the questions that kept running through her mind: *Was Claudene strong? Did she struggle? Just how scared was she?* Instead, she tried to content herself with the knowledge that maybe, just maybe, Claudene's long-lost friend

Mike was with her at the end. Michelle Wilton said she felt like she could feel Claudene somewhere nearby. She still sees her every time a butterfly lands in her yard. Friends and relatives have told Dina and Rex that they are sure Claudene is looking down on them — taking care of them, even. But they feel no such consolation. "We can't feel her at all, no matter how hard we try," Dina wrote on Facebook. "We just keep seeing her fighting alone for her life in the water, then in the morgue. God hasn't taken those sights away yet. They just get worse. Sorry."

4:48 P.M.
Savannah, Georgia
63°F
Barometer: 29.61 inches (rising)
Winds: 21 mph (WNW)
Skies: Partly cloudy

Sean Cross prepared to go out for the last Hurricane Hunter reconnaissance flight. He hadn't seen his four-year-old son, Cooper, in more than a week. Cross wouldn't land until after Cooper's bedtime. He took a few minutes to call. Halloween was just two days away, so they mostly talked about trick-or-treating. Cooper took his first flight on a C-130 in utero. Cross says his son has been obsessed ever since. He was planning on dressing up like his dad for Halloween. Cross even found him what may be the world's tiniest flight suit. He got ready to hang up with their traditional closing.

"What does Daddy say when he goes flying?"

"Let's go find another storm!"

"That's right," said Cross. "Let's go find another storm."

He said good night to his wife, Apryl. She hates to fly, but she agrees to go on the "spousal orientation flights" offered by the Hurricane Hunters every year or so. Cross didn't tell her he was worried. Danger levels increase dramatically as a storm is about to make landfall. That made the stress levels much higher, too.

"Everyone was definitely a lot more on edge," he said. Jon Talbot agreed. "We're going in knowing that people are going to die," said Talbot. "And the storm surge is going to be epic. It's going to disrupt millions and millions of lives."

Talbot wanted to be on this flight, but it was Val Hendry who again drew the straw. She joined the rest of the crew as they stepped out of the hangar in Savannah. They wore their thick leather flight jackets. Even still, the wind cut right through them. Cross turned up his collar and tried to hide a shiver. Temperatures were in the forties. Not a record, but almost. There were reports of snow inland and inside the storm, too. That, says Cross, was the most bizarre thing of all.

"Tropical storm? Snow? Someone's in the wrong neighborhood. It's like the two toughest kids on the block have decided to link arms and beat up on the weak guy."

The C-130 took off and soon retraced the same path up the coast taken by the coast guard SARPAT flight nearly a week earlier. Within minutes, they were encountering 70-mile-per-hour winds. They gusted as high as 86 miles per hour inside. Sandy, says Hendry, had become a kind of weird fun house, snaking and tilting like a tornado.

"That's another first," said Cross.

"Very bizarre," said Hendry. "Very bizarre weather pattern."

Word came from the National Hurricane Center that they needed to go down to five hundred feet to see what was happening inside the storm. There were two goals behind that request, says James Franklin. The first was to determine just how strong the storm really was. The Empire State Building is twelve hundred feet high. The Statue of Liberty is more than three hundred feet. The city has more than two hundred buildings that rise at least five hundred feet high. Some residences are as high as nine hundred feet. The winds were going to be much stronger there. The National Hurricane Center wanted to know just how strong. They also wanted to know whether or not this monster was actually a hurricane. Scientists were going to debate that for decades, Franklin knew. It was already a controversy. And it would have major implications for insurance companies, too.

He didn't explain any of that to the Hurricane Hunters, though they said it wouldn't have mattered if he had. They bristled at the very idea of flying so low in these conditions.

"It's nasty down there. The stakes are incredibly high," said Cross. His primary concern was a microburst — the kind that sank the *Pride of Baltimore* twenty-five years prior. Wind-swept rain screamed against the fuselage, audible even over their headphones. The controls began to shake. *Are we going to make it out of this, or are we going to get pushed into the water?* he wondered. He didn't say it out loud. But Val Hendry did.

"I'm not a big fan," she told him.

Her assertion surprised Cross even more

than the wonkiness of the storm itself. "I've never heard Val ask to bug out of a storm. Ever."

That was enough for him. He regained altitude and fought for a path outside the storm's center. As he did, Hendry was almost apologetic.

"I'm just trying to keep us away from that finger," she said, pointing toward a long, slender band of particularly intense thunderstorms.

"The finger of death," Cross replied. "Kinda like the Grim Reaper sticking his finger out and saying, 'Come back and get some more,' " he said.

"Not today," said Hendry.

Cross thought about Cooper back home in his little flight suit. "Not today," he agreed. "Let's bug out of here and head home."

5:38 P.M.
Ewing, New Jersey
60°F
Barometer: 28.37 inches (falling)
Winds: 42 mph (NE)
Precipitation: Rain

Opening his press conference at the state's Regional Operations Intelligence Center, Governor Chris Christie looked visibly rattled. "For those who are on the barrier islands who decided it was a better idea to wait this out than to evacuate, for those elected officials who decided to ignore my admonition, this is now your responsibility," he said. "If you're still able to hear me, we need you to hunker down and get to the highest point possible in the dwelling that you are in. We will not be able to come help you until daylight tomorrow."

5:59 P.M.
Miami, Florida
70°F
Barometer: 29.78 inches (rising)
Winds: 9 mph (W)
Skies: Scattered clouds

Sandy would be making landfall in just a few hours. The controversy surrounding the storm was still growing. And at the National Hurricane Center, James Franklin was worried. Normally the landfall discussion issued by the NHC is brief — just a few sentences wrapping up the storm and signing off. But the situation surrounding Sandy had become more sensitive than anyone there had imagined. And so, even though the forecasters normally write the discussions, he and Rick Knabb, the NHC director, sat down to do it themselves that evening. They took their time, saying everything they wanted to say, creating what they were certain was a sound rationale for why the storm was no longer a hurricane.

"It was wonderful," said Franklin. "We felt really good about it."

This discussion was about to make history, they knew. Franklin went to hit send. The screen went blank.

"What happened?" asked Knabb.

"We lost it," said Franklin. He tried to call it back up again, but the screen remained blank.

"I was freaking out," said Franklin. "It was this moment of total panic on my part."

They tried to re-create the advisory, to explain why they were calling the storm extratropical: The structure of the storm had deteriorated, they explained. It was being powered by temperature contrasts — a sure sign of transition. Sandy, they said, was becoming absorbed within a larger mid-latitude system.

> ALL OF THESE CONSIDERATIONS LEAD US TO CONCLUDE THAT THE MOST APPROPRIATE CLASSIFICATION AT ADVISORY TIME IS EXTRATROPICAL.

Franklin's hands were shaking. His heart was racing. Knabb, he remembers thinking, looked remarkably calm. He kept typing.

> DESPITE THE RAPID FORWARD MOTION TODAY . . . SANDY IS EXPECTED TO STALL INLAND TOMORROW. THIS . . . COUPLED WITH THE VERY LARGE SIZE OF THE SYSTEM . . . WILL MEAN THAT CONDITIONS WILL BE SLOW TO IMPROVE IN THE AFFECTED AREAS. STRONG WINDS WILL PERSIST ALONG THE COAST AND SPREAD FARTHER INLAND THROUGH AT LEAST TUESDAY. OF PARTICULAR CONCERN ARE THE UPPER FLOORS OF HIGH-RISE BUILDINGS . . . AS RECONNAISSANCE DATA INDICATE THAT WINDS JUST A FEW HUNDRED FEET IN ALTITUDE ARE VERY MUCH STRONGER THAN THOSE NEAR THE SURFACE. EVEN AS SANDY WEAKENS . . . HEAVY RAINS WILL PERSIST OVER A LARGE AREA . . . POSING A VERY SIGNIFICANT INLAND FLOOD RISK.

They went on to explain, one more time, that the local National Weather Service offices would be handling the watches and warnings. Franklin didn't think this version was nearly as good as the first one, and it was twenty minutes late getting out. It was like Sandy wanted one more surprise.

"That is the only time in my fifteen-year career that I've had a forecast disappear on me like that. I still don't know how it happened."

6:10 P.M.
New York, New York
61°F
Barometer: 28.56 inches (steady)
Winds: 42 mph (E)
Precipitation: Rain

The bridges into the city had been closed for an hour. The Holland and Brooklyn-Battery tunnels had already been shut down for hours. At 5:30 P.M., the lights went out in Queens. The Breezy Point neighborhood was completely inundated with water. Now it was also pitch-black. Over the growing winds, you could hear the unmistakable sound of people frantically screaming for help. Others tried calling 911, but calls had long since overwhelmed the switchboard. They were transferred to voice mail and told to leave a message.

The wind grew. One resident near the shore said it sounded like a fleet of freight trains. Another said it was like a nuclear bomb had just gone off. Windows and doors imploded. Glass fell everywhere. Wind gusts of more than 60 miles per hour were reported in Central Park, nestled in behind all the skyscraper windbreaks; 79 miles per hour at Barnegat Light in New Jersey. Water had completely submerged cars on Long Island. No one expected the water to rise so high so fast. They'd pictured a gradual swelling, a seeping. This was walls and walls of water, coming from every possible direction. It rose feet in seconds.

On Staten Island, families became separated. A woman left her mother with a bowl of soup and stepped outside just long enough to start the car. It stalled. She opened the door to waist-high water. A nearby couple saw her, but kept going. They said they had no choice: The water was already up to their vehicle's windows. The woman tried to get back to her mother, but the force of the water was too strong. Around her, others scrambled through the dark and the smoke, dodging downed electrical lines and debris. They could hear a woman scream. "It's coming, it's coming," shouted a panicked male voice. "Get the fuck out!"

Just blocks away, John Paterno's family was trying to get to him as well. His cousin

Frankie drove until his car stalled, then tried repeatedly to dive under the crashing surf. Waves pushed him back each time. A block away, Paterno's pit bull climbed on top of the cockatoo's birdcage. Neighbors never heard him bark. They had no idea Paterno was still inside, trapped in a bedroom quickly filling with water.

Glenda Moore was also panicking. The power had gone out in her house. Damien was still at work. It didn't feel safe to stay put. She made a quick call to her husband, then packed up the boys' Halloween costumes along with some snacks and clothes, and loaded the kids into her SUV. It made sense to her to get to Brooklyn, to her sister's, as fast as she could. She chose a major thoroughfare down by the water. She hadn't made it very far when the car got stuck. She struggled to open her car door, pushing it hard against the surging water. It almost swept her away. She made it to the back door, grabbed Connor and then Brendan, and tried to make it to higher ground. The waves tugged hard at the boys. She lost her grip. She screamed for her sons, but in an instant they were swept away.

6:55 P.M.
Greater New York City Area
61°F
Barometer: 28.56 inches (steady)
Winds: 44 mph (E)
Precipitation: Rain

The National Hurricane Center had just declared Sandy a post-tropical storm. News outlets announced they would drop "Hurricane" from the storm's title. "We are now calling it 'Superstorm Sandy,' " tweeted the Weather Channel. Ashley Robson wasn't following the weather channel. She lived in Westchester County, away from the coast. She was sixteen. Waiting for her driver's license. Excited about volleyball. And exasperated by the storm. She posted a picture of the stairwell in her family's North Salem home, where she and her parents had placed a half dozen or so plastic food containers to collect the rain that was falling. "Thanks Sandy," she tweeted.

Next door, her sister, Caitlin, and younger brother, Michael, were hanging out at the house of Michael's best friend, Jack Baumler. At eleven, Jack was two years younger than Michael, but the boys had been thick as thieves for as long as anyone could remember. The two were playing around in Jack's family room — it was just a normal night for them. Michael was hilarious — always joking. He had mad skills on the ski slope. Ashley called him "kid." Jack idolized him. He was a big-hearted kid who always remembered to tell his mom he loved her.

Jack's mom, Val, had gone through all the routine storm-safety procedures that night. They weren't in a flood zone; they hadn't been told to evacuate. She made a collection of flashlights and bottled water and blankets. There was nothing left to do but wait it out. The wind was howling, yes. But that was no surprise. *Besides,* she thought, *they were all safe and inside. What could go wrong?*

Val was in the kitchen making a pot of soup for dinner when she heard the crash. "It was the loudest noise of my life," she says. "And I didn't know what it was." She called out to the boys. There was no answer. She called again and again. She began to panic. "I didn't hear them and I was screaming for them and I didn't hear them." But, she says, in her heart she knew what had happened. She raced to the family room but couldn't get inside: An enormous, one-hundred-year-old oak had smashed through the roof. Neighbors who had heard the crash came racing over. They broke windows, trying to get inside. They brought saws and chainsaws and tried to cut away sections of the tree. And the whole time, Val was calling the boys' names.

Seventy-five miles to their south, waves were tearing away at the southern tip of Staten Island. The Dresches had just sat down to dinner. Patricia was sure she could feel the dining room floor rising.

"The whole living room is going to take off," she told George.

"No, it's not."

"Yes, it is."

Water started pouring in the front door. They moved to the kitchen. Water was surging in there, too. Just after 7:00 P.M., Patricia called her brother to say that the surge had washed out their landline. She called again to say the addition on the back of the house had been ripped away. *We're going upstairs,* she told him. *To the second floor.* He told her he would call 911. He did, and was promptly placed on hold — one of ten thousand callers trying to get through that hour. Meanwhile, the water continued to rise. The Dresches were crammed in their bathroom, water lapping at Angela's neck. Patricia had one hand on her, the other gripping the bathroom sink. The house began to sway, and they could hear the roof begin to crack, like a hundred shots being fired. And, then, in an instant, the house gave way. George was swept away. She could hear him crying for help. Patricia clung to Angela for a moment, but then a piece of roof hit them both on the head. Patricia lost her grip. Angela went under. At that point, Patricia says, she knew her daughter was gone. In the distance, she could still hear George crying out.

In Brooklyn, Jake Vogelman was staying at his mom's house. The twenty-four-year-old was a lighting and stage designer. He liked black leather coats and college sweatshirts. Everyone who knew him said he went out of his way to be helpful. Just a little after seven, his best friend, Jessie Streich-Kest, called. The two had known each other since middle school. Jessie was a high school special education teacher. She liked to teach learning-disabled kids how to read. She had a two-year-old mutt named Max. Jake told his mom, Marcia, that he was heading over to Jessie's apartment. Marcia told him she didn't think it was a good idea. He told her Jessie needed him. That's all there was to it. He left. A half hour later or so, Jake texted to say that he and Jessie were at her parents' house in Ditmas Park. Jessie's dad, Jon, was a well-known community organizer. He had been diagnosed with liver cancer that summer. Things weren't looking good for him. Jake didn't text to say they were leaving, but not long after, a neighbor saw the two of them walking Max. They looked like they were having a good time, despite the weather.

8:00 P.M.
New York, New York
58°F
Barometer: 28.63 inches (rising)
Winds: 52 mph (E)
Precipitation: Rain

Winds gusted at 90 miles per hour. Waves in New York Harbor were surpassing thirty feet — taller than a two-story house, and the highest waves ever recorded there. They had been driven by wind for hundreds of miles. And they were fierce as sin. They slammed into the coast, sending mountainous white water into the city. Sandy's eye was now just five miles southwest of Atlantic City. Fearing for their underground equipment, Con Edison cut off power to much of lower Manhattan. Five hospitals went dark. They thought backup generators would keep them safe, but those failed, too. NYU's Tisch Hospital began evacuating more than two hundred patients. Across New York, streets and avenues flooded. Cars bobbed down Wall Street. The Hudson River escaped its banks. Torrents poured into the subway tunnels, filling them with swirling white water. More than 43 million gallons of seawater filled each of the Brooklyn-Battery tunnels from floor to ceiling for more than a mile.

"It's worse than my worst fear," said Joseph Lhota, the head of the transportation authority. "And the worst disaster to hit the subway system in its one-hundred-eight-year history."

The storm closed three nuclear power plants, including Nine Mile Point in Oswego, nearly three hundred miles from where the storm made landfall. Water poured into Ground Zero, filling the pit. Governor Andrew Cuomo called it the worst conditions he had ever seen. A transformer exploded in the East Village. Three million people were now in the dark. There was a strange orange glow to the sky, though: All of the Breezy Point neighborhood had become engulfed in flame. Outside the houses there, streets had become deadly, surging streams. Escape was impossible. And so with no other option, people began to pray. By the end of the night, more than one hundred homes burned to the ground.

And still the water kept coming: more than 14 feet in Battery Park in Manhattan; 12 feet on Long Island; 4.7 feet in the financial district; 5 feet in Poughkeepsie; 6 feet at Newark's Liberty International Airport.

Throughout the region, people were trapped in their cars and houses.

Neighbors could hear their cries, but couldn't reach them. Patricia Dresch's brother, who didn't yet know how dire the situation had become, was still on hold. The 911 operators were answering more than twenty thousand calls an hour. One of them came from a distraught man in Queens. His twenty-three-year-old girlfriend, Lauren Abraham, had stepped out of her Richmond Hill home long enough to shoot some pictures of the storm damage. She didn't see the downed power line, and she certainly didn't know it was live. She stepped on it and burst into flames. Emergency personnel arrived at the scene in minutes, but they couldn't get near Abraham, who was alive and burning for at least a half hour. It took Con Edison two hours to turn off the power to the line. Neighbors say they won't ever forget the smell. Across the region, New York Police Department SCUBA and emergency service units were zipping from crisis to crisis in high-speed tenders and on Jet Skis. For every house they could get to, there were an untold number that were blocked by power lines or debris. Police boats managed to get through to Coney Island Hospital. There, the emergency generators shut off, forcing the evacuation of more than two hundred patients. In their place, storm refugees began to congregate in the hospital's makeshift shelter. The driver of the police boat dropped off four rescuees and headed back out into the storm.

By 9:00 P.M., Bellevue Hospital had lost power. Their emergency generators appeared to be working fine, but just before midnight, the fuel pumps failed. They were down to a single emergency generator. Doctors frantically shuffled their most critical patients, trying to get them closer to the single power source. Dozens of staff members formed a human chain in an attempt to get more gas to the basement pumps. They carried it up and down thirteen flights of stairs in the kind of red plastic gas cans you might use to fill a lawn mower. The rest of the hospital was dark. On the nineteenth floor, a psychiatric inmate asked Elizabeth Ford if she would take off his handcuffs when he began to drown.

10:02 P.M.
New York, New York
58°F
Barometer: 28.80 inches (rising)
Winds: 39 mph (E)
Precipitation: Rain

Mayor Bloomberg was on TV, pleading with New Yorkers. "Please, please, please," he began. "We need to keep the roads clear. Do not drive. Let me repeat that, please, do not drive. We have now sent a message to all taxi and livery drivers to get off the roads immediately. As I said earlier, the time to leave has passed. Do not go outside. It is still very dangerous. And from now until the storm is well past, you just have to shelter in place. You need to stay wherever you are. Let me repeat that, you have to stay wherever you are."

Back on Staten Island, Patricia Dresch was drifting. At first, she'd grabbed a few electrical cables. Then part of her bathroom wall. She watched as her neighbors' homes crumbled into the surf around her. And then, in an instant, the water just stopped. She was on dry land. She adjusted her clothes, tried to button up her shirt. She was freezing — very, very cold — but she couldn't feel a thing. Hypothermia had set in. She was in shock, too. Numb, she sat down on a pile of debris and waited. By the time rescuers found her, her temperature had dropped to 81 degrees.

How long she waited, she doesn't know. Eventually, she saw flashlights. A firefighter approached. "You're here to rescue me," she said.

She thanked them and immediately fell unconscious. They sped her to Staten Island University Hospital, where rumors were brewing about the destruction outside their door. For now, though, the hospital was safe.

At the Horizon Care Center and Seaview Manor assisted-living center, administrators had been waiting all day for word about whether or not they should evacuate. Their calls to the emergency management office went unanswered. At Horizon Care Center, the staff moved their patients — all 269 of them — to the second floor and hoped for the best. Within ten minutes of the surge's arrival, their generators had failed. They shivered in the cold and the dark.

They weren't alone. Across the region, people struggled to remain alive, still in disbelief that a storm could do so much damage.

"It was like God looked away for a minute," said one resident.

Afterward

By dawn on Tuesday, entire swaths of the Eastern Seaboard were unrecognizable. And millions of lives had forever changed. For many, the torment continued. Across Appalachia, residents struggled against freezing temperatures and no power. They risked asphyxiation by using camping stoves and gas ovens to keep warm. Nursing home workers swaddled elderly patients in blankets and sleeping bags. The snow continued to fall. Internet service went out throughout the eastern NWS forecasting offices, preventing them from updating critical weather information for the rest of the day. It would be a week before their sites were fully functional.

Meanwhile, 11 billion gallons of sewage flowed into the floodwaters engulfing New York and New Jersey. At Bellevue Hospital, millions of gallons of contaminated water pooled in the basement. It flooded the morgue. As patients continued to die, doctors looked for safe places to keep their bodies. Surviving patients were without water or electricity. The elevator shafts were flooded. Ventilators were running out of the compressed air they needed to function. Critical medical devices drained their last battery power, sounding a chorus of urgent alarms as they shut down. Toilets began to overflow. The smell was already overpowering. Staff members tried to keep the single generator running; they were now assisted by a dozen national guard troops. Doctors wondered aloud why they and their patients were still there.

Up on the nineteenth floor, Ford was getting worried. They were running out of food. Sanitation had become third-worldly. The situation was now a crisis. She approached the corrections officers there.

"I want to bring together all of the patients," she said. "I think it's the only way."

They agreed. Her staff began walking patients one by one. It was dark. The only lights they had were the flashlights they had brought on Sunday.

Once they were all assembled, Ford called for her staff, too. She waited for them to settle in. And then she began to speak. She told them just what they were up against.

She promised to take care of them. "We're all in this together," she said.

They agreed. A therapist went home and made a huge batch of chili. She passed around bags of chips. The lights stayed off. The drinking water dwindled.

Conditions continued to deteriorate. On Wednesday, the backup generator failed, too. Administrators made the decision to evacuate. The hospital, they said, was no longer safe.

They had had plenty of mock disaster drills, but never one in which they had to carry patients down dark stairwells. They fumbled and tripped over one another at first. Two dozen ambulances wrapped around the still-darkened block, waiting to carry the patients to safety. Some of those patients had to walk themselves down flights of stairs; there weren't enough staff members to carry them. The patients weren't supposed to travel without their medical records, but some got lost and the receiving hospitals, already over capacity, struggled to determine the identities of their new patients. On Thursday morning, Dr. Ford was still searching for places that would take twenty-six of her wards. She made phone calls for hours. She began to beg. Eventually a hospital in Utica — 240 miles away

— reluctantly agreed to take them.

The staff helped them change into orange prison jumpsuits. They separated them into small groups and chained their ankles together. Flanked by armed guards, they stumbled their way down dark stairwells, one slow step at a time. No one resisted or acted out. They knew the situation was serious. Ford was proud of them.

At a press conference, Alan Aviles told reporters he'd be lucky to get the hospital up and running again in three weeks. He looked haggard. Almost in shock. "Nothing has happened like this in Bellevue's two-hundred-seventy-five-year history," he said.

Outside, the city was remarkably quiet. Coast guard vessels patrolled the bay, dodging half-sunk boats, roofs of homes, cars, and construction equipment, in an effort to keep the harbor clear. Pleasure boats were strictly prohibited. Commercial vessels were allowed by special permission only. On Staten Island, the only sound was that of helicopters rescuing people from rooftops and police boats patrolling for survivors. They wouldn't begin looking for the dead yet. Not until the waters receded. In Hoboken, New Jersey, the national guard began the dangerous process of rescuing thousands of people who chose not to evacuate and were now stranded by the storm. Officials warned them not to race outside, even when they saw the troops. The water, they said, had been contaminated with raw sewage. Untold active power lines hid below the surface. It was just too dangerous.

In Mantoloking, New Jersey, a broken natural gas line reignited fires that had already destroyed more than a dozen homes during the course of the storm. Firefighters rushed to the scene, but found they were unable to reach the fires: Ironically, the neighborhood was too flooded for their fire engines to get through.

Trees and power lines blocked roads throughout the state, forcing Governor Christie to cancel Halloween by executive order. New York prohibited any vehicle carrying fewer than three people from entering the city — a restriction not imposed since 9/11. Police set up roadblocks to enforce the restriction. Outside the city, cars stacked up by the hundreds around gas stations. New Jersey attempted to implement a rotating system for who could get gas on what days, but residents became confused. Cars with empty fuel tanks began to appear, abandoned on streets. Tempers flared.

Barrier islands, along with entire sections of Staten Island and Long Island, remained without power and water. Residents grew frantic. They had wanted to stay. Now they wanted more than anything to go. Four thousand city buses began removing them — a process that would take days. Those still waiting pled with rescuers to take them next. They cried and screamed. They offered bribes. But it didn't matter; there just weren't enough seats to take them. And if there had been, city shelters had long since filled up.

In some cases, it would take families weeks to track down mentally ill and otherwise compromised patients who had been relocated because of the storm.

By the end of the week, the region looked like it was at war. Amphibious assault vehicles patrolled streets. Navy ships were anchored in New York Harbor. Camouflaged trucks carried emergency rations and refugees. Hundreds of military personnel set up pumps and evacuation centers on street corners. They tried to distribute free gasoline, but quickly aborted the plan after fuel trucks were mobbed by panicky residents. Police patrolled the streets with megaphones, warning people to stay inside. People became distracted, uneasy. One man was killed when he stepped out in front of a military vehicle. The driver never even saw him.

The coast guard continued to search for Robin Walbridge for days, eventually suspending its search on November 2. His body has never been recovered. Claudia is certain it remains in the ship he loved so much.

On that same day, two patients still languished at the otherwise empty Bellevue Hospital. One was in desperate need of heart surgery. The other was too heavy to lift. Doctors told reporters they would be fired if they commented on the conditions there.

Tens of thousands of cars remained abandoned or swamped in the most unlikely of places. Within days, New York City had already towed 3,400 of them, along with more than 180 boats that had washed up into city parks.

It would take much longer for the subways to begin running. City officials soon admitted they were overwhelmed by the damage. And so FEMA sent a plane of engineers and hydrologists from the US Army Corps of Engineers to assist in the recovery process. Together with transit authority employees, they would try to solve the problem of removing water from underground tunnels.

They worked side-by-side with electrical crews, who were toiling to return power to the millions of people still in the dark. Pumps, generators, and hoses flanked buildings, pumping tens of thousands of gallons of dirty water into flooded streets every minute. Piles of rat carcasses mounted. Much of the electrical infrastructure was still under as much as twenty-five feet of water. It was, said one executive of the power company, the worst disaster in their history. A week after the storm, more than a million people were still without power, from West Virginia to Ohio to Connecticut. Power companies told some residents it would be weeks before their power was restored. That included tens of thousands of residents in public housing facilities across the city. They walked down dozens of flights of stairs carrying buckets to collect water from fire hydrants. At night, they congregated in groups, locked themselves in dark apartments, and hoped they'd be safe. They railed against the housing authority for not having a hurricane preparedness plan. Forty thousand residents were now homeless. They said they just had no idea it would be so bad. Officials admitted they had no place to put them: Temporary FEMA housing trailers don't fit on busy city streets. The city offered them blankets and hot meals, but there weren't enough of those to go around, either.

On November 7, the region was rocked by yet another nor'easter, forcing the shutdown of FEMA centers and further crippling those already in peril. "We do not believe it is necessary to evacuate," Mayor Bloomberg again told reporters. Power lines began to snap, sending tens of thousands of people once again into darkness. Winds rocked already damaged homes. Snow piled up in living rooms and the shells of basements and cellars. The death toll began to rise again. And still, residents remained incredulous.

To this day, residents and emergency managers say they were shocked and surprised by the damage Sandy wrought. A full 79 percent of them told researchers that the storm's impact was far more than they expected.

In April 2013, the National Weather Service announced that it would be changing its system of watches and warnings. The next time a storm like Sandy appears, the National Hurricane Center will be able to continue issuing its advisories, regardless what changes occur to the storm. In May 2014, they unveiled an experimental surge map. The next time a hurricane hits a major metropolitan area, they hope to show just where the water will go. And there will be a next time, they promise.

Sandy was the worst-case scenario that was never supposed to happen. New York may have fared better than Haiti, but the storm showed just how vulnerable we all are. Each of us tries to manage risk, to plan for the future, to understand storms. We consult our latest computer models and our most time-tested best practices. But sometimes, that's just not enough. Sometimes, nature breaks all the rules. And it always plays to win.

ACKNOWLEDGMENTS

This book would not have been possible without the generosity of myriad people willing to share their stories. Thank you all. The staff of the National Hurricane Center, the Mt. Holly NWS forecasting office, and the coast guard's Air Station Elizabeth City and Sector North Carolina were especially giving with their time: These are heroic individuals who work tirelessly — and selflessly — every day to keep the rest of us safe, and that makes their willingness to host a journalist for days on end all the more extraordinary. Thanks also to the crew of the *Pride of Baltimore II* for letting me hop aboard, and to the crew of the *Picton Castle,* who found a way to be in touch from the South Pacific whenever I asked.

So many individuals who endured unimaginable loss during the storm agreed to speak with me, and for that I am both humbled and very grateful. Thanks to Oxfam for arranging interviews in the Caribbean, and to everyone from there to Canada willing to talk about how the storm affected them. I'm particularly indebted to the crew, family, and friends of the *Bounty* for their trust. Thanks most of all to Claudia McCann and Michelle Wilton for your hospitality and friendship. It's an honor and privilege to know you both and to learn from your remarkable strength.

This book began with an article I wrote on the sinking of the *Bounty* for *Outside* magazine. Elizabeth Hightower, their features editor, put untold hours into the piece, beginning with my first pitch and continuing through to publication. Every writer should get an opportunity to have such careful shepherding. Thanks also to Jonah Ogles, their associate editor, who checked each fact and made sure we got it right.

It was Murray Carpenter's idea that I should consider a book-length project about the storm, proving once again that his journalistic instincts are razor sharp and his advice always sound. Sarah Moore read and commented on early drafts, and always had invaluable insight. So, too, did David Gessner, one of our country's most important environmental voices. Bill Roorbach, Jeff Thomson, and Camille Dungy inspired me to write better at every turn. Dozens of reporters contributed ideas and information, both in person and through their well-researched stories. It's because of their hard work that I am able to write this narrative. I'm particularly grateful for the late Matthew Power: I dearly miss his competitiveness and collaboration. Thanks also to Michael Kruse, Mario Vittone, and Matt White, who know this story at least as well as I do, and who graciously gave information and camaraderie in equal measure. Tom Di Liberto served as a meteorological advisor for the book, and I am most grateful for his expertise. Any mistakes are mine and not his.

Working with Stephen Morrow and his staff at Dutton is a dream come true. I first met Stephen at the end of an exhausting February day. He sparked a fire in my belly that hasn't abated, and his clarity of vision has turned an assortment of facts and dates into something much bigger (and better). His assistant, Stephanie Hitchcock, is as skilled as she is patient and kind.

Wendy Strothman and Lauren MacLeod remain the very best agents a writer could hope for. I learn something important from them each and every day, and I'm a better person just by knowing them. I'm so glad to have them both in my life.

I was visiting my family in North Carolina when Sandy struck. Thank you, Chris and Dawn, for not holding a grudge about a pork tenderloin that caught fire after I abandoned it to watch the news. Thanks to my parents for the continued support you've given since that auspicious day. Thanks especially to Max and Owen Keller, who helped me brainstorm titles, told the world's best jokes, and crept quietly through the house while I was writing. These two guys rock my world. So, too, does their dad, Ben. His unwavering love and support has buoyed me through helicopter-rescue school, lots of long research nights, and difficult interviews. Writing about tragedy is hard and can definitely take its toll. More than anything, Ben's care and compassion saw me through.

NOTES

I have arranged the notes by chapter with subheadings. Within each subheading section, the notes are in the order of reference. In the main text, wherever possible, I quote individuals in their own words. All statements in direct quotes are either those that an individual remembers saying verbatim or those that could be independently verified. Whenever an individual remembered the gist, rather than the letter, of what was said, those statements appear in italics. I am particularly indebted to the extensive and excellent reporting done by reporters too numerous to list in the New York City metropolitan area around the time of Sunday's landfall. All financial figures appearing in the book are in US dollars. When appropriate, they have been adjusted for inflation using the Consumer Price Index (CPI) provided by the Federal Reserve.

Landfall

Interviews

Lixion Avila, Robbie Berg, Jack Bevin, Eric Blake, Michael Brennan, Joe Bruno, John Cangialosi, Tony Gigi, Dean Iovino, Ray Kruzdlo, Chris Landsea, Kelly McKinney, Joe Miketta, Richard Pasch, Gary Szatkowski

Published Documents

Barron, James, Joseph Goldstein, and Kirk Semple, "Staten Island Was Tragic Epicenter of Storm's Casualties." *The New York Times,* November 1, 2012.

Binkovitz, Leah, "ALL Smithsonian Museums and the Zoo Remain Closed on Tuesday." *Smithsonian Magazine,* October 29, 2012. http://www.smithsonianmag.com/smithsonian-institution/update-all-smithsonian-museums-and-the-zoo-remain-closed-on-tuesday-96299711/

Boyle, Christina, "Staten Island Family Decides Not to Evacuate for Hurricane Sandy After Being Robbed During Irene — and Pays Terrible Price." *New York Daily News,* November 2, 2012.

Italie, Leanne, and Marilynn Marchione,

"NYU Hospital Evacuation: Hurricane Sandy Power Failure Moves More Than 200 Patients." *Huffington Post,* October 30, 2012. http://www.huffingtonpost.com/2012/10/30/nyu-hospital-evacuation-hurricane-sandy_n_2044026.html

Stirling, Stephen, "Sandy Still a Category 1 Hurricane, Still a 'Worst-Case Scenario,' Experts Say." *The Star-Ledger,* October 28, 2012.

Foderaro, Lisa W., "Hurricane Filled New York Aquarium with Dangerous Substance: Water." *The New York Times,* November 7, 2012.

Segar, Mike, "Hurricane Sandy: Staten Island Survivors." *The Atlantic,* November 21, 2012. http://www.theatlantic.com/infocus/2012/11/hurricane-sandy-staten-island-survivors/100410/

Unpublished Documents

Blake, Eric S., et al., "Tropical Cyclone Report: Hurricane Sandy" (AL182012, National Hurricane Center, February 12, 2013). www.nhc.noaa.gov/data/tcr/AL182012_Sandy.pdf

US Department of Commerce, "Service Assessment Hurricane/Post-Tropical Cyclone Sandy, October 22–29, 2012" (May 2013). http://www.nws.noaa.gov/os/

assessments/pdfs/Sandy13.pdf

Sunday

Interviews

Lixion Avila, Chris Barksdale, Katie DePrato, Doug Faunt, Jeff Finston, James Franklin, Jess Hewitt, Dean Iovino, Andrew Jaeger, Sarah Johnson, Kristin Kline, Chris Landsea, Brad Leggett, Claudia McCann, Ralph McCutcheon, Anthony Popiel, Gary Szatkowski, Wendy Sellens, Jon Talbot, Michelle Wilton

Published Documents

Davies, Pete, *Inside the Hurricane: Face to Face with Nature's Deadliest Storms.* New York: Henry Holt, 2000.

Politi, Steve, "Hurricane Sandy Heroes: N.J. Weather Forecaster Is Reluctantly Right." *Star-Ledger,* November 11, 2012.

Williams, Jack, and Bob Sheets, *Hurricane Watch: Forecasting the Deadliest Storms on Earth.* New York: Vintage, 2001.

Unpublished Documents

Blake, Eric S., et al., "Tropical Cyclone Report: Hurricane Sandy" (AL182012, National Hurricane Center, February 12,

2013). www.nhc.noaa.gov/data/tcr/AL182012_Sandy.pdf

"NOAA Historical Background" (NOAA Public Affairs, January 2002). http://www.publicaffairs.noaa.gov/grounders/noaahistory.html

US Coast Guard, "Investigation into the Circumstances Surrounding the Sinking of the TALL SHIP BOUNTY 123 Miles off the Coast of Cape Hatteras, North Carolina, on October 29, 2012, with Loss of One Life and Another Missing and Presumed Dead" (May 2014).

US Department of Commerce, "Service Assessment: Hurricane/Post-Tropical Cyclone Sandy, October 22–29, 2012" (May 2013).

Miscellaneous

Svendsen, John, Sworn Testimony before the US Coast Guard and National Transportation Safety Board (*Bounty* Hearings, March 2013).

Monday

Interviews

Lixion Avila, Chris Landsea, Joe Miketta, Richard Pasch, Gary Szatkowski, Jon Talbot

Published Documents

Toomey, David, *Stormchasers.* New York: W. W. Norton, 2002.

Khain, A., B. Lynn, and J. Dudhia, "Aerosol Effects on Intensity of Landfalling Hurricanes as Seen from Simulations with the WRF Model with Spectral Bin Microphysics." *Journal of the Atmospheric Sciences* 67 (Feb 2010): 365–384.

McQuaid, John, and Mark Schleifstein, *Path of Destruction: The Devastation of New Orleans and the Coming Age of Superstorms.* New York: Little, Brown, 2009.

Miscellaneous

"The Birth of a Monster." "Epic Storm's Puzzling Path." (*Hurricane Hunters,* the Weather Channel, 2013).

Tuesday

Interviews

Mitchell Bandklayder, Chris Barksdale, Katie DePrato, Doug Faunt, Rich Harter, Jess Hewitt, Andrew Jaeger, Todd Kosakowski, Jamie McNamara, Jan Miles, Dan Moreland, Josh Scornavacchi, Claudia McCann, Ralph McCutcheon

Published Documents

Carrier, Jim, *The Ship and the Storm.* New York: Harvest, 2002.

Piddington, Henry, *The Sailors Horn-book.* London: Frederic Norgate, 1889.

Davis, Walter R., "Hurricanes of 1954." *Monthly Weather Review* (Dec. 1954): 370–373.

Dunn, Gordon E., Walter R. Davis, and Paul L. Moore, "Hurricanes of 1955." *Monthly Weather Review* (Dec. 1955): 315–326.

Parrott, Daniel S., *Tall Ships Down.* Camden, Maine: International Marine, 2004.

Tutton, Michael, "Bob Gainey Breaks Silence on Daughter's Death, Seeks Tall Ship Safety Changes." *Canadian Press,* November 27, 2007.

———, "Report Questions Decisions Leading to Laura Gainey's Death." *Canadian Press,* October 29, 2008.

Unpublished Documents

"Accident Overview: History of Flight 191" (Federal Aviation Administration), http://lessonslearned.faa.gov/ll_main.cfm?TabID=1&LLID=32&LLTypeID=2 (Accessed May 11, 2014.)

"Marine Investigation Report M06F0024: Crew Member Lost Overboard Sail Training Vessel PICTON CASTLE 376 nm SSE of Lunenburg, Nova Scotia 08 December 2006" (Transportation Safety Board of Canada, October 27, 2008).

"Safety Recommendations" (National Transportation Safety Board, February 18, 1987).

"Marine Accident Report into the Capsizing and Sinking of the PRIDE OF BALTIMORE" (US Coast Guard, January 21, 1987).

US Coast Guard (Marine Safety Information System [MSIS] printouts MC98033150, MC98013222, MC01000276, MC01007227).

Miscellaneous

Disney Cruise Line Blog: http://disneycruiselineblog.com

Sworn testimony of Dan Cleveland, Laura Groves, Adam Prokosh, and Matt Sanders (USCG/NTSB Hearings into the Sinking of the *Bounty,* March 2013).

Wednesday

Interviews

Eric Blake, Michael Brennan, Millicent Frick, Jamie McNamara, Richard Pasch, Beat Schmid

Published Documents

Associated Press, "Hurricane Sandy, Day by Day." *The Big Story,* October 26, 2012. http://bigstory.ap.org/article/hurricane-sandy-day-day

McFadden, David, "Jamaica Prepares for Tropical Storm Sandy." *The Big Story,* October 23, 2012. http://bigstory.ap.org/article/tropical-storm-warning-jamaica-ahead-sandy

Malkin, Elisabeth, "Yet Another Blow to Haiti from a Natural Disaster." *The New York Times,* October 29, 2012.

Morgan, Curtis, and Jacqueline Charles, "Sandy's Death Toll Rises to at Least 42." *Miami Herald,* October 26, 2012.

"The Day Gilbert Ravaged Jamaica." *Ja-*

maica Observer, September 12, 2013.

Dunn, Gordon E., et al., "The Hurricane Season of 1963." *Monthly Weather Review* 92:3 (1965): 128–382.

Collymore, Jeremy, *The Impact of Hurricane Gilbert on Jamaica: An Assessment of Response and Relief Measures.* Pan Caribbean Disaster Preparedness and Prevention Project, 1989.

Kruse, Michael, "The Last Voyage of the *Bounty.*" *Tampa Bay Times,* October 24, 2013. http://www.tampabay.com/specials/2013/reports/bounty/

Unpublished Documents

Blake, Eric S., et al., "Tropical Cyclone Report: Hurricane Sandy" (AL182012 National Hurricane Center, February 12, 2013). http://www.nhc.noaa.gov/data/tcr/AL182012_Sandy.pdf

Lorenz, Edward N., "Predictability: Does the Flap of a Butterfly's Wings in Brazil Set Off a Tornado in Texas?" (American Association for the Advancement of Science, 1972).

"The Caribbean: Hurricane Sandy Situation Report No. 2" (OCHA, November 19, 2012). http://reliefweb.int/sites/reliefweb.int/files/resources/Situation_Report_351.pdf

"Hurricane Gilbert in Jamaica, September, 1988" (Disaster Reports Number 5, Pan American Health Organization, Emergency Preparedness and Disaster Relief Coordination Program, Washington, D.C.; s.f).

Fordyce, Erin, Abdul-Akeem Sadiq, and Grace Chikoto, *Haiti's Emergency Management: A Case of Regional Support, Challenges, Opportunities, and Recommendations for the Future* (Washington, D.C.: FEMA, 2012).

Reliefweb International, "Haiti Suffers Further Blows Following Hurricane Sandy." http://reliefweb.int/report/haiti/haiti-suffers-further-blows-following-hurricane-sandy (Accessed 11 May 2014.)

Miscellaneous

"Carnival, Royal Caribbean Ships Avoid Tropical Storm Sandy." *Travel Pulse*, October 23, 2012. http://www.travelpulse.com/news/features/carnival-royal-caribbean-ships-avoid-tropical-storm-sandy.html

Thursday

Interviews

Lixion Avila, Chris Barksdale, Robbie Berg, Steve Bonn, Mickey Brown, Dina Christian, Aaron Cmiel, Connie DeRamus, Doug Faunt, Jeff Finston, James Franklin, Gary Kannegiesser, Rich Harter, Jess Hewitt, Dean Iovino, Chris Landsea, Claudia McCann, Ralph McCutcheon, Dan Moreland, Richard Pasch, Jane Pena, Jamie Rhome, Beat Schmid, Josh Scornavacchi, Tracie Simonin, Paul Slovic, Mimi Sprague, Gary Szatkowski, Michelle Wilton, Hernán Zini

Published Documents

David Longshore, *Encyclopedia of Hurricanes, Typhoons, and Cyclones.* New York: Facts on File, 2008.

Smith, Mike, *Warnings: The True Story of How Science Tamed the Weather.* Austin, TX: Greenleaf Book Group Press, 2010.

Junger, Sebastian, *The Perfect Storm.* New York: W. W. Norton, 2009.

Schwartz, John, "Early Worries That Hurricane Sandy Could Be a 'Perfect Storm.' " *The New York Times,* October 25, 2012.

McNoldy, Brian, "Hurricane Sandy Becomes Stronger and Larger than Expected." *Washington Post,* October 25, 2012.

Enten, Harry J., "Hurricane Sandy Barrels Towards the US — Will It Really Be the End of Days?" *The Guardian,* October 25, 2012.

Preston, Jennifer, "Tracking Hurricane Sandy up the East Coast." *The New York Times,* October 25, 2012.

Stirling, Stephen, "Hurricane Sandy on Path to Hit N.J., Latest 'Frankenstorm' Forecast Shows." *The Star-Ledger,* October 25, 2012.

Power, Matthew, "Inside the Coast Guard's Rescue Swimming School." *Men's Journal,* November 2013.

Luce, Stephen Bleecker, and Aaron Ward, *Text-Book of Seamanship.* New York: Van Nostrand, 1884.

Boylan, Desmond, "Cubans Start Cleanup of Hurricane Sandy Destruction." Reuters, October 27, 2012.

Callimachus, *Hymns and Epigrams. Lycophron. Aratus.* Translated by Mair, A. W. & G. R. Loeb Classical Library Volume 129. London: William Heinemann, 1921.

Quaife, Milo M., "Increase Allen Lapham, First Scholar of Wisconsin." *Wisconsin*

Magazine of History 1 (1917–18): 3–15.
Williams, Jack, "When Storms Were a Surprise: A History of Hurricane Warnings." *Capital Weather Gang* (blog), *Washington Post,* August 16, 2013.
Cushman, Gregory T., "The Imperial Politics of Hurricane Prediction: From Calcutta and Havana to Manila and Galveston, 1839–1900," in *Nation-States and the Global Environment: New Approaches to International Environmental History,* eds. Erika Marie Bsumek, David Kinkela, and Mark Atwood Lawrence. New York: Oxford University Press, 2013.
Silver, Nate, "The Weatherman Is Not a Moron." *The New York Times,* September 7, 2012.
Eos, Transactions American Geophysical Union 88:9 (February 2007): 108.
Lau, William K., and Kyu-Myong Kim, "How Nature Foiled the 2006 Hurricane Forecasts."
Cox, Jonathan, Donald House, and Michael Lindell, "Visualizing Uncertainty in Predicted Hurricane Tracks." *International Journal for Uncertainty Quantification* 3:2 (2013): 143–156.
Broad, Kenneth, Anthony Leiserowitz, Jessica Weinkle, and Marissa Steketee, "Misinterpretations of the 'Cone of

Uncertainty' in Florida during the 2004 Hurricane Season." *Bulletin of the American Meteorological Society.* 88:5 (May 2007): 651–667.

Knowlton, Kim, "Irene Approaches, But Climate Change Got Here First." *Switchboard* (NRDC Staff blog), August 25, 2011. http://switchboard.nrdc.org/blogs/kknowlton/irene_approaches_but_climate_c.html

McKibben, Bill, "Global Warming's Heavy Cost." *The Daily Beast,* August 25, 2011. http://www.thedailybeast.com/articles/2011/08/25/hurricane-irene-can-be-tied-to-global-warming-says-bill-mckibben.html

Begley, Sharon, "The Reality of Global Climate Change Is upon Us." *Newsweek,* May 29, 2011.

Knutson, Thomas R., et. al., "Tropical Cyclones and Climate Change." *Nature Geoscience* 3 (2010): 157–163.

Borenstein, Seth, "East Coast Braces for Monster 'Frankenstorm.' " *The Big Story,* Associated Press, October 25, 2012. http://bigstory.ap.org/article/east-coast-readies-Frankenstorm-monster

Zane, D. F., et al., "Tracking deaths related to Hurricane Ike, Texas, 2008." *Disaster*

Med Public Health Prep 5:1 (2011): 23–28.

Lovewell, Mark Alan, "Lost at Sea for 12 Days, Island Captain Returns Mourning Friend, Boat." *Vineyard Gazette,* November 25, 2010.

Fraser, Doug, "Mashpee Man Dies in Sailing Accident." *Cape Cod Times,* November 25, 2010.

Kahneman, D., and A. Tversky, "Choices, Values, and Frames." *American Psychologist* 39:4 (April 1984): 341–350.

Kruse, Michael, "The Last Voyage of the *Bounty.*" *Tampa Bay Times.* Series. October 2013. http://www.tampabay.com/specials/2013/reports/bounty/

Kotsch, William J., and Richard Henderson, *Heavy Weather Guide.* Annapolis: US Naval Institute, 1984.

Unpublished Documents

Geggis, Lorna M., "Do You See What I Mean?: Measuring Consensus of Agreement and Understanding of a National Weather Service Informational Graphic" (Master's Thesis, University of South Florida, 2007).

Masters, Jeffrey, "Hunting Hugo" (*Weather Underground*). http://www.wunderground.com/resources/education/hugo1.asp

———, "Sandy Slams Cuba, Intensifies over the Bahamas." (*Dr. Jeff Masters' Wunderblog*). http://www.wunderground.com/blog/JeffMasters/sandy-slams-cuba-intensifies-over-the-bahamas

"Sinking of S/V RAW FAITH" (Coast Guard Marine Information for Safety and Law Enforcement Report, December 2010).

US Coast Guard, "Investigation into the Circumstances Surrounding the Sinking of the TALL SHIP BOUNTY 123 Miles off the Coast of Cape Hatteras, North Carolina, on October 29, 2012, with Loss of One Life and Another Missing and Presumed Dead" (May 2014). s3.documentcloud.org/documents/1196856/coast-guard-report-on-bounty.txt

"Issac Cline Journal." (Quoted in *The Beginning of the National Weather Service: The Signal Years [1870–1891] as Viewed by Early Weather Pioneers,* edited by Gary K. Grice). http://www.nws.noaa.gov/pa/history/signal.php (Accessed March 1, 2014.)

Roth, David, "Texas Hurricane History" (Camp Springs, MD: National Weather Service).

" 'Frankenstorm' Sandy: Man Made Monster or an Act of God?" *From the Trenches*

World Report, October 25, 2012). http://www.fromthetrencheswordreport.com/frankenstorm-sandy-man-made-monster-or-an-act-of-god/24335

Paul N. Edwards (ed.), "Atmospheric General Circulation Modeling: A Participatory History." *University of Michigan.* http://pne.people.si.umich.edu/sloan/mainpage.html

Blake, Eric S., and Christopher Landsea, "The Deadliest, Costliest, and Most Intense United States Tropical Cyclones from 1851 to 2010 (and Other Frequently Requested Hurricane Facts)." (NOAA Technical Memorandum NWS NHC-6, August 2011).

NOAA/NESDIS Independent Review Team Report, July 20, 2012. http://science.house.gov/sites/republicans.science.house.gov/files/documents/NESDIS_IRT_Final_Report.pdf

Deputy Secretary Decision Memorandum Regarding NOAA/NESDIS Review, September 18, 2012.

Rappaport, Edward, et al., "An Operational Assessment of the Joint Hurricane Testbed's First Decade" (American Meteorological Society, January 2011). https://ams.confex.com/ams/91Annual/webprogram/Paper178802.html

"Atlantic Hurricanes, Climate Variability and Global Warming" (NOAA State of the Science Fact Sheet, May 2012). http://nrc.noaa.gov/sites/nrc/Documents/SoS%20Fact%20Sheets/SoS_Fact_Sheet_Hurricanes_and_Climate_FINAL_May2012.pdf (Accessed November 7, 2013.)

"Hurricane Sandy After Action: Report and Recommendations to Mayor Michael R. Bloomberg" (May 2013). http://www.nyc.gov/html/recovery/downloads/pdf/sandy_aar_5.2.13.pdf

Miscellaneous

Memmott, Mark, "Halloween Horror: Hurricane Sandy Could Be 'Billion-Dollar Storm.' " NPR, October 25, 2012.

Adam Prokosh, Dan Cleveland, Laura Groves, Jess Hewitt, Anna Sprague, John Svendsen (Sworn Testimony before the US Coast Guard and National Transportation Safety Board, *Bounty* Hearings, March 2013).

Friday

Interviews

Eric Blake, Mickey Brown, James Franklin, Millicent Frick, Tony Gigi, Rich Harter, Jess Hewitt, Chris Landsea, Wes McIntosh, Jan Miles, Mike Myers, Ed Rappaport, Gary Szatkowski, Jon Talbot, Hernán Zini

Published Documents

Macock, Denise, "Grand Bahama Hit Hard By Storm." *Tribune 242,* October 29, 2012.

Wemple, Erik, "CNN Bans 'Frankenstorm' Term for Hurricane Sandy." *Washington Post,* October 26, 2012.

Piddington, Henry, *The Sailors Horn-book.* London: Frederic Norgate, 1889.

Calhoun, C. Raymond, *Typhoon, the Other Enemy: The Third Fleet and the Pacific Storm of December 1944.* Annapolis: US Naval Institute Press, 1981.

Preston, Jennifer, Sheri Fink, and Michael Powell, "Behind a Call That Kept Nursing Home Patients in Storm's Path." *The New York Times,* December 2, 2012.

Schwartz, John, "Early Worries That Hurricane Sandy Could Be a 'Perfect

Storm.' " *The New York Times,* October 25, 2012.

Lisberg, Adam, and Dave Goldiner, "Weather Predictors 'Blew It,' Official Says." *New York Daily News,* August 9, 2007.

Unpublished Documents

Norcross, Bryan, "The Sandy Paradox" (*Weather Underground*). http://www.wunderground.com/blog/bnorcross/the-sandy-paradox

"Hurricane Sandy Response After Action Report Notes" (New York State Division of Homeland Security and Emergency Services, July 1, 2013).

"Service Assessment: Hurricane Irene, August 21–30, 2012" (US Department of Commerce, September 2012).

"Service Assessment: Hurricane Katrina, August 23–31, 2005" (US Department of Commerce, June 2006).

Pirani, Robert, and Laura Tolkoff, "Lessons from Sandy: Federal Policies to Build Climate-Resilient Coastal Regions" (New York: Lincoln Institute of Land Policy, 2014).

Miscellaneous

Dan Cleveland, Laura Groves, Jess Hewitt, Adam Prokosh, Matt Sanders, John Svendsen (Sworn Testimony before the US Coast Guard and National Transportation Safety Board, *Bounty* Hearings, March 2013).

Saturday

Interviews

Chris Barksdale, Joe Bruno, Donald Cresitello, Ross Dickman, Cas Holloway, Marc LaVorgna, Brad Leggett, Heather McGee, Kelly McKinney, Jamie McNamara, Jan Miles, Dan Moreland, Bryan Norcross, Jane Pena, Anthony Popiel, Wendy Sellens, Keri Suess, Gary Szatkowski, Michelle Wilton

Published Documents

Chase, G. Anderson, "Lessons of the Bounty." *Wooden Boat Magazine,* July/August 2013.

Biello, David, "The Science Behind Superstorm Sandy's Crippling Storm Surge." *Scientific American,* November 2012.

Navarro, Mireya, "New York Is Lagging as Seas and Risks Rise, Critics Warn." *The*

New York Times, September 10, 2012.

Dixon, Ken, "Malloy: 'This Could Be Bad . . . Really Bad.' " *Connecticut Post,* October 27, 2012.

Auer, Doug, "Flood of Tears: Bodies of SI Boys Found After Being Swept Away by Sandy." *New York Post,* November 2, 2012.

Byrne, Tom, "Gov. Markell Declares Limited State of Emergency, Orders Some Evacuations." *Delaware Public Media* (WDDE 91.1 FM). http://www.wdde.org/32785-gov-markell-declares-limits-state-emergency-orders-evacuations (Accessed 19 May 2014.)

Unpublished Documents

Bowman, M. J., et al., "Hydrologic Feasibility of Storm Surge Barriers to Protect the Metropolitan New York–New Jersey Region." (Final Report to New York Sea Grant, HydroQual, Inc., New York City Department of Environmental Protection, the Eppley Foundation for Research, March 2005).

Vittone, Mario. "Into the Storm: The Final Days and Decisions on *Bounty.*" *gCaptain,* July 22, 2013. http://gcaptain.com/storm-final-days-decisions-bounty/

Miscellaneous

Chris Barksdale, Dan Cleveland, Laura Groves, Jess Hewitt, Adam Prokosh, Matt Sanders, John Svendsen. (Sworn Testimony before the US Coast Guard and National Transportation Safety Board, *Bounty* Hearings, March 2013).

Sunday

Interviews

Chris Barksdale, Steve Bonn, Joe Bruno, Steve Cerveny, Aaron Cmiel, Rich Harter, Don Cresitello, Doug Faunt, James Franklin, Randy Haba, Jess Hewitt, Cas Holloway, Dean Iovino, Jeremy Johnson, Joseph Kelly, Chris Landsea, Claudia McCann, Wes McIntosh, Kelly McKinney, Joe Miketta, Billy Mitchell, Mike Myers, Bryan Norcross, Jane Pena, Jamie Rhome, Josh Scornavacchi, Gary Szatkowski, Jon Talbot

Published Documents

Buckley, Cara, "Panicked Evacuations Mix with Nonchalance in Hurricane Sandy's Path." *The New York Times,* October 28, 2012.

Steenhuysen, Julie, "Sandy Forecasts Were

on Target, but Message Was a Bit Garbled." Reuters, November 1, 2012.

Fairchild, Amy L., James Colgrove, and Marian Moser Jones, "The Challenge of Mandatory Evacuation: Providing for and Deciding For." *Health Affairs* 25:4 (July 2006): 958–967.

Mitchell, Paula Ann, "Ex–Ulster County Resident John 'Jack' Paterno, Lost in Superstorm Sandy, Was Strong-Willed to the End." *Daily Freeman,* November 11, 2012.

Boyle, Christina, "Staten Island Family Decides Not to Evacuate for Hurricane Sandy After Being Robbed During Irene — and Pays Terrible Price." *New York Daily News,* November 2, 2012.

Haggerty, Erin, "When Bellevue Had to Evacuate Its Criminally Insane." *New York Magazine,* October 29, 2013.

Hartocollis, Anemona, and Nina Bernstein, "At Bellevue, a Desperate Fight to Ensure the Patients' Safety." *The New York Times,* November 1, 2012.

InsideVandy.com, "Sandy Hits Vanderbilt Family." November 11, 2012.

Williams, Jack, and Bob Sheets, *Hurricane Watch.* New York: Vintage, 2001.

"Tracking the Storm." *The New York Times, City Room.* October 28, 2012. http://

cityroom.blogs.nytimes.com/2012/10/28/hurricane-sandy-live-updates/
National Research Council, *Weather Services for the Nation: Becoming Second to None* (Washington, D.C.: The National Academies Press, 2012).

Unpublished Documents

Blake, Eric S., et al., "Tropical Cyclone Report: Hurricane Sandy" (AL182012, National Hurricane Center, February 12, 2013).
Blake, Eric S., and Christopher Landsea, "The Deadliest, Costliest, and Most Intense United States Tropical Cyclones from 1851 to 2010 (and Other Frequently Requested Hurricane Facts)." (NOAA Technical Memorandum NWS NHC-6, August 2011).
"Sinking of S/V Bounty" (Coast Guard Marine Information for Safety and Law Enforcement Report, November 2012).
US Coast Guard, "Investigation in the Circumstances Surrounding the Sinking of the TALL SHIP BOUNTY 123 Miles off the Coast of Cape Hatteras, North Carolina, on October 29, 2012, with Loss of One Life and Another Missing and Presumed Dead" (May 2014).

Miscellaneous

Chris Barksdale, Jessica Black, Dan Cleveland, Doug Faunt, Laura Groves, Jess Hewitt, Adam Prokosh, Drew Salapatek, Matt Sanders, Josh Scornavacchi, Anna Sprague, John Svendsen. (Sworn Testimony before the US Coast Guard and National Transportation Safety Board, *Bounty* Hearings, March 2013).

"The Birth of a Monster." "Epic Storm's Puzzling Path." (*Hurricane Hunters,* the Weather Channel, 2013).

Monday

Interviews

Brian Bailey, Chris Barksdale, Robbie Berg, Eric Blake, Steve Bonn, Mike Brennan, Mickey Brown, Joe Bruno, Steve Cerveny, Dina Christian, Aaron Cmiel, Ross Dickman, Doug Faunt, Jeff Finston, James Franklin, Randy Haba, Rich Harter, Cas Holloway, Kristen Jaekel, Jeremy Johnson, Joe Kelly, Chris Landsea, Brad Leggett, Claudia McCann, Shelly McCann, Ralph McCutcheon, Joe Miketta, Jan Miles, Billy Mitchell, Bryan Norcross, Jane Pena, Anthony Popiel, Ed Rappaport, Josh Scornavacchi, Wendy Sellens, Gary Szatkowski,

Michelle Wilton

Published Documents

Carrier, Jim, *The Ship and the Storm.* New York: Harvest, 2002.

Piddington, Henry, *The Sailors Horn-book.* London: Frederic Norgate, 1889.

Meyer, Robert J., et al., "The Dynamics of Hurricane Risk Perception: Real-Time Evidence from the 2012 Atlantic Hurricane Season." *Bulletin of the American Meteorological Society* (early online PDF release 2014). http://journals.ametsoc.org/doi/pdf/10.1175/BAMS-D-12-00218.1

Preston, Jennifer, Sheri Fink, and Michael Powell, "Behind a Call That Kept Nursing Home Patients in Storm's Path." *The New York Times,* December 2, 2012.

Semple, Kirk, and Joseph Goldstein, "How a Beach Community Became a Deathtrap." *The New York Times,* November 10, 2012.

Jorgensen, Jillian, "Staten Island Woman's Spirit Survives After Losing Husband, Daughter to Hurricane Sandy." *Staten Island Live,* December 2, 2012.

Haggerty, Erin, "When Bellevue Had to Evacuate Its Criminally Insane." *New York Magazine,* October 29, 2013.

Unpublished Documents

Blake, Eric S., et al., "Tropical Cyclone Report: Hurricane Sandy" (AL182012, National Hurricane Center, February 12, 2013).

Norcross, Bryan. "Sandy on Track and Serious Trouble." *Weather Underground.* October 29, 2012. http://www.wunderground.com/blog/bnorcross/archive.html?year=2012&month=10

US Department of Commerce, "Service Assessment Hurricane/Post-Tropical Cyclone Sandy, October 22–29, 2012." May 2013.

"Sinking of S/V Bounty" (Coast Guard Marine Information for Safety and Law Enforcement Report, November 2012).

US Coast Guard, "Investigation in the Circumstances Surrounding the Sinking of the TALL SHIP BOUNTY 123 Miles off the Coast of Cape Hatteras, North Carolina, on October 29, 2012, with Loss of One Life and Another Missing and Presumed Dead" (May 2014).

Miscellaneous

News 12 Westchester, "North Salem Boys Lost During Superstorm Sandy Remembered." (Originally aired October 29, 2013.)

Nova, "Inside the Megastorm." PBS. (Originally aired November 18, 2012.)

"Superstorm Sandy Strikes" (*Hurricane Hunters,* the Weather Channel, 2013).

Chris Barksdale, Jessica Black, Dan Cleveland, Doug Faunt, Laura Groves, Jess Hewitt, Adam Prokosh, Drew Salapatek, Matt Sanders, Josh Scornavacchi, Anna Sprague, John Svendsen. (Sworn Testimony before the US Coast Guard and National Transportation Safety Board, *Bounty* Hearings, March 2013).

Afterward

Haggerty, Erin, "When Bellevue Had to Evacuate Its Criminally Insane." *New York Magazine,* October 29, 2013.

Hartocollis, Anemona, and Nina Bernstein, "At Bellevue, a Desperate Fight to Ensure the Patients' Safety." *The New York Times,* November 1, 2012.

Hallman, Ben, "After Sandy, Communication Breakdown Hampered Efforts to Find Evacuated Seniors." *Huffington Post,* November 16, 2012. http://www.huffingtonpost.com/2012/11/16/sandy-communication-evacuated-seniors_n_2141699.html

"Hurricane Sandy: Covering the Storm."

The New York Times, November 6, 2012.

Unpublished Documents

US Department of Commerce, "Service Assessment, Hurricane/Post-Tropical Cyclone Sandy, October 22–29, 2012." May 2013.

ABOUT THE AUTHOR

Kathryn Miles serves as writer-in-residence for Green Mountain College. Her article for *Outside* magazine on one Hurricane Sandy story was named a "must-read" by *The New Yorker, Longform,* and *The Daily Beast.* Her writing has also appeared in publications including *Best American Essays.* She lives in Belfast, Maine.

The employees of Thorndike Press hope you have enjoyed this Large Print book. All our Thorndike, Wheeler, and Kennebec Large Print titles are designed for easy reading, and all our books are made to last. Other Thorndike Press Large Print books are available at your library, through selected bookstores, or directly from us.

For information about titles, please call:

(800) 223-1244

or visit our Web site at:

http://gale.cengage.com/thorndike

To share your comments, please write:

Publisher
Thorndike Press
10 Water St., Suite 310
Waterville, ME 04901